Milady's Standard:
NAIL TECHNOLOGY

4th Edition

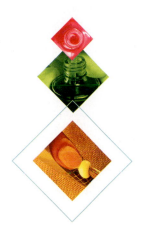

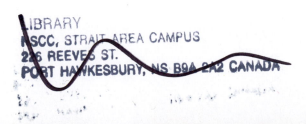

Milady's Standard: NAIL TECHNOLOGY

4th Edition

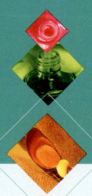

Sue Ellen Schultes

Deborah Beatty

Jewell Cunningham

Lin Halpern

LaCinda Headings

Terri Lundberg

Janet McCormick

Rebecca Moran

Godfrey F. "Oscar" Mix, D.P.M.

Laura J. Mix

Vicki Peters

Douglas Schoon

THOMSON

DELMAR LEARNING™

Australia   Canada   Mexico   Singapore   United Kingdom   United States

THOMSON

DELMAR LEARNING

Milady's Standard: Nail Technology, Fourth Edition

Sue Ellen Schultes, Editor/Contributor

President:
Susan L. Simpfenderfer

Acquisitions Editor:
Pamela Lappies

Developmental Editor:
Judy Aubrey Roberts

Editorial Assistant:
Courtney VanAuskas

Executive Production Manager:
Wendy A. Troeger

Production Coordinator:
Nina Tucciarelli

Executive Marketing Manager:
Donna J. Lewis

Channel Manager:
Stephen Smith

Cover Design:
Spiral Design Studio

Composition:
TDB Publishing Services

Library of Congress Cataloging-in-Publication Data
ISBN 1-56253-882-9

NOTICE TO THE READER

Publisher does not warrant or guarantee any of the products described herein or perform any independent analysis in connection with any of the product information contained herein. Publisher does not assume, and expressly disclaims, any obligation to obtain and include information other than that provided to it by the manufacturer.

The reader is expressly warned to consider and adopt all safety precautions that might be indicated by the activities herein and to avoid all potential hazards. By following the instructions contained herein, the reader willingly assumes all risks in connection with such instructions.

The Publisher makes no representation or warranties of any kind, including but not limited to, the warranties of fitness for particular purpose or merchantability, nor are any such representations implied with respect to the material set forth herein, and the publisher takes no responsibility with respect to such material. The publisher shall not be liable for any special, consequential, or exemplary damages resulting, in whole or part, from the readers' use of, or reliance upon, this material.

CONTENTS

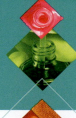

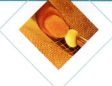

Chapter 11   PEDICURING

Chapter 12   **ELECTRIC FILING**

Chapter 13   **AROMATHERAPY**

PART 4   THE ART OF NAIL TECHNOLOGY

Chapter 14   NAIL TIPS

Chapter 15   NAIL WRAPS

Chapter 16   ACRYLIC NAILS

◉ CONTENTS

Chapter 17 GELS

Chapter 18 THE CREATIVE TOUCH

PART 5   THE BUSINESS OF NAIL TECHNOLOGY

Chapter 19   SALON BUSINESS

Chapter 20   SELLING NAIL PRODUCTS AND SERVICES

PREFACE

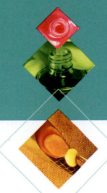

Nail technology is an exciting and rewarding profession. Each year professional nail technicians perform more than $6 billion worth of manicuring, pedicuring, and artificial nail services for millions of fashion-conscious clients. The business of nails has grown enormously over the past five years and will continue to grow. Thus, the need for educated and competent nail technicians is expanding in the same way.

Milady's Standard: Nail Technology is the complete guide to basic nail technology that every professional nail technician needs. When the staff at Delmar Learning began the revision process, we surveyed **you**, the users of the book. Through hundreds of surveys, formal focus groups, and detailed written critiques, you told us what you wanted in a new nail technology book, **and we listened**. We have added two new chapters: one on electric filing and the other on aromatherapy. All other chapters have been updated with cutting edge information in an effort to give you the latest advances in nail technology and the opportunity to realize your full potential as a nail professional.

FEATURES OF THIS EDITION

In response to **your needs**, this exciting new edition of *Milady's Standard: Nail Technology* includes the following features:

- ❖ *Chapters and Parts.* The book is divided into twenty chapters and five parts so it is very easy to use.
- ❖ *Full-Color Art.* All art is in **full color**, with actual photographs to show you step-by-step procedures for manicuring, pedicuring, tips, wraps, acrylic nails, gels, and basic nail art.
- ❖ *Learning Objectives and Review Questions.* Learning objectives provide goals for the students in each chapter. These objectives are reinforced by review questions that assess how well the student has mastered the goals established in the learning objectives. The answers to these review questions are conveniently located at the back of the book. They can be used by students to study for exams.
- ❖ *Actual Photos of Nail Disorders.* Full-color photos are included to help students identify nail disorders more accurately.
- ❖ *Client Consultation Guidelines.* A complete chapter focuses on client consultation and gives suggestions for identifying and meeting the needs of each individual client.
- ❖ *Chemical Safety Coverage.* A complete chapter is devoted to the important topic of chemical safety in the nail salon. Students will learn to identify the chemicals commonly used in the nail salon, how they can cause harm, how to protect themselves and their clients, and how to read a Material Safety Data Sheet (MSDS).
- ❖ *State Licensing Exam Topics.* The topics required for state licensing examinations are presented in a complete, easy-to-read fashion.
- ❖ *Safety Cautions.* Highlighted safety cautions alert students to services that include potentially dangerous procedures. These cautions explain how to avoid dangerous situations and how to provide services in a safe, clean environment.

❖ *Sanitation Cautions.* Highlighted sanitation cautions give specific suggestions for maintaining proper sanitation at all times.

❖ *Tips.* These tips provide hints on the most efficient and effective way to complete step-by-step procedures and help students improve their nail technology skills.

❖ *State Regulation Alerts.* Because state regulations vary, state regulation alerts remind students to check with their instructors for specific regulations in their state.

❖ *Two New Chapters.* Chapter 12, Electric Filing and Chapter 13, Aromatherapy are included to help students secure and expand their knowledge of the entire spectrum of nail technology.

❖ *Business Tips:* These tips help nail technicians improve their business relations to achieve complete customer satisfaction.

❖◆◆ SUPPLEMENTS FOR THE STUDENT AND INSTRUCTOR

Milady's Standard: Nail Technology, fourth edition, features these supplements.

Milady's Standard: Nail Technology Workbook

This workbook is a valuable student supplement that coordinates chapter-by-chapter with the textbook. It strengthens the students' understanding of nail technology by reinforcing the material covered in the textbook. The workbook includes short answer, short essay, sentence completion, matching, definition, labeling, and word review activities. The workbook also includes a final exam review made up of multiple choice questions and a series of situational tests that ask students what they would do in difficult situations if they were the nail technician.

Milady's Standard: Nail Technology Course Management Guide

This step-by-step, simple-to-use course guide has been designed specifically to help the nail technology instructor set up and operate a successful nail technology training program. It includes

❖ guidelines for starting and implementing a nail technology program.

❖ detailed lesson plans for each chapter in the book.

❖ handouts ready for use in the classroom.

❖ transparency masters for easy-to-create visual aids.

❖ a Chemical Safety Program that can be implemented in the nail technology classroom.

❖ the answers to *Milady's Standard: Nail Technology Workbook*

State Exam Review for Nail Technology

This book of exam reviews contains questions similar to those that may be found on state licensing exams for nail technology. It employs the multiple-choice type question, which has been widely adopted and approved by the majority of state licensing boards. Groups of questions are arranged under major subject areas.

Advanced, Reference, and Continuing Education Material

❖ *Airbrushing for Nails,* Elizabeth Anthony—A comprehensive resource that provides components and directions for assembling and maintaining an airbrush system. Application techniques, from color fades and French manicures to detailed nail art picture work, are given in step-by-step instructions through photographs, illustrations, and written procedures.

❖ *Guide to Owning and Operating a Nail Salon,* Joanne Wiggins—Includes well-organized, step-by-step tips for starting a salon, business features specific to nail salons, and tips on developing a long-term plan. (Book also available on audio cassette.)

❖ *Nail Art & Design,* Tammy Bigan—Provides a thorough, detailed resource for creating achievable, wearable, and commercial nail art. Full-color photography and illustrations show techniques in explicit detail and focus. It features the latest trends on glitter art, gold leaf application, pierced nail charms, among others.

❖ *Nail Q & A Book,* Vicki Peters—This book has over 500 questions and answers for nail technicians ranging from nail preparation to business practice tips.

❖ *Nail Structure and Product Chemistry,* Douglas D. Schoon—Topics cross the spectrum of nails from anatomy to salon safety, with particular attention to basic product chemistry and how it affects the nails.

❖ *The Professional's Reflexology Handbook,* Shelley Hess—This handbook offers a full spectrum of treatments using pressure points of the foot, hand, and ear. This guide provides clear, concise instructions and background on how reflexology treatments can be used in selected areas of service.

❖ *Technails: Extensions, Wraps, and Nail Art,* Tammy Bigan—Chapters include preparing for services, nail tips, wraps, gels, repairs, and fill-ins. It also explores the business side of nail services.

❖ *Spa Manicuring for the Salon and Spa,* Janet McCormick—This is the most complete and instructional source of information for any nail technician wishing to treat body, mind, and spirit. Easy to understand, concise, and inspiring, this book takes manicuring, and we as professionals, to a higher level of knowledge. It will change your concept of the spa service.

❖ *The Salon Professional's Guide to Foot Care,* Godfrey Mix, DPM—A licensed podiatrist offers invaluable information on the human foot and its care. Common foot problems and general foot diseases that can affect the foot are discussed. Knowing how and when to consult a medical professional or refer a client will help you better serve your clientele and increase loyalty.

ABOUT THE AUTHORS

Sue Ellen Schultes, Editor/Contributor

Sue Ellen Schultes is an award-winning nail artist and salon owner whose salon has been recognized as one of the top 100 nail salons in the country by *Nails* magazine ten years running. Sue is recognized as one of the leading nail art technology authorities in the U.S. and teaches extensively throughout the United States, conducting workshops and seminars. Sue currently serves as Competition Judge for various trade shows, both nationally and internationally. She was invited this year to serve as judge for the nail competition at the Brighton Beauty Show in Brighton, England. Besides acting as series editor and contributing author for this edition of *Milady's Standard: Nail Technology* for Delmar Learning, Sue also contributes special interest articles to *Nails* magazine, *NailPro, The Beauty News, Nail Shows* magazine, and several newspapers. Sue was commissioned by the Smithsonian Institute's National Museum of American History to create a full set of nails commemorating the United States Presidential Inaugurations.

Janet McCormick, Contributor

Janet McCormick, M.S., is a licensed nail technician and aesthetician, a former salon owner, seasoned instructor of nails and skin care skills, consultant, and author. Janet has achieved status as a CIDESCO diplomat and holds a master's degree in Allied Health Management. She speaks often at industry conferences and has authored over 200 skill and business articles in industry trade magazines. She is author of *Spa Manicuring for Salons and Spas,* published by Delmar Learning, describing a new, profitable focus for the industry: skin care based manicuring. Janet is owner of Salon Techniques Consulting, a spa consulting company in Frostproof, Florida.

Deborah Beatty, Contributor

Deborah has over 32 years of industry experience, which has allowed her to gain and develop a wealth of knowledge that she shares during her educational seminars as well as in her classrooms. With 14 years experience in the educational sector, she enlightens and motivates cosmetologists, instructors, and students with her energetic and interactive approach to teaching. She is presently the Division Chairperson for the Personal Services Division at a post-secondary college. In addition to being a master cosmetologist and licensed instructor, she also holds her master barber license, is a licensed nurse, and is licensed by the Georgia Professional Standards Commission. Deborah is a book and product reviewer for Thomson Learning and is an educator for Milady's Career Institute. She is also a contributing editor for the revision of *Milady's Standard Cosmetology* textbook and *Milady's Standard: Nail Technology*. Deborah is presently pursuing her bachelor's degree in Technological Studies.

LaCinda Headings, Contributor

LaCinda's passion for education has influenced her 15 years in the beauty industry as a cosmetologist specializing in nails. As the Nail Division Manager for Peel's Salon Services of Kansas, LaCinda has helped numerous nail technicians and salons start and grow their nail business. Her varied experience in the industry gives her a unique perspective that allows her to connect with nail technicians in every aspect of the business. LaCinda's background includes 10 years in the salon, manufacturer's top trainer and consultant, school nail instructor, and presently distribution and education. LaCinda has inspired nail technicians all over the world with her motto of "live, laugh, love, and learn."

Lin Halpern, Contributor

A native New Yorker, Lin Halpern has been a nail technician for 39 years. Lin started her professional nail shop business in 1980 and expanded to a full service spa salon in 1981. From 1981 consecutively through 1999, Lin worked as a consultant to four different nail product manufacturers developing acrylics, light-cured gels, and nail coatings. Over the years she has developed numerous new and innovative products from fast-drying top coats, easier to use controlled-flow acrylics to a unique three-dimensional nail tip for which she holds a U.S. Patent. Ms. Halpern is a contributor to *Nails* and *NailPro* magazines, has produced marketing design concepts for advertising photos and posters, and applied the models' nails. Lin has judged many international nail competitions, provides international education on nail product knowledge and nail application techniques, and co-wrote and produced an interactive seminar on acrylic and gel nail product chemistry. Lin has been invited to join other notable nail technicians from varied companies to participate in open talk forums at beauty events around the world. Since closing her spa salon in 1989, she continues to service clients daily as she develops new nail product chemistry to improve our every day work objective.

Douglas Schoon, Contributor

With over twenty-two years experience as a research scientist, international lecturer, author, and educator, Douglas Schoon heads up the most extensive nail research and development laboratory in existence today. As the Director of Research and Development for *Creative Nail Design*, Doug spends much of his time designing state-of-the-art nail enhancement products as well as on computerized testing equipment to aid in his research of nail enhancement products. This gives *Creative Nail Design* research capabilities that exceed even those found at large university and government laboratories.

The author of many video and audio training programs, as well as over 30 magazine articles on salon chemicals, chemical safety, and disinfection, Doug has also written *Milady's Nail Structure and Product Chemistry* with a new edition currently in revision; *HIV/AIDS & Hepatitis: Everything You Need to Know to Protect Yourself and Others*, and is a contributing author to *Milady's Standard: Nail Technology*. Doug often serves as an expert witness in legal cases involving cosmetic safety and health. Additionally, Doug assists in writing books and professional papers concerning fingernails and hair; proving that, without a-doubt, he is one of the world's leading experts on salon products and chemical safety.

As a writer and speaker, Doug is especially popular with nail professionals and cosmetologists due to his unique ability to make even the most complex chemical theories and ideas seem simple and easy to understand. His safety and disinfection lectures present invaluable information for anyone interested in understanding both product chemistry and health. In addition, Mr. Schoon is founder and executive director of Chemical Awareness Training Services (CATS), a chemical consultant to American Beauty Association (ABA), and a member of the Safety and Standards Committee Manufacturer's Council (SSCMC). Doug holds a Master's degree in Chemistry from the prestigious University of California–Irvine. He currently resides in Laguna Beach, California.

Vicki Peters, Contributor

Nailpro's education director, Vicki Peters, is a past competition champion and now a leading competition director, technical educator, and featured business speaker. She is also the author of *The Nail's Q & A Book,* published by Delmar Learning, *Drilltalk, The Competitive Edge*, and *The Nail Healthy Guide*, as well as numerous CDs and tapes. Her artistry has graced the covers of fashion magazines, *TV Guide, DAYSPA*, and *NailPro*. Peters is the director of the *NailPro* Nail Institute continuing education program and producer of Nail Those Profits Cruises. Vicki has also been a keynote speaker for many international beauty shows, including the International Cosmetology Expo and the World International Nail and Beauty Association. She has also worked as a research and development consultant for numerous nail product companies.

Rebecca Moran, Contributor

Rebecca Moran has been a nail technologist and salon owner for the past eight years. Rebecca received her instructor's license and has been a practicing licensed educator in Portland, Maine for the past three years. Currently, Rebecca is the director of education for the school at which she teaches, and has worked as a subject matter expert and expert reviewer for Delmar Learning, in addition to being a contributing author of this edition of *Milady's Standard: Nail Technology.* The proud mom of two daughters, ages 6 and 4, Rebecca finds time to continue her education with classes as often as she can and consults as an educator for a local product distributor.

Terri Lundberg, Contributor

Terri Lundberg has been a nail technology educator in both the professional arena and in the schools since 1990. Beginning her career as the International Education Director for a nail product manufacturer, she not only trained company educators across the world, but developed a "train the trainer" method that is still in use today by many nail manufacturers. Terri also developed a mentoring program, creating a unique curriculum for mentoring nail technicians to a higher skill level, and authored and taught an advanced skills course. In January 2000, Terri opened a fully-licensed cosmetology school with Carolyn R. Kraskey and Hoa T. Phan and developed its nail technician program, which prepares students to be salon-ready at graduation.

Jewell Cunningham, Contributor

Jewell Cunningham has been involved with the beauty industry for over 20 years. As a licensed nail technician, she competed in sculptured nail competitions from 1981 through 1986, winning 25 First Place awards, an industry record, including National Champion and World International Champion. Jewell followed that success as a judge for national and international competitions, writing rules and regulations as well as directing competitions. In 1990, Jewell joined a manufacturer, where she developed over 75 items for the line and designed packaging as well. Jewell is a nationally recognized consultant to day spas, manufacturers, and salon owners, and continues to thrive in the beauty industry.

Laura J. Mix, Contributor

Laura Mix began her career as a clinical laboratory technician for a major metropolitan hospital in California. After a number of years as technician, then as a full time homemaker, Laura returned to work with her husband, Dr. Oscar Mix, in his podiatry practice. The Mixes decided to offer pedicure services to patients, and so Laura began manicuring school in June of 1993. After obtaining her license, Laura has continued working with her husband, providing pedicures and nail services. In November 1998, she opened a specialty day spa, Footworks, Inc., and has worked as a product educator for fiberglass nail enhancement systems. She also consults as a subject matter expert for the Sacramento Bureau of Barbering and Cosmetology. Laura continues to keep her laboratory technician's license current as well, and assists her husband at many of his seminars and classes.

Godfrey F. "Oscar" Mix, D.P.M., Contributor

Godfrey "Oscar" Mix is a Doctor of Podiatric Medicine; a member of the American Podiatric Medical Association, the California Podiatric Medical Association, and the Sacramento Valley Podiatric Medical Society, of which he is a past president. Mix is an Associate of the American College of Foot Surgeons and is Board Certified by the American Board of Podiatric Foot Surgery, as well as the Americn Board of Quality Assurance and Peer Review. Dr. Mix is the author of *The Salon Professional's Guide to Foot Care*, published by Delmar Learning, and currently writes on foot-related subjectrs for *Nails* magazine, continuing to work as a manufacturer's consultant in the professional beauty industry.

◆ ◆ ◆ ACKNOWLEDGMENTS

The staff of Delmar Learning wishes to acknowledge the many individuals and organizations who helped shape the fourth edition of *Milady's Standard: Nail Technology*. Their input enabled us to produce a book that will be a valuable resource for both students and professionals in the field of nail technology. To all those who contributed to this edition we extend our sincere thanks and appreciation.

Fourth Edition Reviewers

Twila R. Adams
   Universal College of Beauty
   Charlotte, North Carolina
Rae Ann Amacher
   Orleans-Niagara BOCES
   Sanborn, New York
Dianne Atchley
   Halfmoon Hair Design
   Bandon, Oregon
Laurie Biagi
   Skyline Community College
   San Bruno, California

Virginia Burge
   Beautique Day Spa and Salon
   Houston, Texas
Pam Garrison
   Vincennes Beauty College
   Vincennes, Indiana
Joseline Glenn
   Skyline College
   San Leandro, California
Chrystal Gutshall
   SUN Area Career and
   Technology Center
   Watsontown, Pennsylvania

Ruby Howard
   Pinecrest High School
   Cameron, North Carolina
Donna McKinney
   Hill College
   Hillsboro, Texas
Martha Phillips
   Ford Beauty Academy
   Lowellville, Ohio
Angela Sharp
   Sharp's Academy of Hairstyling
   Grand Blanc, Michigan

Previous Edition Reviewers

Barbara Abramovitch
New England Hair Academy
Malden, MA

Evelyn Adams
Jan-Mar Beauty Academy
Newport News, VA

Elizabeth Anthony
Progressive Nail Concepts, Inc.
Palatine, IL

Suzanne Arduini
Albany, NY

Jan Austin
Austin Beauty School
Albany, NY

Giselle Bohamde
Austin Beauty School
Albany, NY

Dale Bona
C.H. McCann Vocational
Technical High School
North Adams, MA

Jason Boulla
Albany, NY

Bich Ly
Albany, NY

Teresa K. Bryant
Carousel Beauty College
Middletown, OH

Gayle Bryner
Oklahoma State Board
of Cosmetology
Oklahoma City, Oklahoma

Burmax Co.
Hauppauge, NY

Patricia Castro
College of San Mateo
San Mateo, CA

Alice Ciurlino
P & B Beauty School
Gloucester, NJ

Deborah Clark
Albany, NY

Elizabeth Coleman
Albany, NY

Howard Conlon
Bellaire Beauty College
Bellaire, TX

Suzanne Council
Van Michael Salon
Atlanta, GA

Van Council
Van Michael Salon
Atlanta, GA

Matthew Creo
Austin Beauty School
Albany, NY

Nancy Court
Arnold Beauty College, Inc.
Fremont, CA

Wilma Curry
Bellaire Beauty College
Bellaire, TX

Brenda De Angelo
Daytona Beauty School
Daytona Beach, FL

Arnold DeMille
Milady Publishing Consultant
Continuing Education Specialist
New York, NY

Christine DeRusso
Albany, NY

Peggy Dietrich
Laredo Beauty College
Laredo, TX

Luciano Di Paolo
Euclidian Beauty College Inc.
Euclid, OH

Barbara Dorsey
Baltimore Stud. of Hair Design
Baltimore, MD

Cindy Drummy
Nails Magazine
Redondo Beach, CA

Carol Duffy
Alameda Beauty College
Alameda, CA

Roslyn Duncan
Debbie's School of Beauty Culture
Houston, TX

Dana Ennello
Mechanicville, NY

Barbara Feiner
NailPro Magazine
Van Nuys, CA

Flo Finch
Northland Pioneer College
Holbrook, AZ

Marion Ford
Albany, NY

Laverne Foster
Pat Goins Beauty Schools
Monroe, LA

Nehme Frangie
Albany, NY

Jamal Frangie
Albany, NY

Wadad Frangie
Austin Beauty School
Albany, NY

Anne Fretto
Stanton, CA

Nancy Gallitelli
Albany, NY

Ray Gambrell
South Carolina State Board of
Cosmetology
Greenwood, SC

Anthony Gardy
Albany, NY

Sharon Gil
Garden State Academy
South Bound Brook, NJ

Cynthia Gimenez
Arnold Beauty Colleges, Inc.
Remont, CA

Anne Golloway
Ossining, NY

Aurie Gosnell
National Interstate Council
of Cosmetology
Aiken, SC

Constance Gregg
Boca Raton Institute
Boca Raton, FL

Ann Harrell
St. Petersburg, FL

Linda Harris
Maxims Beauty Academy
Blaine, MN

Danielle Hasberry
Albany, NY

Helen Heine
South Eastern College of
Beauty Culture
Charlotte, NC

Michael Hill
Arkansas State Board of
Cosmetology
Fayetteville, AR

Frances Hoffman
Manatee Area Vocational
Technical Center
Bradenton, FL

Barbara Hogue
Arizona Academy of Beauty
Tucson, AZ

Linda Howe
Pittsburgh, PA

Sally Hudson
Tampa Bay Career Academy
Tampa, FL
Karen Iolli
Ailano School of Cosmetology
Brockton, MA
Frank Jacobi
Citrus Community College
Glendara, CA
Janice Jaynes
Institute of Cosmetology
Houston, TX
Julia Jefferson
Vogue College of Hair Design
Highland Heights, KY
Dorothy Johnson
Yuma School of Beauty
Yuma, AZ
Spring Kelsey
Earlton, NY
Glenn Kewley
Drome Sound Music Store
Schenectady, NY
Paulette Know
Antioch Beauty
Antioch, CA
L. Jean Lake
Elaine Steven Beauty College
St. Louis, MO
Carol Laubach
San Jacinto College
Pasadena, TX
Denise Leach
Oakland Technical Center
South East Campus
Royal Oak, MI
Yvonne Lowenstein
Margate International School
of Beauty
Margate, FL
Inna Lozhkin
Albany, NY
June A. Lyle
Lyle's School of Hair Design
Nashville, TN
Charles Lynch
International Beauty School
Lancaster, PA
Deborah A. Mack
Pivot Point International, Inc.
Chicago, IL
Tina Macki
Albany, NY
Laura Manicho
Nationwide Beauty Academy
Cols, OH

Sharon Matern
Albany, NY
Patricia Mc Daniel
Bellaire Beauty College
Bellaire, TX
Robert McLaughlin
Maine State Board of
Cosmetology
Cape Elizabeth, ME
John Mickelbank
Albany, NY
Louise Miller
Lamson Academy of Hair Design
Phoenix, AZ
Ruth Miller
Quincy Beauty Academy
Quincy, MA
Marcia Miller
Federico Beauty College
Fresno, CA
Peggy Moon
Georgia State Board
of Cosmetology
Lavonia, GA
Pauline Moram
Innerstate Beauty School
Bedford Heights, OH
Mary Ann Morris
House of Heavilin
Blue Springs, MO
Eileen Morrissey
Maison de Paris Beauty College
Haddon Field, NJ
Florence Nebblett
Washington, DC
Neka Beauty Supplies
Albany, NY
Pat Nix
Past President,
National Interstate Council
of Cosmetology
Booneville, IN
Theda O'Brien
Albany, NY
John Olsen
Phagan's Beauty School, NW
Tigard, OR
Stephanie Pedersen
New York, NY
Susan Peters
Lansdale School of Cosmetology
Lansdale, PA
Dino Petrocelli
Albany, NY
Nilsene Privette
College of Beauty and Art

and Science
Sedona, AZ
Lois Purewal
Spring Branch Beauty College
Houston, TX
Irma Quezada
Pipo Academy of Hair Design
El Paso, TX
Sarah Rainey
St. Augustine Technical Center
St. Augustine, FL
Jennifer Rhatigan
Albany, NY
Cleolis Richardson
Philadelphia, PA
Jim Rogers
Milpitas Beauty College
Milpitas, CA
Betty Romesberg
The Head Hunters
Cuyahoga Falls, OH
Sue Sansom
Executive Director,
Arizona State Board of
Cosmetology
Phoenix, AZ
Richard Scher, MD
College of Physicians and
Surgeons
Columbia University
New York, NY
Douglas Schoon
Chemical Awareness Training
Service
Irvine, CA
Regina Schrenko
Northhampton, PA
Joan Sesock
Austin Beauty School
Albany, NY
Tanya Severino
Albany, NY
Sandra Skoney
Toledo Academy of Beauty
Culture
Toledo, OH
Jenny Smith
Vogue Beauty College
Idaho Falls, ID
Kenneth J. Smith
Nail Tech Academy
Brown Deer, WI
Alicia Solazzo
Bronxville, NY
Bertha Stanko
Menands, NY

Linda Stark
Michigan College of Beauty
Troy, MI

Judith Stewart
PJ's College of Cosmetology
Carmel, IN

Alma Tilghman
North Carolina Board of
Cosmetology
Beaufort, NC

Sandy Tirpak
Albany, NY

Mona Townsend
Backscratchers Nail Care Products
Sacramento, CA

Wendy Trainor
Schuylerville, NY

Veda Traylor
Arkansas State Board of
Cosmetology
Mayflower, AR

Peggy Turbyfill
Mike's Barber and Beauty Salon
Hot Springs, AR

Barbara Turman
School of Nail Technology Inc.
Coral Gables, FL

Beverly Venable
Loudonville, NY

Judy Ventura
Greensboro, NC

Dave Welsh
J & D Supply
Albany, NY

Barbara Wetzel
Nail Splash, Inc.
LaGrange Park, IL

Renee Wilson
Argyle, NY

Lois Wiskur
South Dakota Cosmetology
Commission
Pierre, SD

Victoria Wurdinger
New York, NY

Jack Yahm
Milady Publishing Consultant
Emeritis
"Father of Cosmetology
Accreditation"
Lauderdale Lakes, FL

Linda Zizzo
Milwaukee Area Technical College
Milwaukee, WI

Elvin Zook, M.D.
Southern Illinois University
School of Medicine
Springfield, IL

The Milady staff would like to thank the following individuals and organizations for their generous assistance with this project:

Photography and Location:

Salon Location:

Sue Ellen Schultes
Notorious Nails
Green Brook, NJ

All location photos:
Michael Dzaman Photography
©Michael Dzaman/Dzaman
Photography
www.dzamanphoto.com

Cover image; chapter 7 bitten nails,
Fig. 7-17; chapter 10 massage photo,
Fig. 10-54; chapter opener images for
chapters 2, 9, and 20
Paul Castle, Castle Photography, Inc.
Troy, NY
www.castlephtographyinc.com

Photos for Chapters 16 and 17:
Photographs courtesy of NSI - Nail
Systems International. All rights
reserved.

Chapter 8 opener image provided by
the Nanoworld Image Gallery,
Centre for Microscopy and
Microanalysis, The University of
Queensland

Nail disorders photos in chapter 7:
Figs. 7-2, 7-3, 7-4, 7-9, 7-10, 7-13, 7-
14, 7-15, 7-15, 7-18, 7-24, 7-26
Courtesy of Godfrey F. Mix, DPM
Sacramento, CA

Chapter 7, Onycholysis, Fig. 7-25
Courtesy of Orville J. Stone, M.D.
Dermatology Medical Group
Huntington Beach, CA

Chapter 7 opener image and anatomy
iilustrations in chapters 6, 7, and 8
by Joe Chovan, Health Care Visuals

The following chapter opener photos
were provided by PhotoDisc/
GettyImages: Chapter 1, Chapter 6,
Chapter 11, Chapter 13, Chapter 19.
© PhotoDisc/GettyImages.

**For their generous assistance with
supplies, tools, and apparel:**

Gavson Salon Classics
Quality Salon Apparel
Garland, TX
www.gavsonsalon.com

Bianco Brothers International
Hand-honed instruments for the
medical and beauty industries
Brooklyn, NY
http://members.aol.com/biancob/
index.html

Essie Cosmetics, Ltd.
Astoria, NY
www.essieltd.com

Emiliani Enterprises
Union, NJ
www.beauty-net.com

AromaTouch
Encino, CA

**For participation as models in
the photo shoot:**

Sarah Ginsberg
Guy Erceg
Raymond Schultes
Valerie Erceg Pietryak
Allison Parker
Carolyn Gillish
Alison Banks-Moore
Nicole Cedeno
Shannon Ciasulli
Robert Lartaud
Kurt Manz
Lisa Manz
Mylene Quines
Lois S. Robinson
Gladys Schalet

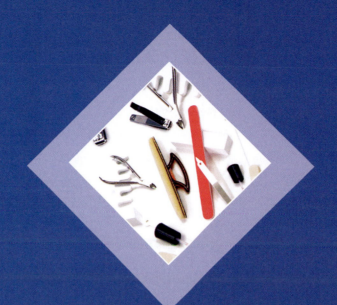

INTRODUCTION

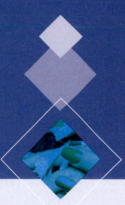

Nail Technology Overview

You have chosen to become a nail technician, one of the fastest-growing and most creative, rewarding, and high-paying professions in cosmetology today. As a nail technician you will use the latest technology to apply artificial nails and use your artistic abilities to create original designs on nails. You will be part of the booming manicuring, pedicuring, and artificial nail industry, with combined sales of more than $6 billion a year. This figure represents a greater than 25 percent increase over previous years in some areas, and continues to climb. Manicuring, as a profession, has gained a great deal of respect. No longer are nail technicians thought of as high school dropouts. The women and men entering the field today are older and wiser, with good work ethics.

◆ ◆ NAIL TECHNOLOGY OVERVIEW

Because nail technology is a complex, changing profession you will want to continue learning even after you receive a license. Education is the key to excelling in the nail industry. In order to be successful, you must always be open to learning about new techniques. If you take advantage of the ever-evolving information made available, you will gain the reputation of being a knowledgeable professional. *A professional nail technician's education never ends.*

You may start your career as a nail technician in a salon. As you develop your knowledge and skills, you may want to move into other career areas in the nail industry, including teaching nail technology in cosmetology schools or demonstrating manufacturer's nail products at trade shows, conventions, or stores. You can become a salon owner or even the personal nail technician for fashion models or actors on the stage, in movies, or on TV. You can write, edit, or be a consultant for nail technology books and magazines.

Nail technology has changed in the 5,000 years since the first manicure was recorded. Manicures used to be a luxury enjoyed only by rulers and the wealthy, and were performed by servants. Today, nail services are enjoyed by millions of fashion-conscious people from many social and economic groups. In most states today, licensed professionals, who have completed up to 500 hours of classroom instruction, perform nail technology services. During instruction, they learn to improve the health of their clients' nails and recognize healthy nails and skin, as well as possible nail and skin disorders. They become skilled in using the latest nail technology while following proper sanitation, disinfection, and safety procedures to protect both themselves and their clients. Today's professional nail technicians learn how to provide services to enhance the look of their clients' hands and feet, and to relieve their stress. They also learn how to handle the business aspects of their profession.

The first manicures did not require formal instruction. The word "manicure" comes from the Latin "manus" (hand) and "cura" (care). The first evidence of nail care recorded in history was before 3,000 B.C. in Egypt and China. Ancient Egyptian men and women of high social rank stained their nails with red-orange dye called henna, which comes from a shrub. The color of a person's nails in ancient Egypt was a sign of importance. Kings and queens wore deep red, while people of lower rank were allowed to wear only pale colors. Around 3,000 B.C. the Chinese developed a nail paint made from beeswax, egg whites, gelatin, and gum arabic. In 600 B.C., Chinese royalty wore gold and silver paint on their nails. In the fifteenth century, leaders of the Chinese Ming Dynasty painted their nails black and red. Military commanders in Egypt, Babylon, and early Rome spent hours before a battle having their hair lacquered and curled and their nails painted the same shade as their lips.

As a twenty-first century nail technician, you can give your clients many more choices for nail care than the privileged people of ancient civilizations. You can offer your clients variations of the manicure and pedicure and information about nail care. They can also choose from a variety of artificial nail services—shaped, colored, and designed specifically to suit their needs. You will become a successful nail technician by studying hard and learning the skills and professional manner to make all your clients feel like twenty-first century kings and queens.

If you are in school and reading this book for the first time, remember that you will learn the basics in school and it is up to you to reach out further to get more experience. Read and reread this book. Use it for reference. Network with other techs, find a mentor, and attend every manufacturer's class you can. Learn about the products available as well as how to use them correctly. Regularly attend trade shows and keep in touch with the trends and industry events by reading trade publications. Get online and communicate with others like yourself. It is your responsibility to gain more knowledge and grow as a professional.

The authors of these pages are just that—professionals. Years of knowledge and skill back the technical information you will read in this book. Sue Ellen Schultes, in her research for this book, reached out to some of the biggest names in the industry to collect the latest information she could for this project. *Nowhere else* will you find a collection of information like this. It does not matter whether you are at the beginning of your career or a seasoned pro, the information in this book is some of the best you can find.

Let's get started studying this exciting field.

Vicki Peters, Nailpro Magazine
Sue Ellen Schultes, Editor

part 1

GETTING STARTED

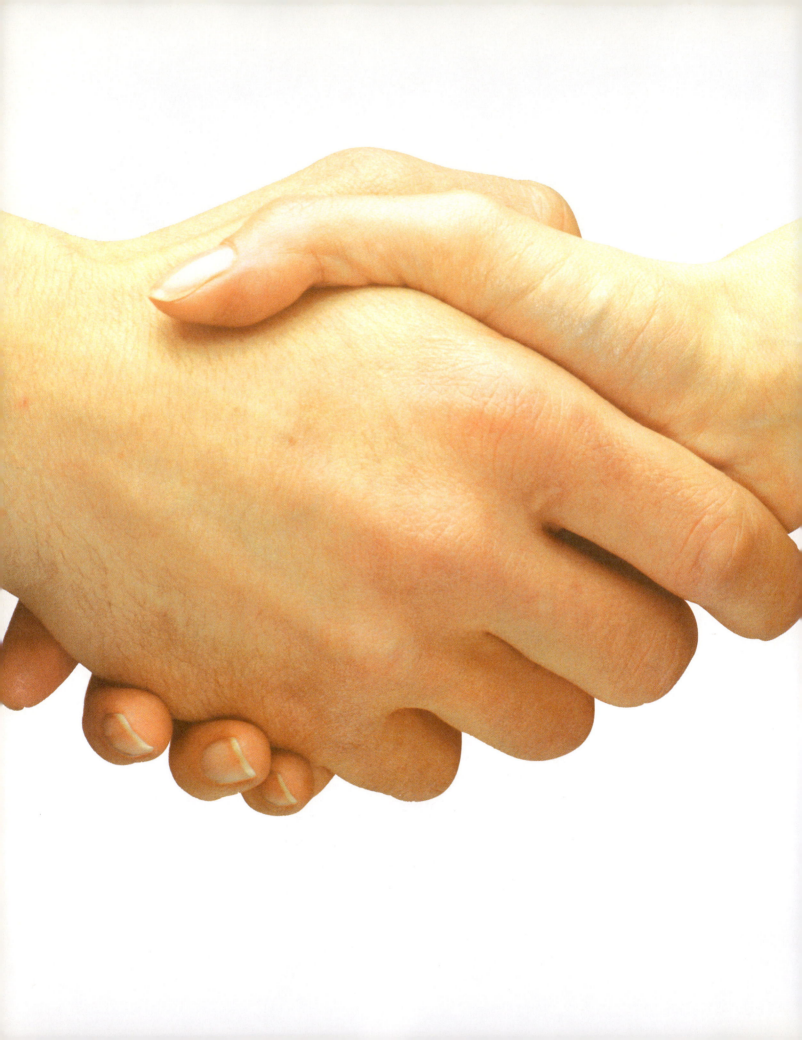

1

YOUR PROFESSIONAL IMAGE

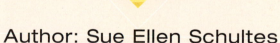

Author: Sue Ellen Schultes

CHAPTER OUTLINE

Professional Salon Conduct

Professional Ethics

Your Professional Appearance

Learning Objectives

After you have completed this chapter, you should be able to:

1 Define salon conduct.

2 Give examples of professional salon conduct toward clients.

3 Give examples of professional salon conduct toward employers and coworkers.

4 Define professional ethics.

5 Give examples of professional ethics toward clients.

6 Give examples of professional ethics toward employers and coworkers.

7 Describe the type of appearance you should have as a professional nail technician.

Key Terms

Page number indicates where in the chapter the term is used.

ethics
pg. 12

salon conduct
pg. 9

Successful nail technicians are able to do more than give an expert manicure, create natural-looking artificial nails, or paint original designs on a client's nail. You need to know how to behave in a professional manner. You will follow the rules for professional behavior with clients, employers, and coworkers. You must develop good personal health and grooming habits. In this chapter, you will learn the rules of professionalism for nail technicians. They include proper salon conduct, professional ethics, and how to present yourself to clients as an attractive and well-groomed representative of the nail technology industry. When you practice these rules, you will quickly build a satisfied clientele and a workplace environment that will lead to your success. This chapter is one of the most important in the book. It has nothing to do with technical competency but everything to do with becoming the best this profession has to offer.

◆ ◆ PROFESSIONAL SALON CONDUCT

Salon conduct is the way you behave when you are working with clients, your employer, and coworkers in a salon. As a professional, your behavior will have a direct impact on how the industry is perceived as a whole. Raising and maintaining a high standard of conduct in the salon will elevate the impression you make on others, thus raising your own self-esteem. This is very important for several reasons. The better you feel about yourself the better job you do, and the more open you are to learning and cooperating with employees and coworkers. We are constantly being evaluated by those around us. Unprofessional behavior could affect promotions, income, and credibility—three things that are vital to enjoying your job while moving toward a successful career. Remember, always maintain a professional attitude.

Professional Salon Conduct Toward Clients

Set high standards for proper salon conduct. You can create an environment in your salon that is relaxed and pleasant for clients and makes them want to come back and bring their friends.

1. **Be on time.** You will appear relaxed, competent, and concerned about your clients' needs by being on time, waiting to serve them when they arrive. Being late can make you appear disorganized or uncaring. It is discourteous and can annoy and inconvenience your clients.

2. **Be prepared.** Before your clients arrive, make sure your station is completely set up with an adequate supply of materials and equipment. Make sure your implements are disinfected and ready to use, and your work area is sanitary. Put a smile on your face.

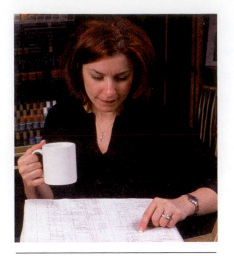

Figure 1–1 Plan your day carefully.

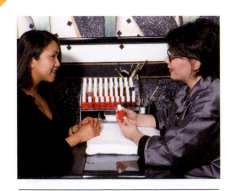

Figure 1–2 Communicate with your client.

3. **Plan your day.** Keep an appointment schedule near you for each day. The schedule should include your client's name, service to be performed, time of appointment, and client's phone number. Call your clients by name when they arrive. When you know what service you are to perform, you can begin without hesitation. This gives your clients a feeling of security and importance (Figure 1–1).

4. **Plan in advance.** Except in emergency situations, nail technicians should not reschedule appointments to accommodate their personal lives. You should know about important events three or more weeks in advance. Be sure to put them on your calendar and set your schedule accordingly. This career offers flexibility in scheduling, if you are organized and can plan weeks in advance.

5. **Arrange appointments carefully.** Schedule your appointments so that each client has enough time. If you schedule too many clients during your day, you won't have time to serve them and some will have to wait or be rescheduled for another day. If the receptionist makes appointments for you, be sure to provide a neat list of the services you offer and the time you need to complete each one.

6. **Keep clients informed of schedule changes.** Contact clients if your appointments are running very late or if you have to reschedule their appointments. They will appreciate your honesty and they will be grateful that you have not wasted their time. If you are running only slightly late, make sure your clients are aware of this and let them know you will be right with them.

7. **Be courteous.** Have a cheerful, friendly, and helpful attitude. This attitude will tell your clients that you care for them. Before you perform any service, you can make your clients feel comfortable and relaxed. Help them take off their coats, show them where to wash their hands, and where to sit for the service. All new clients can be given a tour of the salon and shown where the rest rooms and phones are. You may also tell them how to book future appointments, how to reschedule an appointment, what forms of payment your salon accepts, and what policies your salon has that affect them.

8. **Perform all tasks willingly and efficiently.** Never make your clients feel their appointments inconvenience you.

9. **Communicate with your clients.** Explain the services you will perform for your clients and the retail products needed to maintain these services. Listen to their concerns with undivided attention and answer their questions. If you do not know the answer to a question tell them you will research it and get back to them. No matter how successful you become, always keep your attitude humble when dealing with your clients (Figure 1–2).

10. **Never complain to, or argue with, a client.** Try to keep any conversation on a professional level at all times. While you are performing nail services, you can use the time to explain what you are

doing and why. This builds confidence between you and the client. You can also use this unique time to suggest and discuss other salon services and products that could help your client. If a client gets more than one service or product at your salon, the loyalty factor doubles. If the client has confidence in you and trusts you, the loyalty factor rises again.

11. **Use good judgment.** Do not share personal information about your private life. More importantly, do not share personal stories about other clients, your coworkers, or your employer with your client. Discussion of politics or religion must be avoided. While the nail technician and client or coworker may share the same views, others in earshot may not and may be offended. Concentrate on your client's needs and take this time to address concerns about her nails or to explain more about your procedure.

12. **Never chew gum, smoke, eat, or take personal telephone calls where you can be seen by clients.** These habits can be extremely annoying to clients. Smoking can be dangerous around nail chemicals. Any one of these habits can detract from your professionalism (Figure 1–3).

13. **Smile.** Always treat any client that comes into your salon with a cheerful attitude. If you see someone in need of any type of assistance be mindful of how you can help.

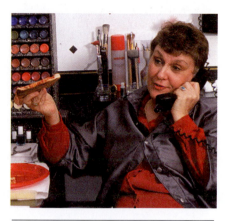

Figure 1–3 Never eat, chew gum, or take personal telephone calls where you can be seen by clients.

Professional Salon Conduct Toward Employers and Coworkers

It is important to work closely with your employer and coworkers because it will help create a strong, successful salon that will eventually secure your future in this industry. To be competitive, the entire staff must work together. You want to create an atmosphere that will make your clients enjoy their visits to your salon so much they will not want to go to another.

Below are guidelines to follow for dealing with employers and coworkers.

1. **Communicate.** Establish an open, honest line of communication between yourself and your employer. Be perfectly honest about your strengths and weaknesses. Make sure your work meets all standards the salon expects.

2. **Be willing to learn.** Keep an open mind and be willing to accept suggestions. Do not automatically assume that your way of doing something is the only correct way. Nail products and services are improved often; be prepared to update your skills.

3. **Making mistakes.** If you are new in a salon, be prepared to learn the salon policies and procedures (and follow them). If you are a new technician or learning a new skill, be prepared to make mistakes. Be determined to get better with each client, each time, each nail. Do not take the correction personally. It is a necessary part of the learning process.

4. **Give credit to others.** Never take credit for another person's ideas. Try to acknowledge contributions made by others.

5. **Respect the opinions of coworkers.** Your ideas and opinions are important, but yours are not the only ones. Frequently, the ideas of many people create the best solution.

6. **Take the initiative.** Never be afraid to offer help or suggestions to make things better or easier for your employer or coworkers. It will be greatly appreciated.

7. **Use good judgment.** If you have a problem or question about your job, discuss it directly with your employer, not with your clients or coworkers.

8. **Leave personal problems at home.** Do not tell your personal problems to your employer, fellow employees, or clients. Personal problems are distractions that interrupt the concentration needed to do a good job. You should not take telephone calls from family or friends while you are working unless it is an emergency.

9. **Differences of opinion.** Never air grievances with your coworkers or employees on the floor of the salon. Have any negative discussions in private.

10. **Never borrow money from employers or coworkers.** This is a practice that can result in a very awkward work situation. Eventually your coworkers may lose respect for you.

11. **Promote the salon.** Learn about the other services offered at your salon, such as hair care, skin care, and cosmetic consultations, so you can promote the entire salon to clients.

12. **Develop your ability to sell.** Explain the benefits of products and services to clients without pressuring them. Products for home care will benefit you and your client because your client will come back with their hands and feet in better condition. The more varied services you perform on a client, the deeper their loyalty becomes.

13. **Follow salon policies and procedures.** To show respect for your employees and coworkers it is important to follow *all* salon policies and procedures. Learning to support your salon team promotes a harmonious working environment.

◆ ◆ ◆ PROFESSIONAL ETHICS

Professional ethics (ETH-iks) is the sense of right and wrong when **you** interact with your clients, employer, and coworkers. The essential values in professional ethics are honesty, fairness, courtesy, and respect for the feelings and rights of others.

Professional Ethics Toward Clients

High ethical standards for treating clients will earn you a good reputation. Your clients will trust you, keep coming back, and bring their friends. Your best source of advertising is through the recommendations of clients who respect and trust you.

1. **Suggest services that meet your clients' needs.** Never suggest or give clients any services they do not need or want, or ones that could harm them. Explain what you recommend for your clients and why, so they will feel comfortable with your services.

2. **Keep your word and fulfill all obligations.** Always do what you have promised the client and what the client wants you to do. Do not take short cuts because you are rushed or substitute other services because they are more convenient for you.

3. **Treat all your clients equally.** Never offer special discounts or services to one client and not to another.

4. **Follow your state regulations for sanitation and safety.** Always follow provisions of the state laws covering nail technology. Regulations may seem inconvenient at times, but they are created to protect you and your clients. To be an ethical nail technician, you must always be knowledgeable about current laws concerning your profession (Figure 1–4).

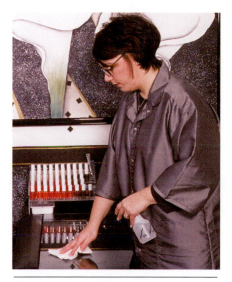

Figure 1–4 Follow your state regulations for sanitation and safety.

5. **Be loyal.** Never complain, gossip, or talk to your client about other clients, your employer, or coworkers. This is unkind and diminishes how your client feels about you and your place of work. Your clients will not trust you if you talk about other people to them because they will think you will talk about them the same way.

6. **Do not criticize others.** Never criticize the services offered by other nail technicians or other salons. Even if the client insists on discussing another colleague's or salon's service, you may listen, but remain neutral in your responses.

7. **Do not abandon your clients.** If you leave the manicuring field or move to another community, give your clients enough notice to find another nail technician or recommend a trusted coworker or colleague. If you have a large clientele, consider training someone to take your place. You want your clients to experience the least amount of discomfort.

Professional Ethics Toward Employer and Coworkers

By using professional ethics to support the efforts and morale of your coworkers and employers, you will help contribute to the success of your salon. As the salon becomes more successful, so will you.

1. **Be honest.** Never blame a coworker for your mistakes. Take responsibility for your own actions.

2. **Fulfill your obligations.** Keep any promises you make to an employer and coworker, such as coming in on your day off to help

with a special client. If you cannot possibly keep a promise, contact your employer or coworker ahead of time and ask if you can help to make other arrangements.

3. **Respect the talents of your employer and coworkers.** Praise them and encourage them when they do a good job. Try not to criticize.

4. **Do not invite criticism of coworkers.** When you hear a client complain about another technician, do not take sides. You do not know all the facts and it is not your business. Suggest that the client speak directly to the coworker involved. Never criticize someone else's work. Let your standards and work speak for themselves. If another's work is exceptionally poor, offer to repair your client's nails without placing blame on another nail technician.

5. **Never gossip or start rumors among coworkers.** Some people think these tactics can get them ahead in business, but they only serve to make you look bad and alienate your associates.

BUSINESS TIP

Know the Competition and Refine Your Skills

Your clients want what's best for their nails, and they rely on you to tell them which products will keep their hands looking beautiful between manicure appointments. In order to reinforce the belief that professional products are best for maintaining nails' health and beauty, you must thoroughly educate yourself about the points of difference between salon and drugstore formulas. You must also be able to explain the differences to your clients. For instance, if you know that mass market emery boards are very abrasive and can cause problems by tearing up layers of nail plate, you'll know to prescribe professional boards, which have a softer abrasive and don't rip the layers.

Plan on attending trade shows, at least once a year, pertaining to your industry. Many manufacturers and suppliers are there in person or have well-trained representatives available to talk to you first hand. They can answer any questions you may have about their professional product and its use. They can tell you how it works and why it is better than other over-the-counter products. Read trade books and magazines so you can get cutting edge information on new products and their procedures. Seek out individuals who excel in any area of interest to you. Take classes and seminars to hone your skills and increase your knowledge.

Videos produced by industry professionals are a great visual aid and a wonderful learning tool. Become familiar with a computer as information is readily available on the Internet and at your discretion at any time. Anything you read, hear, or watch, that will improve your product knowledge and technical skills, or save you time, is an investment in your career.

◆ ◆ ◆ YOUR PROFESSIONAL APPEARANCE

Be a model of good grooming for your clients because you are a member of the beauty industry. Your clients expect you to look your best. You should be pleasant to be around. Be clean and pleasant-smelling so clients will not object to having you touch them while you perform nail services. They should find it pleasant to sit across from you while you perform nail services (Figure 1–5).

1. **Be clean and fresh.** Bathe or shower daily and use an effective deodorant.

2. **Have fresh breath and healthy teeth.** Make sure your breath is fresh at all times. Do not eat garlic or spicy foods that can give you bad breath during the working day. Keep a toothbrush, toothpaste, and mints with you so you can freshen your breath when needed. Keep your teeth and gums healthy by regular brushing and dental check-ups.

3. **Wear clean clothes that are appropriate for the salon.** You should look your best in stylish, professional clothes that reflect your dedication to the industry without inhibiting your ability to work (Figure 1–6).

4. **Pay attention to your hair, skin, and nails.** Make sure your hair is neat, you have on just enough make-up to enhance your natural beauty, and your nails are well-manicured.

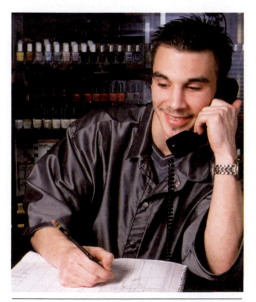

Figure 1–5 A professional male nail technician

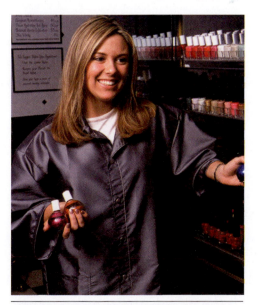

Figure 1–6 A professional female nail technician

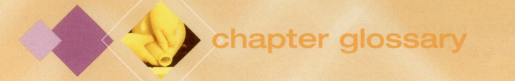

chapter glossary

ethics	The sense of right and wrong when interacting with clients, employers, and coworkers. Honesty, fairness, courtesy, and respect for the feelings and rights of others are the essential values in professional ethics.
salon conduct	The proper way to behave when you are working with your clients, employer, and coworkers.

1

1. What is salon conduct?

2. Give ten examples of professional salon conduct toward clients.

3. Explain why a salon might lose clients if nail technicians do not exhibit professional salon conduct.

4. Give ten examples of professional salon conduct toward employers and coworkers.

5. Define professional ethics.

6. Give seven examples of professional ethics toward clients.

7. Give five examples of professional ethics toward employers and coworkers.

8. Describe the type of appearance you should have as a professional nail technician.

9. Explain why a salon might lose clients if it employs nail technicians who have an unprofessional appearance.

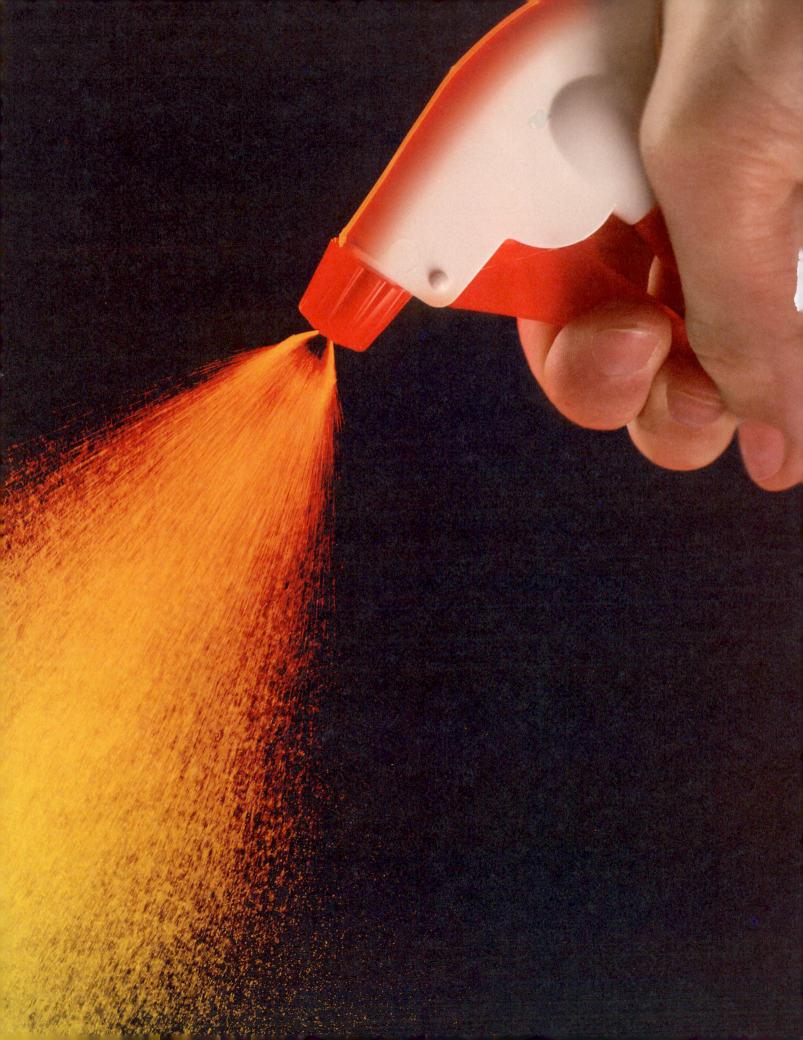

2

BACTERIA AND OTHER INFECTIOUS AGENTS

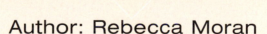

Author: Rebecca Moran

CHAPTER OUTLINE

Bacteria

Viruses and Fungus

Parasites

Understanding Infection

Learning Objectives

After you have completed this chapter, you should be able to:

1 Define and understand bacteria.

2 Explain the difference between pathogenic and nonpathogenic bacteria.

3 Identify and describe the main groups of pathogenic bacteria.

4 Give examples of common infections caused by viruses and bacteria.

5 Understand which types of infections are likely to occur on the fingernail.

6 Name the various types of immunities.

7 Name some common sources of infection in the salon.

8 Identify the steps necessary to protect you and your client from the spread of infection.

Key Terms

Page number indicates where in the chapter the term is used.

Acquired Immune Deficiency Syndrome (AIDS)
pg. 23

asepsis
pg. 22

bacilli
pg. 22

bacteria
pg. 21

cilia
pg. 23

cocci
pg. 22

contagious
pg. 28

diplococci
pg. 22

flagella
pg. 23

fungi
pg. 24

germs
pg. 22

immunity
pg. 26

immunocompromised
pg. 27

infection
pg. 25

microorganisms
pg. 21

mitosis
pg. 23

natural barrier
pg. 27

nonpathogenic
pg. 21

parasites
pg. 25

pathogenic
pg. 22

rickettsia
pg. 25

sepsis
pg. 22

spirilla
pg. 22

staphylococci
pg. 22

streptococci
pg. 22

toxins
pg. 22

viruses
pg. 23

Virtually any type of public service procedure can be completed safely, given the proper precautions. This is definitely true of services performed by *professional* nail technicians. Skilled professionals know that they must operate within certain parameters and guidelines, not only to maintain a high level of consistent quality, but also to safeguard their own longevity in their chosen career. As a professional nail technician you must be knowledgeable and aware of the possible problems infectious agents pose.

Not surprisingly, certain kinds of infections may be transmitted during nail services. In this chapter, you will learn what causes infection and how to prevent its spread. Then you will learn how easy it is to avoid these problems with proper disinfection and sanitation procedures. However, continuing education is a necessary tool for the true professional, and the issues surrounding infectious disease control should be a high educational priority. Public health matters are continually evolving as new findings, recommendations, and laws are released and implemented regularly. Maintaining a well-informed status on these topics is wise. The Food and Drug Administration (FDA), Centers for Disease Control (CDC), and Occupational Safety and Health Administration (OSHA) are just a few agencies the medical, public service, and health care industries consider to be invaluable resources. Remember, the best defense against infectious diseases is knowledge.

◆ ◆ ◆ BACTERIA

Bacteria (bak-TEER-ee-ah), the plural of bacterium, are one-celled **micro-organisms** (meye-kroh-OR-gah-niz-ems) that are so small they can only be seen through a microscope. A microorganism is any living thing that is too small to be seen by the eye. Many bacteria are so tiny that fifteen hundred of them barely cover the head of a pin. For example, one pinch of healthy, fertile soil can harbor over a billion bacteria. A thimble of soil can contain as many as five billion bacteria. Bacteria are the most plentiful organisms on earth. There are 15,000 known species of bacteria, and they can exist nearly everywhere. They multiply at an incredible speed. A single bacterial cell can produce 16,000,000 copies of itself in only half a day.

Bacteria are found in water, air, dust, lint, and decaying matter. They are on the skin of the body, in the secretions of body openings, on clothing, on your manicuring table, on your implements, and under nails. Most bacteria are harmless, but some can cause problems.

Types of Bacteria

Bacteria are classified into two types, depending on whether they are beneficial or harmful.

1. **Nonpathogenic** (non-path-o-JEN-ik) (non-disease-causing) bacteria can not harm us and are often beneficial. About 70 percent of all bacteria are nonpathogenic. Some forms of nonpathogenic bacteria

help produce food and oxygen. Others are used in compost piles to improve the fertility of the soil. In humans, nonpathogenic bacteria are most numerous in the mouth and intestines where they help the digestive process by breaking down food.

2. **Pathogenic** (path-o-JEN-ik) (disease-causing) bacteria are harmful. Though less than 30 percent of all bacteria are pathogenic, they are the most common cause of infection and disease in humans. Pathogenic bacteria are also called **germs**. They invade living plant or animal tissues and feed on living matter. They breed rapidly and spread disease by producing **toxins**, or poisons, in the tissue they invade. **Sepsis** is the presence in the blood or other tissues of pathogenic microorganisms or their toxins, and **asepsis** is freedom from disease-producing bacteria.

Classifications of Pathogenic Bacteria

There are three main groups of pathogenic bacteria. They include:

1. **Cocci** (KOK-si). These are round, pus-producing bacteria. Cocci appear singly or in groups as follows (Figure 2–1):

    a. **Staphylococci** (staf-lo-KOK-si) grow in clusters and are present in local infections, such as abscesses, pustules, and boils (Figure 2–2).

    b. **Streptococci** (strep-to-KOK-si) grow in chains. They cause strep throat and infections or diseases that spread throughout the body such as blood poisoning and rheumatic fever (Figure 2–3).

    c. **Diplococci** (deye-ploh-KOK-si) grow in pairs and cause pneumonia (Figure 2–4).

2. **Bacilli** (bah-SIL-i). These are the most common bacteria. They are rod-shaped and produce such diseases as tetanus, typhoid, tuberculosis, and diphtheria (Figure 2–5).

3. **Spirilla** (spi-RIL-a). These are spiral or corkscrew-shaped bacteria. One example of these bacteria is *treponema pallida* (trep-o-NE-mah PAL-i-dah), which causes syphilis (Figure 2–6).

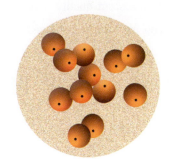

Figure 2–1 Cocci

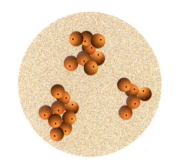

Figure 2–2 Staphylococci

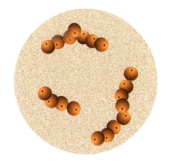

Figure 2–3 Streptococci

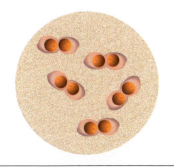

Figure 2–4 Diplococci

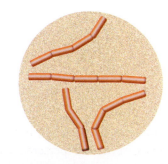

Figure 2–5 Bacilli

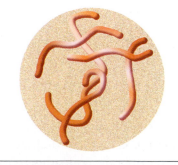

Figure 2–6 Spirilla

Growth and Reproduction of Bacteria

Bacteria live, grow, and multiply best in warm, dark, damp, unsanitary conditions. The drawer of a manicuring table is a perfect place to breed bacteria on dirty implements.

Each bacterium, or bacteria cell, has the ability to grow and reproduce. As bacteria are nourished, each bacterium grows in size. When it reaches maturity, it splits in half and forms two identical cells. This type of reproduction is called **mitosis** (meye-TOH-sus). These two cells will grow and divide again, forming four cells. It is easy to see how one bacterium can reproduce into as many as 16 million bacteria in 12 hours.

When conditions become unfavorable for growth and reproduction, some types of bacteria form a tough outer covering called a spore. Then they remain dormant, or in a state of rest. Some bacteria remain in very harsh conditions for long periods. Spores can be blown about in the dust and they are not harmed by even the most powerful disinfectants. When conditions become favorable, they again begin to grow and reproduce.

Movement of Bacteria

Bacteria travel very easily. They are spread through air or water, or through contact with contaminated objects. Bacilli and spirilla are the only bacteria that can propel themselves. They have hairlike projections known as **flagella** (flah-JEL-ah) or **cilia** (SIL-ee-a), which they move in a whiplike motion to propel themselves in liquid.

◆ ◆ ◆ VIRUSES AND FUNGUS

Viruses

Viruses are pathogenic (disease-causing) agents that are many times smaller than bacteria. Viruses enter a healthy cell, grow to maturity, and reproduce, often destroying the cell. Hepatitis, chicken pox, influenza, measles, mumps, and the common cold are examples of viral infections that can be transferred through casual contact with an infected person. Infection spreads when the person sneezes or coughs.

Acquired Immune Deficiency Syndrome (AIDS)

Acquired Immune Deficiency Syndrome (AIDS) is a disease caused by the HIV virus. HIV attacks, and usually destroys, the body's immune system. The disease usually lies dormant for many years. Some people have been infected for more than 15 years without showing symptoms. Luckily, it is very difficult to transmit HIV. Unlike other viruses, HIV cannot be transferred through casual contact with an infected person, sneezing, or coughing, etc. HIV is passed from one person to another through the transfer of bodily fluids, such as semen or blood.

The most common methods of transmitting HIV are

1. sexual contact with an infected person.

2. the use of dirty hypodermic needles for injectable drugs.

HIV can also be transferred from mother to child during pregnancy and birth. In the early 1980s HIV was transmitted during transfusions of infected blood. However, this rarely happens anymore.

Fortunately, it is virtually impossible to transfer HIV in the salon. HIV is not spread through salon services. You should make sure your clients are aware of this. Many are needlessly frightened and will look to you for reassurance. This does not mean that preventing disease transmission in the salon is not important. It simply means that HIV prevention is NOT the reason for proper sanitation and disinfection.

Fungus and Mold

Fungi (FUN-gi) is the general term for plantlike parasites, including all types of fungus and mold. Both are contagious, but only fungi are a risk to clients receiving nail services. Fungi can spread from nail to nail on the client.

Nail Fungal Infections

Certain common types of fungus may appear as white or discolored areas under the nail plate. They may appear to spread toward the cuticle. As the condition matures, the discoloration becomes darker. Fungus may affect the hands, feet, and nails. Clients with nail fungus must be referred to a physician (Figure 2–7).

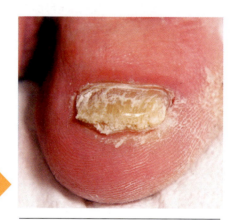

Figure 2-7 An example of nail fungus

Mold and Mildew

One of the biggest misconceptions in the nail industry is that molds or mildews can infect fingernails. These organisms rarely, if ever, appear on the fingernails. They are generally confused with the more common greenish bacterial infections (*Pseudomonas* bacteria). Improperly prepared nail plates harbor bacteria which survive on the moisture and oils found between an unsanitized natural nail and enhancements.

A bacterial infection can be identified in the early stages as a yellow-green spot that becomes darker in advanced stages. The green is caused by the bacteria's waste products. These wastes stain the nail plate causing a green discoloration long after the bacteria is gone. If the infection is destroyed, the green stain will remain.

If the nail has been infected for a period of time, the discoloration becomes black and the nail may soften or smell bad. Neglect is the major reason that this condition advances to this stage. Clients should be warned that the infection could become serious. A qualified medical doctor can quickly treat the problem.

Exposing the Natural Nail

You should not provide nail services for a client who has nail fungus or other infections, but the client may want you to remove any artificial nail covering to expose the natural nail. After the natural nail is exposed, the client should be referred to a physician.

You should wear gloves during removal of artificial nails and follow the manufacturer's directions for removal. When the artificial nail has been removed, discard orangewood sticks, abrasives, and any other porous product used. Disinfect all other implements and the table surface before and after the procedure.

Prevention

Bacterial and fungal infections are easily avoided by following sanitary precautions. In most cases, these problems are caused by the nail technician. Do not perform nail services for a client who has discoloration on his or her nails. Do not take short cuts or omit any of the sanitation steps when performing an artificial nail service. If you find that your clients are suffering from such infections you should reexamine your procedures and application techniques for the cause. No one should suffer from nail infections. These problems are bad for the client, a poor reflection on your services, and a black eye for the entire nail industry.

◆ ◆ ◆ PARASITES

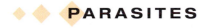

Parasites (PAR-ah-syts) are tiny, multi-celled animal or plant organisms that live off living matter without providing any benefits to their hosts. An example of plant parasite infection is ringworm. Animal parasites are responsible for such contagious diseases as scabies, itch-mite, and pediculosis (lice).

Rickettsia

Rickettsia (rik-ET-see-ah) are much smaller organisms than bacteria, but larger than viruses. They cause typhus and Rocky Mountain spotted fever. Fleas, ticks, and lice carry rickettsia.

◆ ◆ ◆ UNDERSTANDING INFECTION

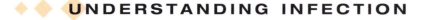

An **infection** occurs when body tissue is invaded by disease-causing microorganisms such as bacteria, viruses, and fungi. Microorganisms establish themselves and multiply in body tissue to produce tissue damage. At first, the infection is usually localized. Infection that spreads to the bloodstream is called a general infection. Blood poisoning is a type of general or systemic infection.

SAFETY CAUTION

During the removal process of some artificial nail products, your client has her hands soaking in a container of acetone. Place a clean terry cloth towel over her hands and the container. This helps to minimize the fumes from the acetone rising into your client's face (Figures 2–8a and 2–8b).

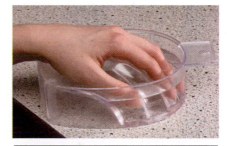

Figure 2–8a Soaking in acetone to remove artificial nails can produce strong fumes.

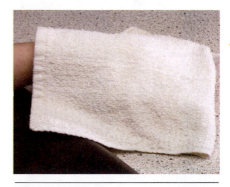

Figure 2–8b Placing a towel over the hand and bowl protects the client from fumes.

Immunity to Infection

All living organisms have defenses or immunity against infection. Immunity (i-MYOO-ni-tee) is the ability of the body to resist disease and destroy microorganisms when they have entered the body. Immunity against disease is a sign of good health. Immunity can be natural, naturally acquired, or artificially acquired.

1. **Natural immunity.** By keeping our bodies healthy, we are able to fight off microorganisms before they can grow and cause disease. Our bodies fight infection in three ways.

    a. We have a protective layer of unbroken skin.

    b. We naturally secrete perspiration and digestive juices that discourage the growth of pathogens.

    c. Our blood contains white blood cells that kill pathogens.

2. **Naturally acquired immunity.** After fighting off a disease, antibodies (a type of protein molecule) remain in the bloodstream ready to fight another attack of the microorganisms should they return.

3. **Artificially acquired immunity.** This immunity is one produced by the injection of a serum or vaccine. The injection introduces a small dose of dead or disabled pathogens into the body. This small dose fools the immune system into making antibodies that can fight that particular disease.

How Infections Breed in the Salon

Most bacteria, viruses, fungi, and other pathogens enter the body through the nose, the mouth, and small breaks in the skin. They can also enter the body through your eyes or ears. You are at risk of becoming infected or transmitting infection to your clients because you come in constant contact with pathogens in the salon. Some of the common sources of infections include:

1. **Contaminated manicuring tools and equipment.** Bacteria and other pathogens multiply at a very rapid rate in places such as dirty nail files, cuticle nippers, manicuring tables, trash cans, and towels (Figure 2–9).

2. **Your clients' nails, hands, and feet.** Each client who walks into the salon brings in a whole new set of microorganisms and possibly parasites. When you perform a service on this client, you risk being infected. When you perform artificial nail services, you risk trapping pathogens between the natural nail plate and the enhancement or overlay.

3. **Your clients', coworkers', and your own mouth, nose, and eyes.** Anyone in the salon who has a cough, is sneezing, or has a runny nose is like a fountain of bacteria or viruses.

4. **Open wounds or sores on you or your client.** Infected fluids can be transferred from one person to another through open wounds.

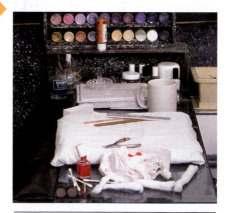

Figure 2-9 Bacteria multiply rapidly on a messy manicuring table.

5. **Objects throughout the entire salon.** Pathogens collect on chairs, telephones, cash registers, tables, towels, bottles, brushes, and everything else that is exposed to the air in the salon. They also collect on the fixtures in the rest room—especially the door handle.

Who Is Most At Risk?

Several factors contribute to the contracting or spreading of infectious diseases. Broken skin, poor hygiene, poor diet, being very young, old, or **immunocompromised** (having an impaired or injured immune system; unable to fight off disease) are factors that can influence the susceptibility of an individual. Frequent traveling, especially global travels, and exposure to visitors from other countries can influence one's susceptibility, as well as community factors, such as limited access to proper health care and immunizations, poor housing, and cultural customs.

Occupational factors can play an important role in susceptibility to infectious diseases. Health care workers, service workers, and those who work closely with the public are more susceptible than those who work in a more closed, non-exposed environment. Nail technicians fall into the categories of service workers and those who work with the public, so they must work defensively, utilizing every precaution for their own protection from the contraction of diseases, and for the protection of their clients from the spread of disease.

Broken skin interferes with two of the many **natural barriers** we have against infection—the skin and its mantle. When the skin is broken or the mantle is reduced or it's acidic balance changed, it is said to be compromised. This means its barrier function is not working as it should. When this happens, non-desirable materials can enter, such as pathogenic bacteria or viruses, and infection can be the result.

Poor hygiene on the part of the professional allows direct client exposure to disease-producing bacteria. Rapid growth of bacteria is then transferred to the client. A client who is immunocompromised is especially susceptible to disease after this transfer. Of course, poor hygiene on the part of the client can allow the transfer of pathogenic bacteria to the professional, though it can be prevented. Stringent sanitation activities and the use of protective equipment, such as gloves or masks, will help protect the wise professional.

Poor diet prevents any person from having a full arsenal of protection from an invading pathogenic microorganism. It can also allow a person's immune system to become compromised, allowing more susceptibility to disease. A working professional must eat properly for protection from disease. Proper nutrition helps the body produce a sufficient supply of antibodies (disease fighters) and maintain a high level of energy for a defense against infection. Any person with an immune system that is not working properly will be more susceptible to disease. These bodies will not respond properly, with less vigor to fight off disease. The very young, due to their immature immune system, and the very old, due to their weakened immune system, are also considered more susceptible to diseases.

2

Travelers to other countries and climates are at an increased risk because they may have unknowingly been exposed to infectious diseases to which their bodies are unfamiliar. Their bodies have no natural immunity to these invading infections and cannot fight off the disease. Many of these diseases will not become apparent for quite some time after their return, due to lengthy incubation periods. For that reason, clients who have recently traveled out of the country are at a higher risk for contracting and carrying infectious diseases.

Never assume that someone who looks and appears healthy does not present a risk. Regular and correct hand washing with a liquid soap and a thorough drying with paper towels is important in preventing the transfer of disease.

How Nail Technicians Can Fight Infections

As a professional, you are responsible for keeping yourself and your clients safe from infection. Here are the steps to take.

1. **Learn proper sanitation and disinfection procedures and follow them.** Chapter 3 in this book describes the procedures to follow for proper sanitation. It is your professional responsibility to learn these procedures and follow them faithfully. If you decide to short-cut sanitation and disinfection, you could easily become infected or transmit infection to your clients.

2. **Do not work in contagious conditions.** You should not work with clients while they are **contagious** (kon-TAY-jus), or have an infection that can easily be transmitted from one person to another. Someone with a severe cold, influenza, or chicken pox, for example, should not receive nail services. The same holds true for nail technicians. You should also stay home and rest if you are contagious. Working with the public, you could easily start your own local flu or cold epidemic.

3. **Do not work near an open wound.** Refer clients who have an open wound to a physician and make sure they return with a written release before you perform any services for them.

4. **Do not cause wounds.** Be very careful when you are performing nail services. It is easy to cut a client while manicuring cuticles or to break the skin if you file too deeply. Overfiling with heavy abrasives and files can also cause wounds and bruises to the sensitive nail bed.

5. **Eat properly and get the rest your body needs.** Proper nutrition and a sufficient amount of rest are very important. They will help your body fight infection and give you the energy you need to do a great job.

It is your job to provide a safe haven for your clients. You can only do this if you understand how. In the next chapter you will learn how to ensure that you are protecting the health of every client, as well as yourself.

BUSINESS TIP

Reassuring Your Clients About Safety

Your clients belong to today's "protection generation": at the doctor's office they are examined with a gloved hand and when they go to the dentist office they see individually-wrapped tarter scrapers. As a result, clients are interested in knowing what precautions you are taking to prevent the spread of harmful bacteria, viruses, and fungi that grow in the salon and can affect their health. Reassure them by showing them the sanitation measures that you take. When speaking with your clients, remember, you're trying to create a feeling of security. Say something like, "This is how I disinfect my tools and wipe down my table for your safety."

chapter glossary

Acquired Immune Deficiency Syndrome (AIDS)	A disease caused by the HIV virus that can lie dormant for many years, but then attacks and usually destroys the body's immune system.
asepsis	Blood that is free of disease-producing bacteria.
bacilli	The most common, rod-shaped bacteria that produces such diseases as tetanus, influenza, typhoid, tuberculosis, and diphtheria.
bacteria	(Plural of bacterium); small, one-celled microorganisms that can only be seen through a microscope.
cilia	Hairlike projections on bacilli and spirilla that move in a whiplike motion to propel the bacteria in liquid.
cocci	Round, pus-producing bacteria that appear singly or in groups.
contagious	Having a disease that is easily transmitted from one person to another.
diplococci	Cocci that grows in pairs and can cause pneumonia.
flagella	Hairlike projections on bacilli and spirilla that move in a whiplike motion to propel the bacteria in liquid.
fungi	The general term used to describe plantlike parasites that can spread easily from nail to nail.

germs	Disease-causing bacteria.
immunity	The ability of the body to resist disease and destroy microorganisms when they have entered the body. Immunity can be natural, naturally acquired, or artificially acquired.
immunocompromised	Having an impaired or injured immune system; unable to fight off disease.
infection	Contamination that occurs when body tissue is invaded by disease-causing microorganisms such as bacteria, viruses, and fungi.
microorganisms	Any living things that are too small to be seen by the eye.
mitosis	Cell reproduction in which cells grow and split in half to form two identical cells. These two cells grow and split again, forming four cells. This process continues to repeat itself, creating millions of cells.
natural barrier	The protective barrier furnished by the eponychium tissue, protecting against bacteria and other invaders.
nonpathogenic	Non-disease-causing; not harmful.
parasites	Tiny, multi-celled animal or plant organisms that live off living matter without providing any benefit to their host.
pathogenic	Disease-causing; disease-producing; harmful.
rickettsia	Organisms carried by fleas, ticks, and lice that are much smaller than bacteria, but larger than viruses and cause typhus and Rocky Mountain spotted fever.
sepsis	The presence in the blood or other tissues of pathogenic microorganisms or their toxins.
spirilla	Spiral or corkscrew-shaped bacteria that can cause such diseases as syphilis.
staphylococci	Cocci that grows in clusters and are found in local infections such as abscesses, pustules, and boils.
streptococci	Cocci that grows in chains and can cause such diseases and infections as strep throat, blood poisoning, and rheumatic fever.
toxins	Poisonous substances produced by some microorganisms.
viruses	Pathogenic (disease-causing) agents, much smaller than bacteria, that enter a healthy cell, grow to maturity, and reproduce, often destroying the cell.

2

1. What are bacteria? What do bacteria look like?

2. Are all bacteria harmful? Give examples to explain your answer.

3. What are the three main groups of pathogenic bacteria? Describe them.

4. Why can bacteria reproduce so quickly?

5. Give examples of common infections caused by viruses.

6. Is it likely that salon services can cause AIDS?

7. Describe the appearance of bacterial infection on the nail plate.

8. Do molds and mildew grow on or under the nail plate?

9. What is immunity? Name three types of immunity.

10. Name five common sources of infection in the salon.

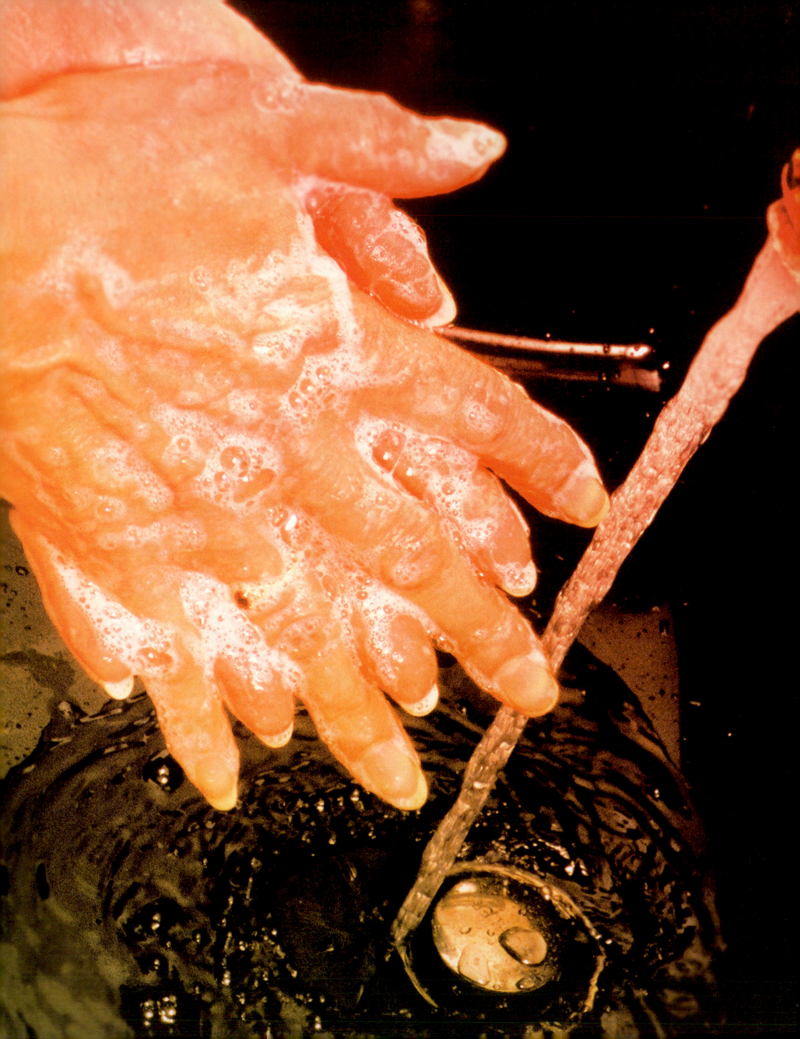

3

SANITATION AND DISINFECTION

Author: Rebecca Moran

CHAPTER OUTLINE

**Contamination Control • Sterilization • Sanitation • Disinfection
Implements and Other Surfaces • Ultraviolet Ray Sanitizers • Bead "Sterilizers"
Beware of Formalin • Blood Spills • Disinfectant Safety • Universal Sanitation**

PROCEDURE

Procedure 3-1 Pre-service Sanitation

Learning Objectives

After you have completed this chapter, you should be able to:

1 Understand contamination control and identify common salon contaminants.

2 Explain why sterilization is not important in the professional salon.

3 Define sanitation and disinfection and know when each is appropriate.

4 Know how to effectively use disinfectants on implements and hard surfaces.

5 Perform Universal Sanitation procedures in your salon.

Key Terms

Page number indicates where in the chapter the term is used.

allergic sensitizer
pg. 43

antiseptics
pg. 36

bactericides
pg. 38

contaminant
pg. 35

contaminated
pg. 35

decontamination
pg. 35

disinfectants
pg. 37

disinfection
pg. 37

disinfection containers
pg. 38

formaldehyde
pg. 43

fungicides
pg. 38

hospital-level disinfectant
pg. 38

Material Safety Data Sheet (MSDS)
pg. 38

pathogens
pg. 35

phenolics
pg. 39

quaternary ammonium compounds (quats)
pg. 39

sanitation (sanitizing)
pg. 36

sterilization
pg. 35

viricides
pg. 38

wet sanitizers
pg. 38

hen you become a nail technician, you are licensed to apply professional products to the hands, feet, and nails of the general public. Whenever you work with the public there is the possibility of infection or injury to you and your clients. The risks are much greater if your implements and work area are not properly cleaned or you do not use disinfection products correctly. States have strict rules for sanitation and disinfection procedures at manicuring work stations. These regulations are in place to protect both you and your clients.

In this chapter, you will learn the proper procedures to enable you to pass state licensing exams and become a licensed nail technician. However, you will learn much more. You will learn why and when you should sanitize or disinfect and what the consequences are if you do not.

◆ ◆ ◆ CONTAMINATION CONTROL

What do floors, door knobs, table tops, and implements have in common? Each of these has a surface. The problem with a surface is that eventually it will become contaminated. Any surface that is not completely free of all foreign substances is **contaminated**. A substance that causes contamination is called a **contaminant**.

Filings and dust are contaminants. Even liquid monomer in a towel is a contaminant. Implements may appear to be clean when, in fact, they are covered with bacteria.

In the last chapter you learned that disease-causing microorganisms are called **pathogens**. Your duty as a professional is to control pathogens. **Decontamination** is the elimination of contaminants, including pathogens, from implements or other surfaces. There are three types of decontamination.

1. sterilization
2. sanitation
3. disinfection

◆ ◆ ◆ STERILIZATION

Sterilization destroys all living organisms on an object or surface. Sterilization is a difficult, multi-step process. Some sterilization techniques are far too dangerous to be used in the salon. It is impractical and virtually impossible to sterilize tools and surfaces in the salon. Sterilization is only required for surgical procedures.

The word "sterilize" is often used incorrectly. For instance, it is impossible to sterilize the nail plate or cuticle. Sterilizing would destroy the nail plate and kill the skin. There is no need to sterilize anything in the salon. It is not possible to kill all microorganisms in the salon, nor should you try. You only have to control pathogens so they cannot cause infection or illness.

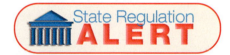

You must obey the rules issued by your local Health Department and your state cosmetology regulatory agency. Be alert for changes in the rules and regulations in your area. For your own safety and that of your clients, it is extremely important that you obtain and obey sanitation/ disinfection rules and regulations.

3

◆ ◆ SANITATION

The lowest level of decontamination is called **sanitation** or **sanitizing**. Sanitation will significantly reduce the number of pathogens on a surface. Normally, low levels of pathogens are considered safe, so sanitation can be a very effective form of decontamination.

Cleaning with detergent and water is an example of sanitizing. Putting antiseptics on skin or nail plates is sanitizing. **Antiseptics** reduce the number of pathogens in a cut and the immune system kills those that remain. So, antiseptics are sanitizers that help prevent skin infections.

Hand washing is also a form of sanitation (Figure 3–1). Frequent hand washing is an important way to control the spread of dangerous organisms. Hand washing removes many types of contaminants. Dirt, oils, monomer, other product residues, and pathogens are all removed by frequent hand washing. Always use a liquid soap, following the manufacturer's directions. Generally, you need to actively wash for a minimum of 15 to 20 seconds for complete cleansing action.

Sanitation is a vital routine that must not be ignored. Sanitation is a critical part of maintaining a professional establishment. Below are some simple guidelines that will help keep the salon clean and sanitary.

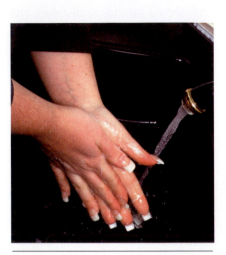

Figure 3–1 Hand washing is a form of sanitation.

❖ Floors should be swept clean whenever needed.

❖ Deposit all waste materials in a metal waste can with a self-closing lid.

❖ Waste cans must be emptied regularly throughout the day.

❖ Mop floors and vacuum carpets every day.

❖ Dust and nail filings can carry pathogens so they must be controlled.

❖ Windows, screens, and curtains should be clean.

❖ Salons need both hot and cold running water.

❖ Rest rooms must be clean and tidy (Figure 3–2).

❖ Toilet tissue, paper towels, and liquid soap must be provided.

❖ Wash hands after using the rest room and between clients.

❖ Clean doorknobs often, especially in the bathroom.

❖ Clean sinks and drinking fountains regularly.

❖ Separate or disposable drinking cups must be provided.

❖ The salon must be free from insects and rodents.

❖ Salons should never be used for cooking or living quarters.

❖ Food must never be placed in refrigerators used to store salon products.

❖ Eating, drinking, and smoking in the salon is prohibited by federal regulations.

❖ Employees must wear clean, freshly washed clothing.

❖ Always use a freshly laundered or disposable table towel for each client.

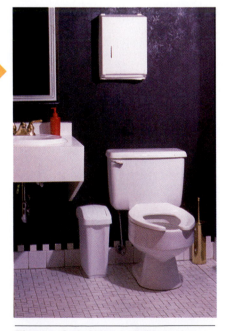

Figure 3–2 Clean and tidy rest room

❖ All containers must be clearly marked, tightly closed, and properly stored.

❖ The outside of all containers, pumps, and dappen dishes should be kept clean.

❖ Soiled linen is to be removed from the workplace and properly stored for cleaning. Then it must be washed at 160°F for a minimum of 25 minutes or it can be effectively sanitized at a slightly lower temperature with carefully controlled amounts of detergent and bleach.

❖ Do not place any implements or tools in your mouth or pockets.

❖ Implements must be properly cleaned, disinfected, and stored *after each use.*

❖ Professionals should avoid touching their face or eye area during services.

❖ Wash hands before touching the face, eyes, eating, or using the rest room.

❖ No pets or animals should ever be allowed in salons, except for trained, seeing eye dogs.

These are only a few of the things you must do in order to safeguard yourself and clients. Contact your local State Board of Cosmetology or Health Department for a complete list of regulations.

◆ ◆ ◆ DISINFECTION

Sterilization is not practical in salons and sanitation may not kill all pathogens. How can nail technicians prevent the spread of dangerous organisms? Disinfection is the answer! **Disinfection** controls microorganisms on nonliving surfaces, such as implements. Disinfection is the second level of decontamination. It is a much higher level than sanitation and is almost identical to sterilization, except disinfection does not kill bacterial spores. Fortunately, bacterial spores cause no harm in salons. Therefore, disinfection is just as effective in the salon as sterilization, but without the expense, danger, and hassle.

Disinfectants are substances that destroy pathogens on implements and other nonliving surfaces, but are not safe for use on skin or nails. Disinfectants are designed to kill pathogens. Substances powerful enough to destroy pathogens will certainly damage skin. Disinfectants are serious, professional-strength tools that may cause irritation and skin damage with prolonged or repeated contact.

Of course, manufacturers of these products are careful to make disinfectants as safe as possible. However, disinfectants are potentially dangerous if used incorrectly, and like all of your tools, must be used properly. Disinfectants are only safe if used *exactly* as the manufacturer instructs and definitely kept out of the reach of children. Federal law requires that you be given directions for proper use, safety precautions, a list of active ingredients, and a list of the virus that the product is effective against. You must also receive a **Material Safety Data Sheet (MSDS)**. More information on the MSDS is provided in Chapter 4.

Effective Use of Disinfectants

Each disinfectant is different. The best way to learn about them is to **read the manufacturers' instructions.** You should also periodically review these directions in case new information is added.

High quality disinfectants must perform a variety of special jobs in the salon. They must be

bactericides (to kill harmful bacteria).

viricides (to kill pathogenic viruses).

fungicides (to destroy fungus).

A **hospital-level disinfectant** must perform all of these functions and pass special EPA registration tests. EPA registered, hospital-level disinfectants are perfect for salons. In fact, they exceed requirements for salon disinfection. Unless you are cleaning up blood spills, no other disinfectant is required.

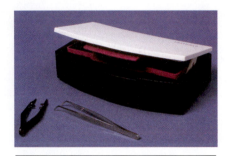

Figure 3-3 Disinfection container

Always clean implements before placing them into the disinfectant. Dirty implements will contaminate the disinfecting solution. Nail filings, oils, and lotions will lessen the effectiveness of the solution. The glass, metal, or plastic jars or containers used to disinfect implements are often incorrectly called **wet sanitizers**. They should really be called **disinfection containers** (Figure 3–3). The purpose of these containers is not to sanitize, but instead, to disinfect.

Cloudy disinfectant solution must be changed immediately. Change the solution according to manufacturer's instructions regardless of its appearance. If you think that using cloudy, contaminated disinfectant is "better than nothing," think again! Microorganisms can live in contaminated disinfectant solutions. Besides, if clients see implements in a jar of cloudy liquid, they will not think highly of you. Also, be sure that the implement is properly placed in the disinfecting solution. The EPA recommends that implements be *fully immersed for a minimum of ten minutes.* The extent of killing of the bacteria is based on these factors.

1. correct concentration of the disinfectant

2. type and amount of bacteria

3. time of contact in the solution

4. temperature of the solution

5. correct pH of the solution

6. presence of foreign matter, such as hair, skin, and nails

Types of Disinfectants

Quats

There are several types of salon disinfectants. **Quaternary ammonium compounds (quats)** are the most commonly used. Quats have the advantage of being safe and fast-acting. Most disinfectants of this type are blends of many different kinds of quats. This dramatically increases effectiveness. Quats are the most cost effective of all professional disinfectants. Most quat solutions disinfect implements in ten minutes with total immersion. A 1:1000 solution of quats requires a one- to five-minute immersion time. Leaving them in for too long may damage metal implements. However, most formulas contain corrosion and rust inhibitors. Quats are also very effective for cleaning table and counter tops.

Phenolics

Like quats, **phenolics** have been used for many years to disinfect implements. They too can be safe and extremely effective if used according to instructions. Some materials, such as rubber and certain plastics, are not compatible with these disinfectants. Phenolics can soften and destroy these materials over time. Care should be taken to avoid skin contact with phenolics. The concentrated liquid can cause serious skin irritation and is corrosive to the eyes. Avoid uncontrolled spraying of phenolic-type disinfectants. Inhalation of the mists can be extremely irritating to the sensitive lining of the nose, throat, and lungs. Phenolics are highly effective, but they are the most expensive of all common, professional salon disinfectants. Some states have expressed concern over disposal of phenolic disinfectants because of their high alkaline pH (usually greater than pH 11). You should check your state regulations to see if special disposal restrictions exist for phenolic disinfectants. As with all disinfectants, you must exactly follow manufacturer's instructions.

Alcohol and Bleach

Common alcohol and bleach are sometimes used for disinfecting implements. To be effective disinfectants, implements must be completely immersed for ten to twenty minutes. A simple wipe with alcohol is completely ineffective as a disinfectant. There are many disadvantages to using alcohol and bleach. Alcohol is extremely flammable, evaporates quickly, is slow acting and less effective than professionally designed disinfectant systems. They cannot be diluted below 70 percent or concentrated much above 80 percent, or they lose effectiveness. Alcohol needs hydration to work, but can easily be diluted too much. It will corrode tools and cause sharp edges to become dull. Household bleach is effective as a disinfectant, but shares some of the same drawbacks of alcohol. Neither bleach nor alcohol are professionally designed and tested for disinfection of salon implements. Bleach can discolor some materials and has almost no cleaning power. Bleach was used extensively in the past, but has since been replaced by more advanced and effective technologies. Some states have specific time requirements, while others do not allow the use of alcohol or bleach as a disinfectant at all. Be guided by your instructor.

IMPLEMENTS AND OTHER SURFACES

There are many things that require disinfection, for example, table and counter tops, mirrors, telephone receivers, door handles, etc. Implements such as clippers, nippers, cuticle pushers, scissors, reusable forms, and manicure and pedicure bowls must be disinfected between each client.

Some files and buffers can be disinfected. Check with the manufacturer for disinfection recommendations. Buffers, files, porous drill bits and wooden sticks that absorb water cannot be disinfected. Brushes used in applying acrylics and gels do not require disinfection.

To decontaminate other surfaces such as counter tops, wash them thoroughly with a detergent, then spray or wipe on a disinfectant recommended for this purpose. Wipe up the disinfectant and spray again. Then allow the surface to air dry. Be sure to wear gloves while disinfecting surfaces. Also, if using a spray bottle, wear a mask and take care to avoid inhalation of the mists.

ULTRAVIOLET RAY SANITIZERS

Once implements are properly disinfected, they must be stored where they will remain free from contamination. Ultraviolet (U.V.) sanitizers are useful storage containers, but the types sold to salons *will not disinfect salon implements.* They are not very effective against viruses and cannot reach into crevices. Never use these devices to disinfect! However, they make useful storage cabinets for properly disinfected implements (Figure 3–5). Another alternative is to store your implements in an airtight container, i.e. Rubber Maid™ or Tupper Ware™, etc.

BEAD "STERILIZERS"

These devices do not sterilize or disinfect implements. They only give users a false sense of security. Sterilizing an implement with dry heat would require heating to 325°F for at least 30 minutes. These units cannot even come close to doing this. Also, to be effective, the entire implement, including handle, would have to be buried in the beads. These devices are a waste of money and a gamble with your client's health. Do not be fooled by claims suggesting that these are FDA registered devices. This means absolutely nothing. The FDA does not require any testing or proof; therefore, FDA registration is meaningless to salon professionals.

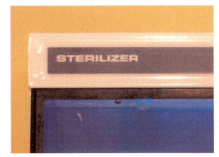

Figure 3–5 Ultraviolet (U.V.) sanitizer

3

PROCEDURE

3-1

Pre-service Sanitation

Before your service begins you should perform the following steps.

1. **Wash implements.** Rinse all implements with cool running water, then thoroughly wash them with soap and warm water emulsifying the dirt and breaking the surface tension. Brush grooved items if necessary, and open hinges (Figure 3–4a).

2. **Rinse implements in plain water.** Rinse away all traces of soap with plain water. The presence of soap, in most disinfectants, can cause them to become inactive. Soap is most easily rinsed off in warm-as-possible water. Dry thoroughly with a clean or disposable towel (Figure 3–4b).

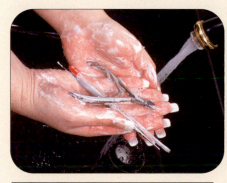

Figure 3–4a Wash implements.

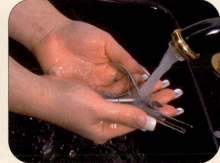

Figure 3–4b Rinse implements in clear water.

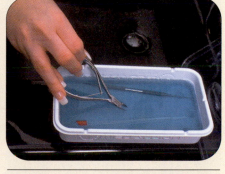

Figure 3–4c Immerse implements in disinfectant.

3. **Completely immerse implements in disinfectant solution.** It is very important that the surface tension is broken prior to immersion into the disinfecting solution, or the implement will remain contaminated. It will, additionally, contaminate the disinfectant solution. Immerse implements in a container holding an EPA registered, hospital-level disinfectant for the required time (usually ten minutes). If it is cloudy, the solution is contaminated and must be replaced. Make sure to avoid skin contact with all disinfectants by using tongs or rubber gloves (Figure 3–4c).

4. **Wash hands with liquid soap.** Thoroughly wash your hands with liquid soap, rinse, and dry with a clean or disposable towel. Liquid soaps are far more sanitary than bar soaps and are required by law in most states. A soap dish can also breed bacteria (Figure 3–4d).

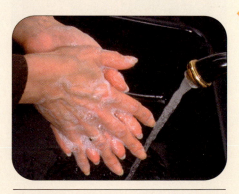

Figure 3–4d Wash hands with a liquid soap.

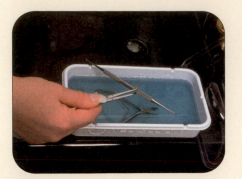

Figure 3–4e Remove implements with tongs or wearing rubber gloves and rinse.

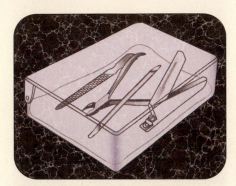

Figure 3–4f Store sanitized implements in a covered container.

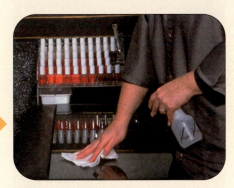

Figure 3–4g Sanitize table.

5. **Rinse implements and dry with a clean or disposable towel.** Remove implements from disinfectant solution with tongs or while wearing rubber gloves, rinse well in water, and wipe dry with a clean or disposable towel to prevent rusting (Figure 3–4e).

6. **Follow approved storage procedure.** Follow your state regulations for storage of sanitized manicuring implements. The regulations will tell you to store sanitized implements in sealed containers, or to keep them in a cabinet sanitizer until ready to be used (Figure 3–4f).

7. **Sanitize table.** To sanitize, wipe manicuring table with disinfectant or sanitizing solution (Figure 3–4g).

8. **Disinfect surface.** To disinfect, spray surface with any EPA registered disinfectant that is allowed by your state regulations. Allow surface to remain wet for ten minutes and wipe dry, then spray again and let air dry (Figure 3–4h).

9. **Wrap client's cushion in clean towel.** Put a clean towel over your manicuring cushion. Be sure to use a clean towel for each client (Figure 3–4i).

10. **Refill disposable materials.** Put a new emery board, a new orangewood stick, cotton balls, and other disposable materials on your manicuring table. These materials are discarded after use on *one* client (Figure 3–4j).

11. **Use a sanitizing hand wash.** Clients like to see that you practice sanitation. Make a ceremony of this and they will trust you. When the client sits at your table use a waterless hand sanitizer gel or wipe on your hands. Ask your client to do so, too. Be sure to make an effort to regularly rehydrate your hands, as you will be doing this often and some dryness may occur (Figure 3–4k).

Now you are ready to begin your service.

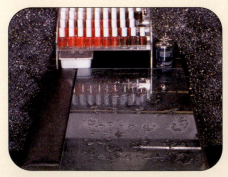

Figure 3–4h Disinfect the surface of your table.

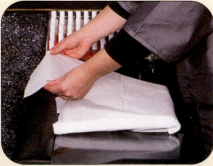

Figure 3–4i Wrap cushion in a clean towel.

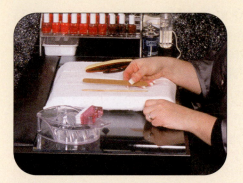

Figure 3–4j Replenish disposable materials.

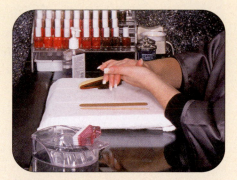

Figure 3–4k Use a sanitizing hand wash.

◆ ◆ ◆ BEWARE OF FORMALIN

For many years, formalin was used as a disinfectant and fumigant in dry cabinet sanitizers. Formalin *is not safe for salon use* and cannot be used in some states. Formalin contains large amounts of formaldehyde, a suspected human cancer-causing agent. It is poisonous to inhale or touch and is very irritating to the eyes, nose, throat, and lungs. It can also cause skin irritation, dryness, and rash. Formaldehyde is a strong allergic sensitizer. Prolonged or repeated exposure can cause allergic reactions similar to chronic bronchitis or asthma. These symptoms may take months to appear and then worsen over time with continued exposure.

◆ ◆ ◆ BLOOD SPILLS

There are several pathogens (i.e., hepatitis B) that can be found in blood. Since health care professionals regularly deal with seriously ill people, they must be very careful cleaning up blood spills. Many health care regulations have been written about cleaning up blood. Many State Cosmetology Boards have borrowed from these hospital regulations and have mandated handling procedures concerning accidental cuts and blood exposure. In addition to your state board requirements, OSHA has adopted the standard of mandatory reporting of blood exposure incidents, by the employee to the employer.

If a blood spill occurs, many state boards require the use of a tuberculocidal disinfectant to clean up the *visible* blood. These disinfectants are considered to provide a little extra protection where blood spills are involved. This does not mean that other disinfectants are weak. Any EPA registered, hospital-level disinfectant will easily exceed all normal salon requirements.

Here's a Tip:
After each procedure that involves artificial nails, discard your plastic trash bag. This will prevent the release of vapors from products you've used.

3

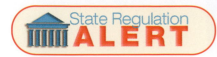
Tuberculocidal disinfectants will not prevent the spread of TB in salons. It is impossible to transmit TB on a salon implement. Tuberculocidal disinfectants are safe, but must be used with extra caution. Most are based on phenolic compounds. The potential hazards of such materials were described earlier in this chapter.

Most cuts occur from new files or emery boards. One way to prevent this is to rub the edges of new files against the abrasive side of another file. This will "break in" the file and soften sharp edges. If you are careful, you will rarely cut a client. But, accidents will happen. If you do cut a client with a file… never try to disinfect it! Tell your client that you are sorry and give them the file to take home. They will see it as a nice gift, but you have just gotten rid of a difficult disinfection problem. Remember, alert your employer.

DISINFECTANT SAFETY

Be sure to read and follow exactly the instructions provided with any professional salon product. Wear *gloves* and *safety glasses* when mixing and using any product, especially disinfectants (Figure 3–6). Do not reuse disposable gloves, as the protective barrier they provide is compromised when used the first time, especially if chemicals are involved. They offer little or no protection after the initial use. Reuse puts both you and your client at risk. *Never* stick your fingers into a disinfectant. Your skin is a barrier between you and microorganisms. Keep that barrier healthy by wearing gloves and avoiding skin contact. Never pour alcohol, bleach, or other disinfectants over your hands. This foolish practice can cause skin disease and increase the chance of infection. Wash your hands with liquid soap and dry them thoroughly.

Carefully measure everything when mixing disinfectants. Otherwise, you cannot expect peak performance. Never place any product or other chemical in an unmarked bottle. This is an invitation to accidents and could have disastrous consequences. Always use clean tongs to remove implements from disinfection solutions. Store all professional products away from food and in a cool, dark, dry location. Be sure they are tightly closed and out of the reach of children.

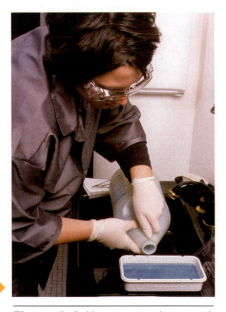

Figure 3–6 Always wear gloves and safety glasses when mixing products, especially disinfectants.

UNIVERSAL SANITATION

To make your salon a safe haven you must use gloves and safety glasses, disinfectants and detergents, personal hygiene and salon cleanliness practices, sanitizers and antiseptics. When all of these things are performed together, it is called *Universal Sanitation*. You're doing it all! Universal sanitation is one of many responsibilities you have as a salon professional. You have the responsibility to protect your clients from harm. They depend on your training and expertise. Today, more than ever, clients are concerned about safety and health. You also have a responsibility to yourself to protect your safety. Do not take short cuts when it comes to sanitation and disinfection. These important measures are also designed to protect you!

Finally, you have a responsibility to your profession. When anyone acts unprofessionally in the salon, everyone's image is tarnished. Clients expect to see you act in a professional manner. This is how trust and respect are earned!

BUSINESS TIP

Promote Nail Health

Clients come to you not only for beautiful-looking hands, but to solve nail problems, such as strengthening too-soft tips or doing something about brittleness and cracking. This is why, in addition to learning about nail anatomy and growth, it's important to know how various circumstances affect nails—from pregnancy to diet to prescription drug use. Medical texts offer a good source of information about conditions affecting nails, as do dermatology and nutrition publications. Being knowledgeable about nail health lets you custom-tailor a manicure to solve an individual's problems and allows you to prescribe personalized homecare regimens. Your clients will appreciate your professional knowledge and your work will appear that much nicer on strong, healthy nails.

chapter glossary

allergic sensitizer	A substance that causes serious allergic reactions due to prolonged or repeated exposure.
antiseptics	Sanitizers that help prevent skin infections by reducing the number of pathogens in an opening in the skin.
bactericides	Disinfectants that kill harmful bacteria.
contaminant	A substance that causes contamination.
contaminated	Made impure by contact; tainted or polluted.
decontamination	Elimination of contaminants, including pathogens, from any surface. Three types of decontamination include sterilization, sanitation, and disinfection.
disinfectants	Substances that destroy pathogens on implements and other nonliving surfaces; not safe for use on hands or nails.
disinfection	Process used to destroy contaminants on implements and other nonliving surfaces; a higher level of decontamination than sanitation.
disinfection containers	Glass, metal, or plastic jars or containers used to disinfect implements.
formaldehyde	A suspected human cancer-causing agent found in formalin.
fungicides	Disinfectants that destroy fungus.
hospital-level disinfectant	Disinfectant that must kill harmful bacteria and pathogenic viruses, destroy fungus, and pass special EPA registration tests.
Material Safety Data Sheet (MSDS)	A document supplied by product manufacturers, and available to anyone who uses the product, that contains basic safety and handling information about a product.
pathogens	Any disease-causing microorganisms.
phenolics	Highly effective, concentrated liquid disinfectants used in salons; can be destructive to certain materials and is very expensive.
quaternary ammonium compounds (quats)	Safe and fast-acting salon disinfectants commonly used to clean implements, tables, and counter tops.
sanitization (sanitizing)	The lowest level of decontamination possible; used to reduce the number of contaminations on a surface or implement.
sterilization	A difficult, multi-step process used to destroy all living organisms on a surface or implement.
viricides	Disinfectants that kill pathogenic viruses.
wet sanitizers	Covered receptacles, large enough to hold a disinfectant solution, in which objects to be sanitized can be completely immersed.

3

1. What is the difference between disinfection and sanitation?

2. Disinfection is almost identical to _____ except, disinfection does not kill bacterial spores.

3. What is an antiseptic?

4. What is the best type of disinfectant to use in a salon?

5. What are the two most commonly used types of disinfectants?

6. Once implements are properly _____, they must be stored where they will remain free from _____.

7. Formaldehyde is a strong _____ _____.

8. What must you use to remove implements from disinfectant containers?

9. Describe Universal Sanitation in your own words.

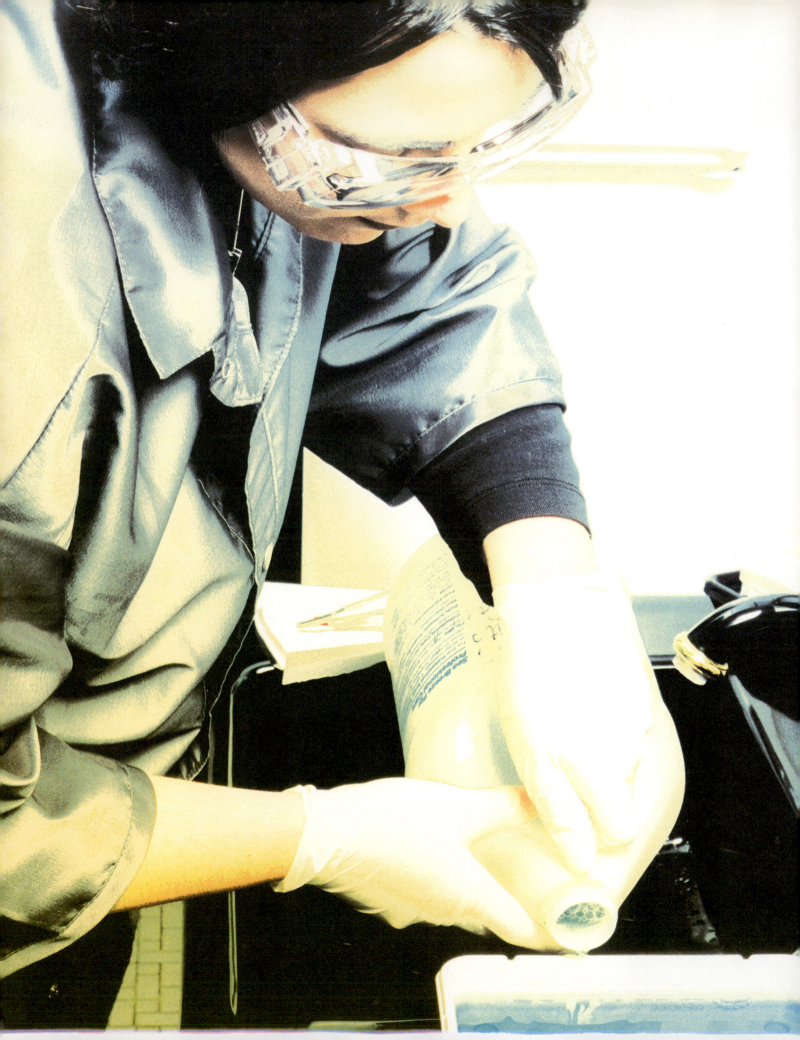

4

SAFETY IN THE SALON

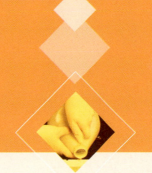

Author: Rebecca Moran

CHAPTER OUTLINE

Common Chemicals Used by Nail Technicians
Learn About the Chemicals in Your Products
OSHA Hazard Communication Standard CFR 1910.1200
Avoiding Overexposure is Easy! • A Dangerous Misconception
Protect Your Eyes • Cumulative Trauma Disorders

Learning Objectives

After you have completed this chapter, you should be able to:

1 Understand and identify the early warning signs of overexposure.

2 Read and use Material Safety Data Sheets (MSDS).

3 List all three chemical "Routes of Entry."

4 Know how to achieve proper ventilation in the salon.

5 Avoid the risks of overexposure to vapors and dusts.

6 Recognize and avoid cumulative trauma disorders (CTDs).

Key Terms

Page number indicates where in the chapter the term is used.

breathing zone
pg. 59

carpal tunnel syndrome
pg. 62

cumulative trauma disorder (CTD)
pg. 62

local exhaust
pg. 59

Material Safety Data Sheet (MSDS)
pg. 52

overexposure
pg. 51

Today anyone can have long, beautiful nails thanks to the advances of chemistry and artistic talents of nail technicians. We can make short nails long, long nails strong, and we can turn anyone's nails into a work of art.

Most nail technicians are skilled in services such as nail tips, nail wraps, acrylic nails, and gel nails. For each of these services you will use "hi-tech" chemicals that could cause harm to both you and your clients. No product *need* harm your health, but all of them *can*. The key to working safely is in understanding your chemical tools.

In other chapters, you will learn step-by-step procedures for giving your clients advanced nail services. But first, you must learn to work safely with professional products. In this chapter, you will learn some basic rules for using nail chemicals wisely.

COMMON CHEMICALS USED BY NAIL TECHNICIANS

If you perform advanced nail services, your manicuring table is full of chemical products including:

- ❖ nail polish and nail polish remover.
- ❖ liquid and powder for acrylic nails.
- ❖ primer for acrylic nails.
- ❖ temporary dehydrators.
- ❖ light-cured gel nail supplies.
- ❖ no-light gels and activators.
- ❖ cuticle oils and creams.
- ❖ adhesives for fabric wraps and much more.

All of these products can be safe, but all can be dangerous if used incorrectly. Luckily, you need not be afraid of these chemicals. Simply coming in contact with a chemical will not harm you. Overexposure is a danger you need to avoid. **Overexposure** for prolonged periods causes most of the problems. How can you tell if you have been overexposed? Your body will usually give you some *early warning signs of overexposure*. Some of these include:

- ❖ rash and other skin irritation.
- ❖ lightheadedness.
- ❖ insomnia.
- ❖ runny nose.
- ❖ sore, dry throat.
- ❖ watery eyes.
- ❖ tingling toes.
- ❖ fatigue.
- ❖ irritability.
- ❖ sluggishness.
- ❖ breathing problems.

If you do suffer from any of these problems, there is good news. You don't have to take it! All of these are easily avoided and will completely reverse themselves in a short time, if you do your part. Working correctly and safely will eliminate these side effects and allow you to work comfortably. That is what working safely is all about.

◆ ◆ LEARN ABOUT THE CHEMICALS IN YOUR PRODUCTS

Manufacturers try to make products as safe as possible. But they can only do so much. Their best efforts can be undone by a single careless act. It's up to you to learn about the chemicals in your professional products and how to handle them safely.

One excellent way to learn about working safely with a chemical is to read the *Material Safety Data Sheet (MSDS)* for that product.

What Is an MSDS?

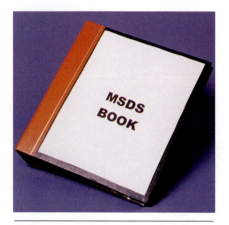

Figure 4–1 Refer to your MSDS book.

The United States government requires that product manufacturers make **Material Safety Data Sheets (MSDS)** available to people who use their products (Figure 4–1). Each MSDS must contain basic items of information. The MSDS is written for everyone, not just nail technicians. Doctors, fire fighters, postal employees, truckers, and many others use the MSDS. Federally mandated by OSHA, they are required to be kept for every chemical located in or on business property. They must be filed in a conspicuous, accessible location at all times. While looking at the MSDS you will discover that there is no standard format. However, each MSDS must contain the following information:

1. **Identity of chemicals presenting physical or chemical hazards.** You can get information concerning potentially hazardous ingredients found in each product.

2. **Physical hazards.** You learn about how the product reacts with other chemicals, potential for explosion, fire hazards, and how easily it will evaporate into the air.

3. **Health hazards.** You can learn the signs and symptoms of overexposure, illnesses that might be caused by the product, and existing medical conditions that might be made worse. There is also information concerning overexposure on the skin, eyes, and respiratory system, as well as problems caused if the product is accidentally swallowed. Both the short- and long-term health effects of overexposure (if any) are listed.

4. **Primary routes of entry into the body.** This explains how the product's ingredients may enter your body. Usually chemicals gain entry through the skin, mouth, or lungs. The MSDS will warn you of any such risks so that you can prevent overexposure.

5. **Permissible exposure limits.** The MSDS must provide recommended safe limits in the air to prevent overexposure by inhalation.

6. **Carcinogen hazard of the chemical.** Information about whether any ingredient over 1/10th percent is suspected of causing cancer must be available.

7. **Precautions and handling procedures.** Tips on safe handling of the product to prevent overexposure and how to properly clean up leaks or spills must be listed.

8. **Control and protection measures.** This explains how to protect yourself and clients against the potential hazards of the product, suggested ventilation needed, type of glove and eye wear protection required, and so on.

9. **Emergency and first aid procedures.** This includes what to do in case of accidents and how to respond in emergencies related to product use. This section is one of the most important since it will give information for treating problems. Emergency first aid advice and emergency phone numbers are given.

10. **Storage and disposal information.** You learn the best and safest way to get rid of old or unused products without causing injury to yourself, others, or the environment. Also, you can get information on proper and safe storage.

Additional information, which could be included on the MSDS, follows:

1. **Emergency phone number.** Your local poison control center may not have information on your product. Therefore, a number is supplied for a similar company who will have the specific information you need.

2. **Hazard rankings.** These are assigned in a uniform manner.

   0 – Least Hazardous,   1 – Slight,   2 – Moderate,
   3 – High,   4 – Extremely Hazardous

3. **Fire control methods.** Some chemicals need specific extinguishing methods to be effective.

   Extinguishers are rated.   **A** – trash, wood, paper, and plastic
   B – grease, liquids, alcohol, and acetone
   C – electrical

   There are combinations of two or all three, such as the **ABC**, which is multi-purpose. Using the correct fire extinguisher is crucial. **A** is water-based, **B** is foam, dry chemical or carbon dioxide, **C** is dry chemical or carbon dioxide.

4. **Specific gravity.** This is the basic weight of the product as it compares with water. The specific gravity of water is one. If the product in question has a specific gravity rating less than one, then it means that the chemical will float to the top of the water that may have been thrown on it. That allows the product to reignite upon exposure to an ignition source. If the product weighs more than one, then it will stay under the heavier water, snuffing it out. The problem is that when water is thrown on a lighter substance, the fire will spread at least as big as the puddle of water on which it is floating.

How You Can Get Material Safety Data Sheets

Your local distributor of beauty supplies is required by federal law to supply you with an MSDS for each product you buy from them (Figure 4–2). It is your legal responsibility to collect these sheets and keep them available for reference. If you have difficulty collecting the MSDS you need, send a formal written request to the distributor.

◆ ◆ ◆ OSHA HAZARD COMMUNICATION STANDARD CFR 1910.1200

In addition to requiring all businesses to have MSDS for all chemicals located in or on business property, OSHA mandates that each business fulfills specific requirements regarding training, inventory control, and written policies and procedures for the handling of hazardous materials. These are all clearly outlined in the OSHA Hazard Communication Standard CFR 1910.1200, which is available on their Web site and at their offices located throughout the United States.

Training is required to be adequately provided by the employer, specifically addressing 11 issues:

1. location of the written hazard communication training materials, for unlimited access at all times

2. location of the all-hazardous chemicals in or on business property

3. location of the MSDS material, for unlimited access at all times

4. copy of the provisions of the Hazard Communication Standard, for unlimited access at all times

5. proper steps in the detection and identification of hazardous chemical presence and or release

6. location of any possible monitoring information regarding actual real-time employee exposure to hazardous chemicals

7. access to information about employee safe-working procedures, job safety analysis information, and employee protection via the use of personal protective equipment, such as gloves, safety glasses, and dust masks

8. physical location of materials and health hazards relevant to the chemicals present

9. handling of non-routine tasks safely, and the location of all written policies and procedures pertaining to the same, with unlimited access at all times

10. when applicable, information necessary to correctly identify chemicals in unmarked or poorly labeled pipes

11. information regarding the business's warning label and MSDS systems and any other labeling system used by the business

Material Safety Data Sheet

May be used to comply with
OSHA's Hazard Communication Standard,
29 CFR 1910.1200. Standard must be
consulted for specific requirements.

U.S. Department of Labor

Occupational Safety and Health Administration
(Non-Mandatory Form)
Form Approved
OMB No. 1218-0072

IDENTITY *(As Used on Label and List)*	Note: Blank spaces are not permitted. If any item is not applicable, or no information is available, the space must be marked to indicate that.

Section I

Manufacturer's Name	Emergency Telephone Number
Address *(Number, Street, City, State, and ZIP Code)*	Telephone Number for Information
	Date Prepared
	Signature of Preparer *(optional)*

Section II - Hazard Ingredients/Identity Information

Hazardous Components (Specific Chemical Identity; Common Name(s))	OSHA PEL	ACGIH TLV	Other Limits Recommended	% *(optional)*

Section III - Physical/Chemical Characteristics

Boiling Point		Specific Gravity (H$_2$O = 1)	

Figure 4-2 MSDS sheet

Vapor Pressure (mm Hg.)		Melting Point	
Vapor Density (AIR = 1)		Evaporation Rate (Butyl Acetate = 1)	
Solubility in Water			
Appearance and Odor			

Section IV - Fire and Explosion Hazard Data

Flash Point (Method Used)		Flammable Limits	LEL	UEL
Extinguishing Media				
Special Fire Fighting Procedures				
Unusual Fire and Explosion Hazards				

Section V - Reactivity Data

Stability	Unstable		Conditions to Avoid
	Stable		
Incompatibility (Materials to Avoid)			
Hazardous Decomposition or Byproducts			
Hazardous Polymerization	May Occur		Conditions to Avoid
	Will Not Occur		

Section VI - Health Hazard Data

Route(s) of Entry:	Inhalation?	Skin?	Ingestion?
Health Hazards (Acute and Chronic)			
Carcinogenicity:	NTP?	IARC Monographs?	OSHA Regulated?
Signs and Symptoms of Exposure			

Figure 4-2 MSDS sheet (continued)

Medical Conditions Generally Aggravated by Exposure	
Emergency and First Aid Procedures	

Section VII - Precautions for Safe Handling and Use

Steps to Be Taken in Case Material is Released or Spilled
Waste Disposal Method
Precautions to Be taken in Handling and Storing
Other Precautions

Section VIII - Control Measures

Respiratory Proctection *(Specify Type)*		
Ventilation	Local Exhaust	Special
	Mechanical *(General)*	Other

Protective Gloves	Eye Protection
Other Protective Clothing or Equipment	
Work/Hygienic Practices	

Figure 4-2 MSDS sheet (continued)

OSHA requires that all businesses adopt and enact a written policy to comply with their labeling mandates. Simply stated, all containers having chemicals in them must be clearly labeled, with the appropriate warning intact and accurate. If a chemical is placed in an unmarked container, other than for one time or immediate use by an employee, a label must be affixed to it, clearly stating the identity of the contents and all relevant hazard warnings. Symbol labels are widely available, and are considered satisfactory by OSHA when used correctly.

OSHA also mandates that a complete chemical inventory list be kept for quick reference. It must clearly refer to the related MSDS and its location. Many computer programs are now available for tasks such as this. A written program of policies and procedures must also be developed, enacted, and enforced by employers directly addressing the requirements of the Hazard Communication Standard and how the business will comply with its requirements. It must detail the methods used to educate employees about the hazards of non-routine duties (such as cleaning and disposal of empty monomer or acetone bottles). It must describe the hazards encountered when using chemicals in unlabeled containers, how to handle chemicals used in numerous work places, the special precautions for each chemical handled, where to access the MSDS at each work place, and how the employer will supply or make available the written program of policies and procedures to and for each employee.

In addition to the requirements of OSHA, the policies and procedures should address fire, accident, first-aid, work place injury, and violent crime issues.

AVOIDING OVEREXPOSURE IS EASY!

It is easy to work safely. Remember, health hazards are created by overexposure. You only have to learn how to avoid overexposure and you will be able to work safely.

Luckily, products can only enter your body in three ways:

You breathe them (*inhalation*).

You absorb them through your skin (*skin contact*).

You eat them (*ingestion*).

If you control these routes of entry, you will greatly lessen the chance of overexposure.

Ventilation Control

Always work in a well ventilated area! This is one of the most important safety rules of nail technology. Your ventilation system must remove vapors and dusts from the building. Most systems just circulate them around the salon, for example, fans, open doors, windows, ceiling vents, air cleaners, and so on. The only effective way to ventilate in the salon is to vent vapors and dust to the outside. Vented manicuring tables are almost completely ineffective. Their flimsy charcoal filters absorb as much vapors as they can hold after about twenty hours of use. You cannot wash or shake these vapors out, the filter must be discarded. Devices that are designed to "clean the air" are ineffective and not practical in salons. The only sure method of removing vapors and dusts is to vent to the outside.

There is one place on earth that is more important to you than any other. That place is called your breathing zone. Your **breathing zone** is an invisible sphere about the size of a beach ball that sits directly in front of your mouth. Every single breath you take comes from your breathing zone. Your health and safety depend on what occurs in this small area. This is the real reason for ventilation.

Excessive inhalation of vapors is a problem for nail technicians. These vapors come from the evaporation of liquids. All liquid nail products evaporate and contribute to the total vapors in the air, even odorless acrylics, wraps, and light-cured gels. Odors are not the reason to ventilate. Ventilate to control vapors and dusts. What can you do to lower your exposure to vapors? Luckily, some of the most effective ways to eliminate vapors are the easiest and least expensive.

❖ Tightly seal all product containers immediately after use.

❖ Use a covered dappen dish or pump to limit the vapors in the air.

❖ Avoid using pressurized sprays. They create finer mists and are difficult to control.

❖ Empty your waste container often. It is one of the best sources of vapors.

Local Exhaust

The only complete answer to salon vapor and dust control is **local exhaust**. These devices are based on a simple concept. They capture vapors and dusts at the source and expel them from your breathing zone. Local exhaust uses an exhaust vent, hose, or tube to capture vapors, dusts, and mists. A moveable exhaust tube can be placed where needed, for example, over your open containers or beside the hand while you file. Specially designed blowers pull contaminants from the breathing zone down the exhaust tube, and expel them from the building (Figure 4–3). An exhaust system should completely ventilate and replace the air volume in a treatment area four to six times per hour. Fresh air should be brought in through a fresh air intake located at least 25 feet from the exhaust outlets. The exhaust outlets should be a least six feet above the ground and three feet above the roof level.

Although venting to the outside is preferred, it is not always possible. If your salon has no outside access, the vapors and dusts can be filtered through a HEPA filter and at least a five gallon canister packed with activated charcoal. If you can vent to the roof, make sure your exhaust pipe is at least fifteen feet from any intake vents, especially your neighbor's. The

Here's a Tip:
Proper ventilation protects your breathing zone and is a requirement for using professional products. Before you decide to work in a salon, you should make sure they have a good ventilation system.

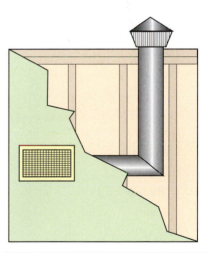

Figure 4-3 Outside venting is preferred to clear air of dust and vapors.

Here's a Tip:
Don't buy systems that just ventilate odors. Eliminating odors doesn't mean the air is clean. Vapors and dusts are what need to be removed and controlled. Do this properly and there will be no odor problem.

higher it is above the roof, the better. This will prevent odors from being drawn into nearby homes or businesses.

Custom systems based on these principles can be built fairly inexpensively. An expert capable of building such a system is as close as your phone book. Look under heating or air conditioning for a specialist that understands proper ventilation. You'll be surprised at how affordable a well designed local ventilation system can be.

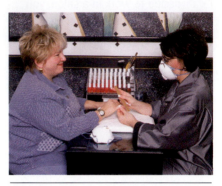

Figure 4-4 Wear a dust mask when filing and offer one to your client.

Preventing Overexposure to Dusts

Prolonged inhalation of excessive amounts of nail filings may be harmful. Not that nail filings are especially dangerous, but breathing large amounts of *any* dusts for long periods may be harmful, even house dust! Our bodies can remove many of the dusts that are inhaled. Problems occur only if you continually inhale more than the lungs can handle. Wearing a dust mask can prevent this (Figure 4–4). Nothing you can buy will do a better job of protecting your lungs against dusts. The large, visible particles are less harmful since they fall on the table top and are easily removed. The smaller, invisible dusts are far more hazardous. Smaller particles lodge deeper in the lungs, increasing the risks. Dust masks filter air from your breathing zone before it enters the mouth. Never use these masks to prevent inhalation of vapors. They cannot block any of the vapors in the salon.

Here's a Tip:

Always wear a dust mask when filing, especially if you use a drill. Drills make much smaller, more hazardous dust particles than files or abrasive boards. Also, throw away dust masks every few days. They're disposable and become ineffective if used too long.

4

◆ ◆ ◆ A DANGEROUS MISCONCEPTION

Many believe that they can tell how safe or dangerous a chemical is by its odor! A chemical's smell has absolutely nothing to do with its safety. Some very dangerous substances have sweet, pleasant fragrances. Products or ventilation systems that "cover-up" or "remove" odors will not protect your health. Odors are really the nail technician's friend. Odors can warn against overexposure danger. Odors are caused when vapors touch sensitive detectors in the nose. After the vapors leave the nose and enter the lungs, their odor is not important. You are asking for trouble if you use odor to judge product safety. The same is true for nice smells. Overexposure to nice smelling vapors can cause harm too!

◆ ◆ ◆ PROTECT YOUR EYES

Accidents involving the eyes are a serious danger in salons. Solvents in the eye can be very painful and may cause severe damage. Primer, wrap monomers and adhesives, or phenolic disinfectant solutions in the eyes are worse! Each of these can cause permanent eye injury or blindness. Imagine what it is like to be blind! It could happen if you are not careful to protect your vision.

Always use eye protection whenever there is the slightest chance that a liquid product could get into your eyes (Figure 4–5). Eye injuries account

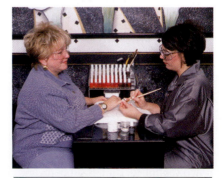

Figure 4-5 Wear safety glasses and give your client a pair.

for approximately 45 percent of the cosmetic related injuries seen in hospital emergency rooms. Many of these are students and salon professionals.

Wearing contacts in the salon is risky. Vapors will collect in soft contacts and make them unwearable. Even if you wear safety glasses, vapors are still absorbed. The contaminated lens can irritate the surface of the eye and cause permanent damage. Should an accidental splash occur, the liquid will "wick" under the lens. This will make proper cleaning of the eye more difficult.

> **Here's a Tip:**
> Always wear approved safety glasses whenever you work with anything that can get into the eyes.

◆ ◆ ◆ OTHER TIPS FOR WORKING SAFELY

1. **Don't smoke in the salon.** Since nail technicians work with many flammable solvents and products, it is wise to take precautions to prevent fires in the salon. One way is by not allowing smoking in the salon. Smoking near flammable solvents is very risky.

2. **Always avoid skin contact.** Never touch any acrylic liquids, wraps or adhesives, light-cured gels, etc., to the skin. This is one of the leading causes of service breakdown, lifting and allergic reactions. More will be said about adverse skin reactions in Chapter 5. The best rule to follow is, "if it isn't designed for skin application, keep it off the skin!"

3. **Never eat or drink in the salon area.** A cup of coffee is an excellent place for nail dust and vapors to collect. Hot liquids, like coffee and tea, can absorb vapors from the air. Dusts settle in any open container. The cup of coffee you or your client is drinking may be filled with contaminants (Figure 4–6).

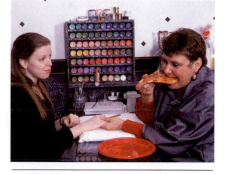

Figure 4-6 Never eat or drink in the salon area. You may find that you are ingesting nail chemicals.

4. **Store and eat your lunch in a separate area of the salon.** When you eat, you should leave the building or eat in a lunchroom that is separated from the rest of the salon by walls and a door. Federal law forbids eating in any area where professional chemicals are being stored or used.

5. **Always wash your hands before and after eating.** When someone offers you a piece of chocolate or when you dodge into the kitchen for a cookie, do you wash your hands first? If you forget to wash your hands before you grab a snack or eat lunch, you will probably end up eating the chemicals that are on your hands.

6. **Label all containers.** Every container, spray bottle, squeeze bottle, or tube in the salon must be properly labeled. This includes all cleaning products and any bulk purchased products in storage. Be sure the label is waterproof. If the container isn't labeled, *do not use it* (Figure 4–7).

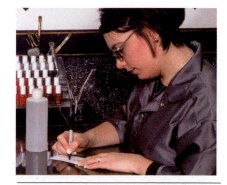

Figure 4-7 Label all containers. If the container is not labeled, do not use it.

7. **Store your products in a cool area.** Never store your professional products in a car trunk, by a window, or near a pilot light, such as those for gas heaters or furnaces. Excessive heat will ruin them and some are more flammable than gasoline.

8. **Empty your trash can regularly.** Use a metal can with a self-closing lid as a trash container. Vapors will escape from open trash and fill your air with vapors. Empty the trash several times a day and dispose of it properly. A metal can will also lessen the risk of fire.

9. **Keep caps on all products.** It may seem easier to leave caps off your products, but it isn't wise. Uncapped bottles on your table are very easy to spill. Keep your product containers closed to reduce the amount of vapor that escapes into the air. Capping will also make your products last longer. Uncapped nail polish thickens, solvents evaporate, and wrap glue starts to harden. (You will find that marbles are just the right size to cover the small dishes you use for acrylic powder and liquid.)

10. **Be prepared to handle accidents.** Do not wait until after an accident has happened to figure out how to handle it. Have the poison control center number and other emergency numbers near the phone (Figure 4–8). Have a fire emergency plan, a chemical spill plan, and a personal injury plan available. Take a first-aid class and have someone in the shop trained in CPR, if possible. Each employee should have assigned tasks. Keep the MSDS for each product in a convenient place. At salon meetings, discuss what you would do in case of an accident. With each plan, panic and confusion are reduced.

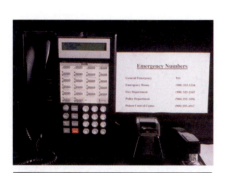

Figure 4-8 Post important numbers close to the telephone.

◆ ◆ ◆ CUMULATIVE TRAUMA DISORDERS

Cumulative trauma disorder (CTD) is also known as repetitive motion disorder. CTDs are the fastest growing type of injury for all occupations. CTDs cause painful and crippling illness that may become permanent if not treated. **Carpal tunnel syndrome** is the most common CTD. This illness affects the hands and wrists of many nail technicians. The carpal tunnel is a small passage in the wrist that carries a nerve from the fingers to the arm. Repetitive motions can create damaging pressure on the nerve.

Injury is usually caused by repetitive motions such as filing nails. Constant vibration from drills may also cause or aggravate the condition. Pain and numbness often spread into the arm and fingers. If ignored, the situation usually becomes worse. Continued injury can permanently damage the nerve. Other things can cause CTDs. Sitting or working in the same position, awkward reaching, stretching, or twisting may damage the carpal tunnel nerve or similar nerves in the neck and back.

Symptoms of CTDs are

❖ pain.   ❖ stiffness.   ❖ weakness.

❖ numbness.   ❖ tingling.   ❖ swelling.

❖ aching.

If you experience any of these symptoms, pay close attention to how you work and report it to your employer immediately. You can usually tell which repetitive motion is causing the pain. It is best to seek medical attention immediately before it is too late to correct the problem.

What to Do?

There are many things nail technicians can do to avoid CTDs.

* Always sit in a natural, unstrained position.

* Don't hunch over the client's nails. Change positions often.

* Stretch frequently, every 20 to 30 minutes, even if only for a few seconds (Figure 4–9).

* Avoid using tools that vibrate excessively.

* Hold wrists straight and avoid bending them while filing or using a brush.

* Stop work and stretch or shake out your hands.

* Do frequent strengthening exercises.

Most importantly, take your time. Rushing through a service is hard on you and the client's nails. Quality is more important than speed! Do not sacrifice your health and your client's nails by rushing through a nail service. It is better to raise your prices and do great work on fewer clients.

Ice and ibuprofen or aspirin will ease the pain, but if you think you have a CTD see a doctor! Your doctor will be able to make prevention recommendations that you might not think about.

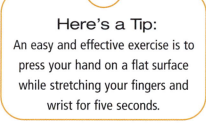

Here's a Tip:
An easy and effective exercise is to press your hand on a flat surface while stretching your fingers and wrist for five seconds.

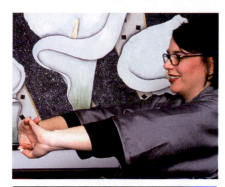

Figure 4–9 Stretching exercises can help to prevent CTDs.

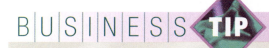

Express Yourself Safely

Have a little fun with your safety goggles by turning them into a professional tool for nail art (Figure 4–10). They're a great vehicle for individual expression and they're sure to attract attention. Add hand-painted designs to goggle frames or edges and change them frequently to reflect seasonal themes, color trends, and personal preference. For mini test-marketing, determine which designs generate the most interest, then offer to create those designs on your client's nails. The bottom line is that you boost your profits and create interest in nail art while promoting safety.

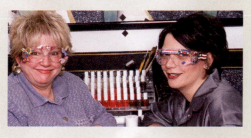

Figure 4–10 Decorated safety glasses

breathing zone	The invisible sphere of air, about the size of a beach ball, that sits directly in front of your mouth.
carpal tunnel syndrome	The most common cumulative trauma disorder (CTD), affecting the hands and wrists.
cumulative trauma disorder (CTD)	Also known as repetitive motion disorder; an occupational disability that can cause pain and crippling if not treated.
local exhaust	A device used to capture salon vapors and dust and expel them from a technician's breathing zone through an exhaust vent.
Material Safety Data Sheet (MSDS)	A document supplied by product manufacturers, and available to anyone who uses the product, that contains basic safety and handling information about a product.
overexposure	Dangerously prolonged, repeated, or long-term contact with certain chemicals.

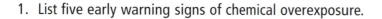

review questions

1. List five early warning signs of chemical overexposure.

2. What does MSDS stand for?

3. Name four simple and inexpensive things you can do to reduce vapors in the salon.

4. Define breathing zone.

5. Describe how a local exhaust system works. Why is it best?

6. What is the best and least expensive way to prevent excessive inhalation of dusts?

7. Why should products be stored away from heat and pilot lights?

8. Why should smoking not be allowed in the salon?

9. What is CTD? Explain how this happens.

10. List seven symptoms of CTD.

part

2

THE SCIENCE OF NAIL TECHNOLOGY

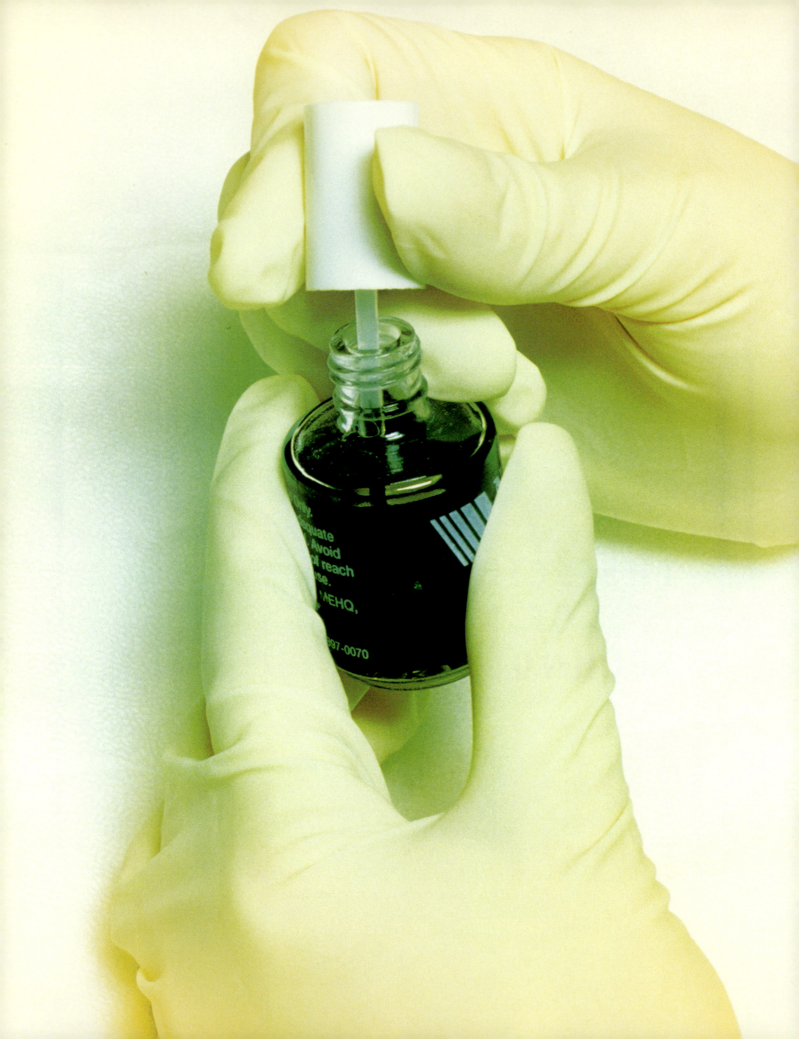

5

NAIL PRODUCT CHEMISTRY SIMPLIFIED

Author: Douglas D. Schoon

CHAPTER OUTLINE

**Understanding Chemicals • Adhesion and Adhesives
Fingernail Coatings • Avoiding Skin Problems
The Overexposure Principle**

Learning Objectives

After you have completed this chapter, you should be able to:

1 Understand the basic chemistry of salon products.

2 Explain adhesion and how adhesives work.

3 Identify the two main categories of nail coatings.

4 Describe the basic chemistry of all enhancements.

5 Determine the cause and prevention of skin disorders.

Key Terms

Page number indicates where in the chapter the term is used.

adhesion
pg. 74

adhesive
pg. 74

catalyst
pg. 72

chemical
pg. 71

chemical change
pg. 71

chemical reaction
pg. 72

coatings
pg. 76

corrosive
pg. 74

cross-linker
pg. 78

dermatitis
pg. 79

elements
pg. 71

energy
pg. 71

evaporate
pg. 71

gas
pg. 72

histamines
pg. 81

initiator
pg. 77

matter
pg. 71

molecule
pg. 71

monomers
pg. 77

overexposure
pg. 79

physically changed
pg. 71

polymerizations
pg. 76

polymers
pg. 76

primers
pg. 74

saturated
pg. 73

sensitization
pg. 80

simple polymer chains
pg. 77

solute
pg. 73

solvent
pg. 73

ultraviolet (U.V.) light
pg. 78

vapor
pg. 72

Why do nail technicians need chemistry? Almost everything you do depends on chemistry. Even if you just want to "do nails," your success depends on having an understanding of chemicals and chemistry.

◆ ◆ ◆ UNDERSTANDING CHEMICALS

It is incorrect to think all chemicals are dangerous or toxic substances. Most chemicals are completely safe. Everything around you is made of chemicals. The walls, this book, food, vitamins, even oxygen is a chemical. In fact, everything you can see or touch, except light and electricity, is a **chemical**.

Nail plates are 100% chemical. They are mostly protein made from chemicals called amino acids. Amino acids are composed of the chemicals carbon, nitrogen, oxygen, hydrogen and sulfur. The chemical sulfur is responsible for the sulfur cross-links that create strong natural nails. Nail plates also contain traces of iron, aluminum, copper, silver, gold and other chemicals.

Matter and Energy

Everything in the world is either matter or energy. **Matter** takes up space or occupies an area. For instance, books occupy space, therefore a book is made of matter. Very few things don't take up space. Even microscopic bacteria use a small amount of space.

Light, radio waves, and microwaves are examples of things that don't occupy space. These are not made of matter—they are **energy**. Energy has no substance. However, energy can affect matter in many ways.

Molecules and Elements

A **molecule** is a chemical in its simplest form. A water molecule can be broken down into hydrogen and oxygen, but it wouldn't be water any longer. Some molecules cannot be broken down at all. These are called **elements**. Oxygen and hydrogen are two of the 106 known elements.

Forms of Matter

Matter can exist as a solid, liquid, or gas. Water can be frozen into a solid, melted to a liquid, and evaporated into a gas or even a vapor. When water freezes, thaws, or evaporates it is **physically changed**. The water is simply changing form or appearance. It is not chemically altered.

Matter can be chemically changed, too. Burning sugar or paper makes a black substance. This is an example of a **chemical change** or one chemical changing into a completely different chemical substance.

Chemical molecules are like tiny tinker toys. They can be arranged and rearranged into an unlimited number of combinations. Petroleum oil can be chemically converted into vitamin C. Acetone can be changed into water or oxygen. Paper can be made into sugar. The possibilities are endless. In medieval times, alchemists searched in vain for ways to turn lead into gold. Today, even this is possible.

Most people are very familiar with the definition of solid and liquid. It is easy to see that something liquid is not a solid. However, since people cannot easily see the differences between **gas** and **vapor**, these terms are often confused. There is a very important difference between these two terms. Gases are very different from vapors. Vapors are formed when liquids **evaporate** into the air. Any substance that is liquid at room temperature will form vapors. The higher the temperature, the faster vapors will form. Also, vapors will turn back into liquids, if they are cooled again. Water, alcohol, and acetone form vapors. All types of nail enhancement systems will form vapors. Monomer liquids (even odorless monomer), U.V. gels, wrap resins, and adhesives all form vapors, not gases. Gases only become liquids when they are put under high pressures (e.g., pressurized butane gas bottles) or if they are cooled to sub-zero temperatures (-70° C or colder). Oxygen, nitrogen, propane, and the air we breathe are examples of gases.

Gases, liquid, vapors, and solids have one thing in common. They are all made of molecules. But what makes them so different? In the case of gases, the molecules are spread very far apart. The molecules of a vapor are closer together and those of a liquid are tremendously closer to each other. The thicker the liquid or gel, the closer the molecules are to each other. In solids, the molecules exist closest together.

Chemical Reactions

Under the right conditions a molecule can chemically change. This is called a **chemical reaction**. In general, a chemical reaction requires energy to occur. Most chemical reactions get this energy from heat or light. Artificial nail enhancements can use either heat or light energy to create the finished product.

Catalyst

A **catalyst** is a chemical that can make a chemical reaction go faster. Different chemical reactions require different catalysts. Catalysts are very important chemical tools. Many chemical reactions happen very slowly. For instance, graphite (pencil lead) will slowly change into diamond, but would take many thousands of years. Obviously, a graphite to diamond catalyst would be an important invention, if it were ever discovered.

Trillions of chemical reactions occur in our bodies every day. Most of these happen very quickly because of catalysts. Nail technicians use catalysts to make wraps, overlays, and sculptured nails. Catalysts are found in both U.V. gels and monomer liquids. In the case of wraps, the catalyst is applied with a spray, dropper, or brush.

Solvents and Solutes

A **solvent** is anything that dissolves another substance. Solvents are usually liquid. The substance that is dissolved is called a **solute**. Generally, solutes are solids, gels, or oils. Water is a very good solvent. In fact, water is called the "universal solvent" because it will dissolve more substances than any other solvent. Acetone is frequently used as a polish remover and to dissolve nail enhancements. It is an extremely safe solvent to use for this purpose.

Solvents dissolving solutes is one of the most important concepts in the professional nail industry. How can your understanding of solvents and solutes help nail professionals? Lots of ways! For example, acetone is a *good solvent* for nail polish (the solute), but it is also a good solvent for the oils in your natural nails. So, it makes sense that excessive use of acetone (removing polish two or three times per week) can make the nail plates look dry and brittle. This can happen when too much of your natural nail oils are stripped away. *Solution:* Adjust the solvent strength of the acetone with water (10%–15% water). The acetone will become a slightly weaker solvent, so it will remove less natural nail oil. The diluted acetone will still be strong enough to remove nail polish, but will reduce the loss of natural nail oil.

Solvents only dissolve a certain amount of solute before they become **saturated**. Solvents become saturated with solute much like a mop becomes saturated with water. In other words, a saturated solvent cannot dissolve any more solute. Saturated solvents are very ineffective. Using a saturated solvent is a waste of time since fresh, clean solvents work much faster. For example, when removing artificial nail enhancements, the solvent remover will work much more quickly if a larger amount is used. If the enhancement is barely covered with solvent it can become saturated with dissolved product. Removal slows down because there is not enough solvent. A good rule of thumb is: the level of solvent should cover the fingers to the bottom of the knuckle.

Gently warming solvents will also make them faster acting. This is especially true for removing artificial nail enhancements. Warming the solvent to 100–105°F max (warm to very hot, similar to Jacuzzi temperature) will dramatically speed up the removal process. Of course, warming highly flammable solvents such as acetone must be done properly and with special care. Flammable solvents should only be warmed in a bowl filled with hot tap water. Be very sure to slightly loosen the cap to prevent pressure from building up and bursting out of the container. Never warm any flammable substances on a flame, stove, or in a microwave oven. This is important to understand. Serious accidents have occurred when these rules were broken. Also, cover the dish and hand with a damp cloth while soaking to reduce vapors in the air. The product's manufacturer will provide you with more safe handling information.

5

◆◆ ADHESION AND ADHESIVES

Adhesion is a force of nature that makes two surfaces stick together. Adhesion is caused when the molecules on one surface are attracted to the molecules on another surface. Paste sticks to paper because its molecules are attracted to paper molecules. Oils, waxes, and soil will contaminate a surface and block adhesion. This is why a clean, dry surface will give better adhesion.

Adhesives

An **adhesive** is a chemical that causes two surfaces to stick together. Adhesives allow incompatible surfaces to be joined. Scotch® tape is a plastic that is coated with a sticky adhesive. Without the adhesive the plastic would not stick to paper. The sticky adhesive layer acts as a "go between." It holds the tape to the paper. Adhesives are like a ship's anchor. One end of the anchor holds the ship, the other end attaches to the ground.

There are many types of adhesives. Different adhesives are compatible with different surfaces. Glue is actually a very old term for any adhesive made by boiling animal hides, hooves, and bones. Your childhood paste and glue may have been of this sort. Today, glue is used for many types of adhesives, ranging from epoxy resins to the high-tech cyanoacrylate adhesives used by nail technicians. Even though they are called glue, adhesive is a more accurate term.

Primers

Primers are substances that improve adhesion. Nail polish base coats are primers. Why? Base coats make nail polish adhere better. Base coats act as the "go-between" or "anchor." They improve adhesion.

Other types of primers are sometimes required with artificial nail enhancements. They are especially useful if the client has oily skin. Primers act like double-sided sticky tape (Figure 5–1). One side sticks well to the enhancement and the other side holds tightly to the nail plate. A common misconception is that nail primers "eat" the nail. This is completely false. Nail clippings can soak for many years in primer without dissolving. Still, nail primers must be used with caution. Some are very corrosive to soft tissue. A **corrosive** is a substance that can cause visible and possibly permanent skin damage. Nail primers, like most professional nail products, should never touch the skin! Primers are acids and can cause painful burns and scars to soft tissue. This is why corrosive primers are required to be kept in containers with child-resistant caps. It is also why corrosive acid primers should be kept away from children.

Even though primers will not damage the nail plate, they can burn the nail bed tissue. Overfiling the natural nail will excessively thin the nail making it more porous. If too much primer is used, the nail plate can become saturated. Small amounts may reach the nail bed causing

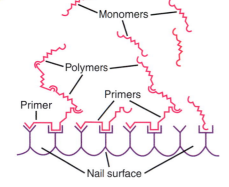

Figure 5–1 Primers act as "double-sided sticky tape" to anchor monomers firmly to the surface of the natural nail plate.

sensitivity and painful burns. It may also lead to separation of the nail plate from the bed. Use primer sparingly! One very thin coat is enough for most clients. If you find that you rely on two or more coats to prevent lifting, something is wrong! Check your nail preparation and application procedure for problems. Primer can become a crutch, covering up improper application or inadequate nail plate preparation. In the long run, it is better to get to the root of the problem and improve your technique rather than rely on excessive amounts of primer.

Not all primers are corrosive to skin. Non-corrosive primers, sometimes called *non-acid primers*, do not contain an ingredient called methacrylic acid. Non-acid primers may actually contain other acids, but they are non-corrosive to skin and, therefore, will prevent burning of the soft tissue. They must be used with caution and skin contact must be avoided (Figure 5–2). Prolonged and repeated skin contact is caused by improper application. Over time, repeated contacts with the product may lead to an allergic reaction. If you never contact the skin, it is extremely unlikely the client will become allergic to the product. Product vapors do not cause skin allergies. These types of allergies are caused by repeated product skin contact. Avoid all contact with soft tissues.

A Clean Start

Good adhesion depends on proper technique and high quality products. The best way to ensure success is to start with a clean, dry surface. Washing the hands and scrubbing the nail plate removes surface oils and contaminants that interfere with proper adhesion. Scrubbing also gets rid of the bacteria that cause most fingernail infections. Skipping this important step is a major contributor to fingernail infections and can lead to product lifting, mainly at the cuticle. However, improper nail preparation is a leading cause of most types of enhancement product lifting.

A nail dehydrator temporarily removes surface moisture from the nail plate. Moisture on the surface of the plate can interfere with product adhesion, just as surface oils can. Some dehydrators remove both moisture and oil. But, within thirty minutes, your normal, natural oils and moisture will begin to return to the nail plate. How is that information useful? It should suggest that for problem lifters, it might help to dehydrate only one hand at a time, very thoroughly, and after a good scrubbing.

It is a myth that enhancements and tips do not stick unless you "rough up the nail." This is absolutely false and very harmful for clients. Adhesion is best when the nail plate is clean and dry. Heavy abrasives, heavy-handed filing, and drills (electric files) can strip away the natural nail plate. The thinner the nail plate, the weaker it will be. Thinner nail plates are a weaker foundation, or base, for artificial nails than thicker nail plates. Keeping the nail plate thick, strong, and healthy is the professional nail technician's first duty!

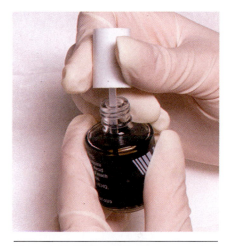

Figure 5–2 Wear gloves when using primers, adhesives, wrap and acrylic monomers, and gels.

When artificial nails are removed, clients can see the damage caused by heavy filing. They mistakenly blame primers and nail enhancements for what they see. Rough filing damages both the nail plate and bed. Also, heavy abrasives and overfiling may cause the nail plate to lift and separate from the nail bed. Once this occurs, clients often develop infections under the nail plate.

Overfiling the nail plate causes more problems for nail technicians than you might realize. Overfiling is one of the leading causes of enhancement service breakdown. It can lead to lifting, breaking, free-edge chipping, and free-edge product separation or "curling." It also can promote allergic reactions and may cause painful friction burns to the soft tissue of the nail bed. Roughing up the plate causes potentially dangerous, excessive thinning of the nail plate. It must be avoided at all costs.

If you think you need to rough up the nail plate to get good adhesion then something is wrong! Many nail technicians have great success without roughing up the nail plate. Why? The answer is simple, they properly prepare the nail plates by removing all dead tissue, bacteria, oil, and moisture. They use correct application techniques and high quality, professional products. Lifting problems can usually be traced back to one of those key areas.

◆ ◆ ◆ FINGERNAIL COATINGS

As a nail technician, you must perform many tasks. The most important of these is to apply coatings to the nail plate. **Coatings** are products that cover the nail plate with a hard film. Examples of typical coatings are nail polish, top coats, artificial enhancements, and adhesives. The two main types of coatings include:

1. coatings that cure or polymerize (chemical reaction).
2. coatings that harden upon evaporation (physical reaction).

Nail polish and top coats are examples of coatings created by evaporation. Artificial enhancements are examples of coatings created by chemical reactions.

Monomers and Polymers

Creating a nail enhancement is a good example of a chemical reaction. Trillions of molecules must react to make just one sculptured nail. Durable and long-lasting coatings or enhancements are all created by chemical reactions. All monomer liquid and powder, U.V. gels, no-light gels, wraps, and adhesives work in this fashion.

The molecules in the product join together into extremely long chains, each chain containing millions of molecules. These gigantic chains of molecules are called **polymers** (POL-uh-murs). Polymers can be liquids, but they are usually solid. Chemical reactions that make polymers are called **polymerizations** (puh-lim-uh-ruh-ZAY-shuns). Sometimes the terms *cure*, *curing*, or *hardening* are used, but they all have the same meaning.

There are many different types of polymers. Teflon®, nylon, hair and wood are polymers. Proteins are also polymers. Nail plates are made of a protein called keratin. So, nail plates are also polymers.

The individual molecules that join to make the polymer are called **monomers** (MON-uh-murs). In other words, monomers are the molecules that make polymers. For example, amino acids are monomers that join together to make the polymer we call keratin (Figure 5–3).

Understanding Polymerizations

If you understand the simple basics of polymerizations, you will be able to prevent many common salon problems. Liquid and powder systems, gels or no-light gels, wraps—they each seem very different, but they are actually quite similar. Each type of product is made from a different, but closely related monomer. Monomers are like track runners mingling around the starting line, patiently waiting for the race to begin. The race starts when the proper signal is given. Once given, the runners don't stop until they reach the finish line.

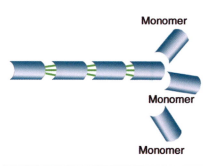

Figure 5–3 A simple polymer chain grows in one direction by adding monomers in a head-to-tail fashion.

The same is true for monomer molecules. They are like the runners, waiting for something to trigger the polymerization. This is done by a special ingredient called an **initiator**. Initiator molecules energize! They carry extra energy. Each time an initiator touches a monomer, the initiator excites it with a boost of energy. But, the monomer molecules do not like the extra energy and try to get rid of it. They do this by attaching themselves to the tail-end of another monomer and passing the energy along. The second monomer uses the same trick to get rid of the energy. As this game of tag continues, the chain of monomers gets longer and longer. A billion monomers can join in less than a second!

Soon, the many growing monomer chains begin to get in each other's way. They become tangled and knotted, which explains why the product starts to thicken. Eventually, the chains are much too long and crowded to freely move around. The product has become a teeming mass of microscopic-sized strings. When this occurs, the surface is hard enough to file, but it will be several days before the chains reach their ultimate lengths. This explains why enhancements become stronger during the first forty-eight hours.

Simple vs. Cross-linking Polymer Chains

Normally, the head of one monomer reacts with the tail of another, and so on. The result is a long chain of monomers attached head to tail. These are called **simple polymer chains**. Wraps and tip adhesives form this type of polymer. In these polymers, the tangled chains are easily unraveled by solvents, which explains why they are easily removed. Polymer chains can also be unraveled by force. Products with simple polymer chains are easily damaged by sharp impacts or heavy stresses. Dyes and stains can also get lodged between the tangled chains. Nail polishes, marker ink, foods and many other things may cause unsightly stains on the surface.

To overcome these problems, U.V. gels and liquid and powder systems use small amounts of special monomers called cross-linkers. A **cross-linker** is a monomer that joins different polymer chains together. These cross-links are like rungs on a ladder. Cross-links create strong net-like polymers. The result is a three-dimensional structure of great strength and flexibility, which we call nail enhancements.

The nail plate and hair also contain cross-links, which create a tough, resilient structure. Other than increasing the strength of both natural and artificial nails, cross-links make them more resistant to staining. Cross-links are also more resistant to solvents. This explains why cross-linked artificial nails take longer to remove in acetone than uncross-linked products such as wraps and tip adhesives.

Light and Heat Energy

Energy is the final key to understanding nail enhancement chemistry. Previously, you learned that monomers are energized by initiator molecules. Where does the initiator get the energy? You will recall that catalysts are used to make reactions happen more quickly. Catalysts give the initiator molecule its energy. Some catalysts use heat as an energy source while others use light. Whatever the source, catalysts absorb energy like a battery. At the appropriate time, they pass this energy to the initiator and the reaction begins. Light-cured enhancements generally use **ultra-violet** or **U.V. light**. All other products use heat energy. The heat from the room and client's hand is enough.

You can see why it is important to protect U.V. curing products from light. Sunlight and even artificial room lights can start polymerization in the container. The same can happen when heat-curing monomers are put in a hot car trunk, a store window, or other warm area. The high heat may also cause polymerization in the container. Products that require normal "incandescent" light bulbs are *not* light-curing monomers. They are using the extra heat released from the light bulb to speed evaporation of solvents.

Evaporation Coatings

Nail polishes, top coats, and base coats also form coatings. However, these products are entirely different. They do not polymerize. No chemical reactions occur and they contain no monomers. These products work strictly by evaporation. The majority of the ingredients are volatile or quickly evaporating solvents. Special polymers are dissolved in these solvents. These polymers are not cross-linked polymers, so they dissolve easily.

As the solvents evaporate, they leave behind a smooth polymer film. This film can hold pigments which give color. Artist paints and hair sprays work in the same fashion. Of course, the strength of uncross-linked polymers is much lower than cross-linked enhancement polymers. This explains why polishes are prone to chipping and are so easily dissolved by removers. Now you can see for yourself the great difference between coatings that cure or polymerize and those that harden upon evaporation.

"Better for the Nail" Claims

Some believe that certain types of enhancement products are "better" for the natural nail. This is absolutely false! No one type of nail enhancement product is better for the nail plate than another. What is better for the nail? That is easy to answer. The best thing for the natural nail is highly skilled, educated, and conscientious nail professionals. They are the natural nail's best friend. Good nail technicians protect and nurture the nail plate and watch for natural nail damage and infections. These problems are usually caused by improper nail plate preparation, improper application or maintenance, or improper removal. Fully educate yourself about the product you are using and its application. Any product can be applied and removed safely. It is up to you to use your knowledge and skill to see that it happens. Educate your clients to routinely maintain their enhancements. Work as a team for a healthier nail environment. **Be informed and caring.** Take control of your profession and its responsibilities.

◆ ◆ AVOIDING SKIN PROBLEMS

Skin problems are common in every facet of the professional salon industry. Nail, skin, and hair services all can cause problems for the sensitive client. Fortunately, the vast majority of fingernail-related problems can be easily avoided—if you understand how!

Dermatitis

Dermatitis is a medical term for abnormal skin inflammation. There are many kinds of dermatitis, but only one is important in the salon. *Contact dermatitis* is the most common skin disease for nail technicians. Contact dermatitis is caused by touching certain substances to the skin. This type of dermatitis can be short-term or long-term. Contact dermatitis can have several causes. The skin may be irritated by a substance. This is called *irritant contact dermatitis*. It is also possible to become allergic to an ingredient in a product. This is called *allergic contact dermatitis*.

Prolonged or Repeated Contact

Allergic reactions are caused by prolonged or repeated direct skin contact. This type of skin problem does not occur overnight. Acrylic liquids, wraps, and U.V. light gels are all capable of causing allergic reactions. In general, it takes from four to six months of repeated exposure before sensitive clients show symptoms.

Nail technicians are also at risk. Prolonged, repeated, or long-term exposures can cause anyone to become sensitive. This is called overexposure. Simply touching monomers does not cause sensitivities. It requires months of improper handling and overexposure. The most likely places for allergies to occur are

1. between a technician's thumb and pointer finger.
2. on the nail technician's wrist or palm.

3. on the nail technician's face, especially the cheeks.

4. on the client's cuticles, finger tips, or the sensitive tissues of the underlying nail bed.

If you examine the area where the problem occurs, you can usually determine the cause. For example, nail technicians often smooth wet brushes with their fingers. This is both prolonged and repeated contact! Eventually the area becomes sore and inflamed. The same occurs when technicians lay their arms on the towels contaminated with U.V. gel, monomer, or filings. The palms are overexposed by picking up containers that have traces of monomer on the outside. Small amounts of product on your hands are often transferred to the cheeks or face. Direct product contact to the skin is the cause of these facial irritations, not the vapors. Nail enhancement product vapors will not cause a skin allergy.

Touching a client's skin with any monomer or U.V. gel has the same effect. This is the most common reason for client sensitivities. With each service the risk of sensitization increases. **Sensitization** is a greatly increased or exaggerated sensitivity to products. It is extremely important that you always leave a tiny, free margin (approximately 1/16") between the product and the skin. The most important rule of being a good nail technician is: **Never touch any nail enhancement product to the skin.**

Improper product consistency is the second most common reason for allergy. If too much liquid monomer is used, the result is an overly wet bead. Many technicians do not realize that the initiator in the polymer powder can only harden a certain amount of the liquid monomer. Wet beads are incorrectly balanced. Beads with too wet of a consistency will harden with monomer trapped inside. This extra monomer eventually works its way down to the nail bed and may cause an allergic reaction. The same thing occurs with gel enhancements. Many things can cause gels to harden incorrectly.

❖ applying product too thickly
❖ too short of a time under the light
❖ dirty bulbs in the lamp unit
❖ old bulbs that should be changed

Several thin coatings and long exposures lead to the best and most complete cure. If the U.V. bulb is dirty or old, it does not give enough energy to fully cure the enhancement. U.V. bulbs remain blue for years, but they lose effectiveness after four to six months of use. They should be cleaned daily and will work best if changed three times per year. The enhancement product will set more thoroughly, last longer, and be less likely to cause an allergy if you take these precautions. Filings can also be too rich in uncured U.V. gel or liquid monomer. If the nail technician's arm, wrist, hands, or fingers are overexposed to these dusts, an allergic reaction to these areas may result.

It is critical to use medium consistency beads. Never use a wet consistency. Beads that flatten out or have a ring of liquid around them are much too wet. A proper consistency bead should form a smooth dome when placed on the natural nail or tip. It should not flatten out, nor should it be runny.

The gooey layer on top of gel enhancements is mostly uncured gel. It must never come in contact with soft tissue. Also, never dip back into the dappen dish to get more liquid or clean up around the cuticle with monomer. If you do, chances are your clients will begin to develop skin problems in those areas. Avoid using extra large or oversize brushes. They usually make overly wet beads that are difficult to control. The belly of these large brushes can carry enough liquid for **four** normal size beads. Brushes that are too large don't save time—they cause allergic reactions.

Mixing product lines or custom blending your own "special" mixture can also create chemical imbalances, which leads to allergic reactions. Do not take unnecessary risks. Always use products exactly as instructed and never mix your own products. If you do, don't be surprised when you or your clients develop skin problems.

Skin disorders of the hands affects more than thirty percent of all nail technicians sometime during their careers. Skin problems and allergies force many good nail technicians to give up successful careers. Unfortunately, once you or a client become allergic to an ingredient, you are sensitive for the rest of your life. This is especially sad, because it is completely avoidable. No one should suffer from any work related allergy or irritation.

Irritant Contact Dermatitis

Irritating substances will temporarily damage the epidermis. Corrosive substances are examples of irritants. When the skin is damaged by irritating substances the immune system springs into action. It floods the tissue with water, trying to dilute the irritant. This is why swelling occurs. The body is trying to stop things from getting any worse. The immune system also tells the blood to release chemicals, called **histamines**, that enlarge the vessels around the injury. Blood can then rush to the scene more quickly and help remove the irritating substance.

You can see and feel all the extra blood under the skin. The entire area becomes red, warm, and may throb. It is the histamines that cause the itchy feeling that often accompanies contact dermatitis. After everything calms down, the swelling will go away. The surrounding skin is often left damaged, scaly, cracked and dry. Fortunately, irritations are not permanent. If you avoid repeated and/or prolonged contact with the irritating substance, the skin will usually quickly repair itself. However, continued or repeated exposure may lead to permanent allergic reactions.

Surprisingly, tap water is a very common salon irritant. Hands that remain damp for long periods often become sore, cracked, and chapped. Avoiding the problem is simple. Always completely dry the hands. Regularly use moisturizing hand creams to compensate for loss of skin oils. Frequent hand washing, especially in hard water, can further damage the skin. Cleansers and detergents worsen the problem. They increase damage

5

by stripping away sebum and other natural skin chemicals. Prolonged or repeated contact with many solvents will strip away skin oils, leaving the skin dry or damaged. Sometimes it is difficult to determine the cause of the irritation. One way to identify the irritant is by observing the location of the reaction. Symptoms are always isolated to the contact area. The cause will be something that you are doing to this part of the skin.

Remember These Precautions

* *Never* smooth the enhancement surface with more liquid monomer.
* *Never* use monomer to "clean up" the edges, under the nail or sidewalls.
* *Never* touch any monomer liquids, U.V. gels, or adhesives to the skin.
* *Never* touch the hairs of the brush with your fingers.
* *Never* mix your own special product blends.
* *Always* follow instructions—exactly!

Once a client becomes allergic, things will only get worse if you continue using the same products and techniques. It is best to discontinue use until you figure out what you are doing wrong. Otherwise, more clients will eventually be affected. Medications and illness do not make clients sensitive to nail products. These are just excuses. Only prolonged and repeated contact causes these allergies.

Protect Yourself

Take extreme care to keep brush handles, containers, and table tops clean and free from product dusts and residues. Repeatedly handling these items will cause overexposure if the items are not kept clean. Enhancement products are not designed for skin contact! If you avoid contact, neither you nor your client will ever develop an allergic reaction.

Many serious problems can be related to contact dermatitis. Don't fall into the trap of developing bad habits.

◆ ◆ ◆ THE OVEREXPOSURE PRINCIPLE

We usually think of toxic substances as dangerous poisons. We hear the term "toxic" often, but should nail technicians try to avoid products that are toxic? The answer to this question may surprise you.

Paracelsus, a famous fourteenth century physician, was the first to use the word "toxic." He said, *"All substances are poisons; there is none which is not a poison. Only the dose differentiates a poison and a remedy."*

The **Overexposure Principle** is the modern day interpretation of what Paracelsus learned. This important principle says that *overexposure* determines toxicity. Scientists have found that Paracelsus is correct.

Everything is a poison! Do we have to avoid everything, including cuticle oils and skin creams? Isn't anything nontoxic? Scientists define toxic and nontoxic differently than the terms are commonly understood. They consider a chemical relatively nontoxic only if drinking a quart or more will not cause death.

Next time someone tells you a product is "nontoxic" think about this definition. Salt water is very toxic to drink. Still, we can safely swim in the ocean without fear of poisoning. Rubbing alcohol is also quite toxic, but we manage to use it quite easily.

B U S I N E S S TIP

Retail As You Work

A manicure provides the perfect opportunity to sell nail care products. If, during a hand massage, the client comments that the lotion you're using feels good, selling it to her should be easy—just explain the lotion's benefits and ask her if she'd like some for home use. Even if the client seems uninterested in the products you are using, you can still sell her items. Show her something you are about to apply to her nails and try saying something like: "This is our latest high-shine top coat" (or whatever else you'd like to sell). Use it as part of the service, then at the end of the manicure place the item in her hand and ask if you can add it to her ticket. This last step is crucial to close the sale. If you make a recommendation early in the appointment but don't pursue it at the end, the client often forgets about it.

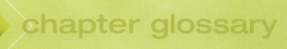
adhesion	A chemical reaction resulting in two surfaces sticking together.
adhesive	An agent that causes two surfaces to stick together.
catalyst	Any substance having the power to speed up a chemical reaction.
chemical	Relating to chemistry; any substance of chemical composition.
chemical change	Alteration in the chemical composition of a substance in which a new substance, with properties different from the original, is formed.
chemical reaction	A chemical change in a molecule, usually as a result of heat or light.
coatings	Products, including nail polish, top coats, artificial enhancements, and adhesives, that cover the nail plate with a hard film.
corrosive	A substance that has the power to eat away or destroy another substance.
cross-linker	A monomer that joins together different polymer chains.
dermatitis	An abnormal inflammation of the skin. Different types include *contact dermatitis*, *irritant contact dermatitis*, and *allergic contact dermatitis*.
elements	The simplest forms of basic matter; substances that cannot be broken down into simpler forms without loss of identity.
energy	Internal or inherent power or capacity for performing work.
evaporate	To change from liquid to vapor form.
gas	A state of matter different from a liquid or solid because of its low molecular density; should not be confused with vapor, as it does not evaporate in the air like vapor.
histamines	Chemicals in the blood that enlarge the vessels around an injury so that blood can get to a site quickly and help remove any irritating substance.
initiator	A special ingredient in a monomer molecule that triggers a boost of energy used to create a monomer chain (polymer).
matter	A substance that occupies space; has physical and chemical properties; and exists in either solid, liquid, or gas form.
molecule	The smallest possible unit of any substance that retains its original characteristics.
monomers	Individual molecules that join together to make a polymer.
overexposure	Dangerously prolonged, repeated, or long-term contact with certain chemicals.
physically changed	A substance that is changed in form or appearance only, without chemically altering it to create a new substance.
polymerizations	Chemical reactions that create polymers; also called curing or hardening.
polymers	Substances formed by combining many small molecules (monomers), usually in long, chain-like structures.
primers	Substances that improve adhesion.
saturated	Became soaked or completely penetrated; absorbed all that a substance can possibly hold.

5

sensitization	A greatly increased or exaggerated sensitivity to certain chemicals or products.
simple polymer chains	The result of long chains of monomers that are attached from head to tail.
solute	The dissolved substance in a solution.
solvent	A substance, usually liquid, that dissolves another substance without any change in chemical composition.
ultraviolet (U.V.) light	Invisible rays of the color spectrum that are beyond the violet rays; shortest and least penetrating of the light rays.
vapor	The gaseous state that is formed when liquid is heated and evaporates into the air.

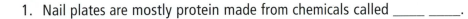

review questions

1. Nail plates are mostly protein made from chemicals called _____ _____.

2. Define molecules.

3. What are catalysts and why are they important to nail chemistry?

4. A _____ is anything that dissolves another substance called a _____.

5. True or False? Primers can eat the nail plate. Explain your answer.

6. Define monomers.

7. What are the two main differences between irritations and allergic reactions?

8. What six things can you avoid or do to ensure that clients never suffer from a product allergy?

9. Only _____ and _____ skin contact can cause a client to become allergic to products.

10. In your own words explain what Paracelsus discovered about toxic substances. How can you use this knowledge to work safely?

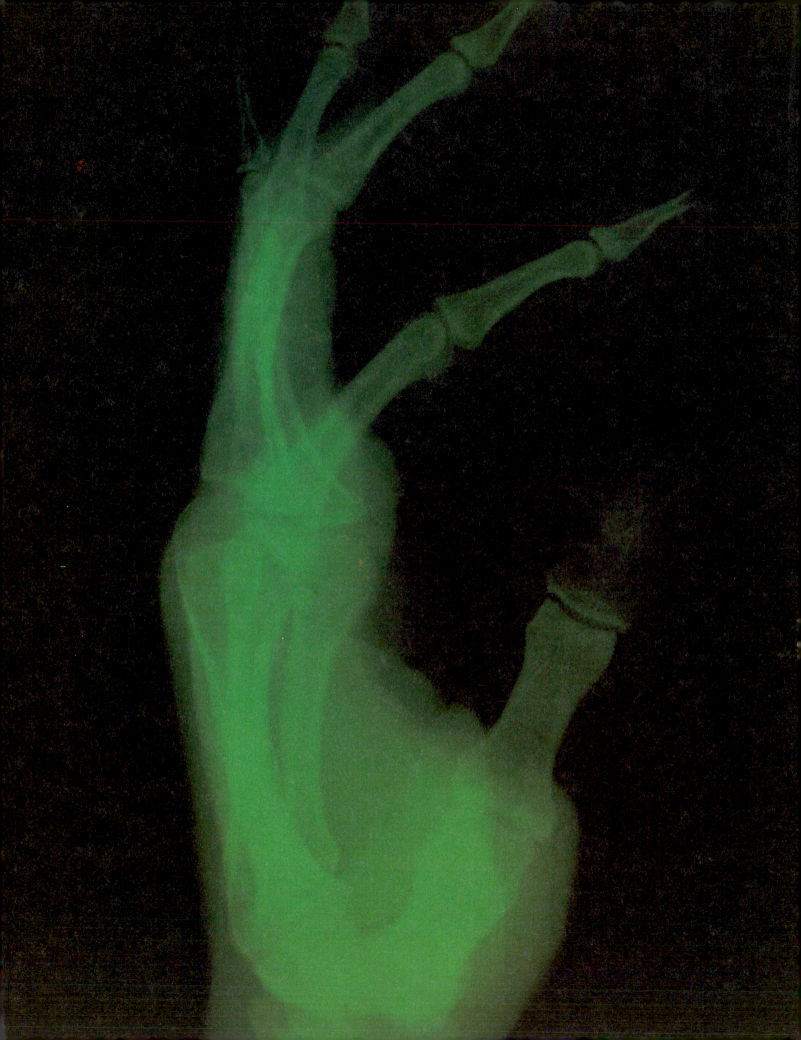

6

ANATOMY AND PHYSIOLOGY

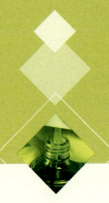

Author: Godfrey Mix, DPM

CHAPTER OUTLINE

Learning Objectives

After you have completed this chapter, you should be able to:

1. Explain how an understanding of anatomy and physiology will help you become a better nail technician.

2. Describe the purpose of cells within the human body.

3. Describe cell metabolism and explain the difference between the two phases of metabolism.

4. Name the different types of body tissue and explain the function of each type.

5. Name the most important organs of the body and explain the function of each organ.

6. Name the systems that make up the human body and explain the function of each system.

7. List the ways in which muscles are stimulated.

8. Name the types of muscles that are affected by massage.

9. Name the divisions of the nervous system and explain the function of each division.

10. Identify the chief functions of the blood.

Key Terms

Page number indicates where in the chapter the term is used.

blood
pg. 103

blood-vascular system
pg. 101

cells
pg. 89

circulatory (vascular) system
pg. 101

digestive system
pg. 106

endocrine system
pg. 104

excretory system
pg. 105

integumentary system
pg. 92

lymph
pg. 104

lymph-vascular (lymphatic) system
pg. 101

metabolism
pg. 90

muscular system
pg. 95

myology
pg. 95

nerves
pg. 100

nervous system
pg. 99

neurology
pg. 99

neuron (nerve cell)
pg. 100

organs
pg. 92

osteology
pg. 93

pulmonary circulation
pg. 103

reflex
pg. 100

respiratory system
pg. 105

skeletal system
pg. 93

systemic (general) circulation
pg. 103

systems
pg. 92

tissues
pg. 91

Although you may have groaned when you saw a chapter on anatomy and physiology, these are important subjects in the practice of nail technology. A basic understanding of the structure of the human body and the functions it performs will give you a scientific background for many of the nail services you will learn. This background will help you decide which service is best for a client's nail or skin condition, and how to adjust and control the service for the best results.

Very generally, anatomy is the study of the structure of the body and what it is made of—for example, bones, muscles, and skin. Histology is the microscopic study of the small, individual structures of the body, such as hair, nails, sweat glands, and oil glands. Physiology is the study of the functions or activities performed by the body's structures.

Although the names of bones, muscles, arteries, veins, and nerves are seldom used in the nail salon, an understanding of body structures will help make you more proficient in performing many services, such as hand and arm massage. Your study of anatomy and physiology will include cells, tissues, organs, and systems of the human body.

CELLS

Cells are the basic units of all living things, including bacteria, plants, and animals. The human body is made up entirely of cells, fluids, and cellular products. As the basic functional units of all living things, the cells carry on all of our life processes. Cells also have the ability to reproduce, providing new cells that enable us to grow and that replace worn or injured tissues.

Cells are made up of **protoplasm** (PROH-toh-plaz-em), a colorless, jellylike substance that contains food elements such as protein, fat, carbohydrates, and mineral salts. The protoplasm of the cells includes the nucleus (NOO-klee-us), cytoplasm (SEYE-toh-plaz-em), centrosome (SEN-tro-sohm), and cell membrane.

The **nucleus** is made of dense protoplasm and is found in the center of the cell within the nuclear membrane. It plays an important role in cell reproduction.

Cytoplasm is found outside of the nucleus and contains food materials necessary for the growth, reproduction, and self-repair of the cell.

The **centrosome**, a small, round body in the cytoplasm, affects the reproduction of the cell.

The **cell membrane** encloses the cytoplasm. It controls the transportation of substances in and out of the cells (Figure 6–1).

Cell Growth

As long as the cell receives an adequate supply of food, oxygen, and water; eliminates waste products; and is maintained at the proper temperature, it will continue to grow and thrive. However, if these conditions do not exist

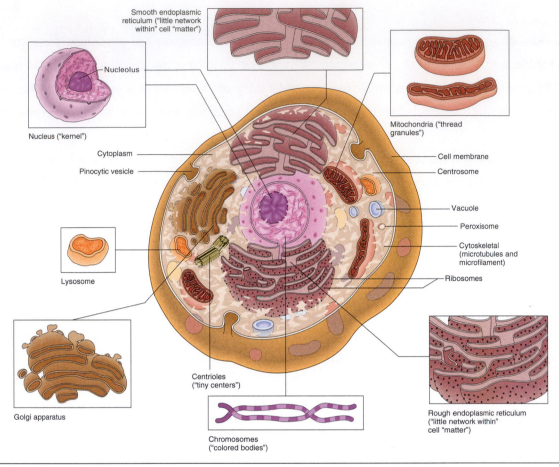

Smooth endoplasmic
reticulum ("little network
within" cell "matter")

Nucleolus

Nucleus ("kernel")

Cytoplasm

Pinocytic vesicle

Lysosome

Golgi apparatus

Centrioles
("tiny centers")

Chromosomes
("colored bodies")

Mitochondria ("thread
granules")

Cell membrane

Centrosome

Vacuole

Peroxisome

Cytoskeletal
(microtubules and
microfilament)

Ribosomes

Rough endoplasmic reticulum
("little network within"
cell "matter")

Figure 6–1 Cells consist of protoplasm and contain essential elements.

and toxins (poisons) or pressure are present, then the growth and health of the cells are impaired. Most of our body cells are capable of growing and repairing themselves during their life cycle. Cells also reproduce themselves through a process of division known as **mitosis** (Figure 6–2).

Cell Metabolism

Metabolism (meh-TAB-o-liz-em) is a complex chemical process whereby the body cells are nourished and supplied with the energy needed to carry on their many activities. There are two phases of metabolism.

1. **Anabolism** (ah-NAB-o-liz-em) is the process of building up larger molecules from smaller ones. During this process the body stores water, food, and oxygen for the time when these substances are needed for cell growth and repair.

2. **Catabolism** (kah-TAB-o-liz-em) is the breaking down of larger substances or molecules into smaller ones. This process releases energy that can be stored by special molecules for use in muscle contraction, secretion, or heat production.

Anabolism and catabolism are carried out at the same time and happen continuously. Their activities are closely regulated so that the breaking down, energy-releasing reactions are balanced with the building-up,

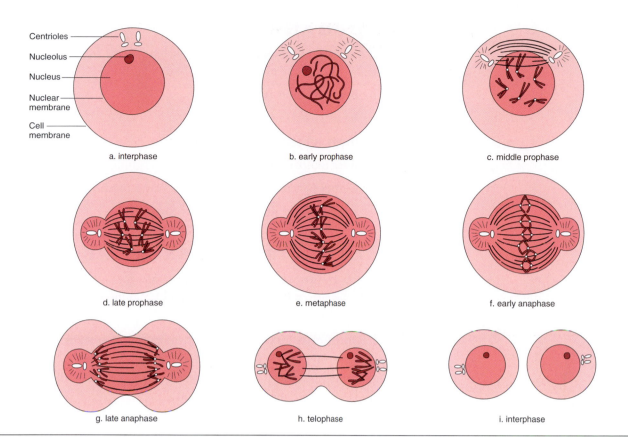

Figure 6-2 Mitosis—indirect division of the human cell

energy-consuming reactions. Therefore, **homeostasis** (ho-me-oh-STAY-sus) (the maintenance of normal, internal stability in the body) is achieved. However, if we use less energy than we manufacture, we may notice a weight gain. The molecules of energy that are not used may turn to fat. To get rid of built-up fat, we must use more energy by exercising or take in less energy by eating less.

◆ ◆ TISSUES

Tissues are composed of groups of cells of the same kind. Each tissue has a specific function and can be recognized by its characteristic appearance. Body tissues are classified as follows:

1. **Connective tissue** serves to support, protect, and bind together tissues of the body. Bone, cartilage, ligament, tendon, fascia (which separates muscles), and fat tissue are examples of connective tissue.

2. **Muscular tissue** contracts and moves various parts of the body.

3. **Nerve tissue** carries messages to and from the brain, and controls and coordinates all body functions.

4. **Epithelial** (ep-i-THE-le-al) **tissue** is a protective covering on body surfaces, such as the skin, mucous membranes, linings of the ear, digestive and respiratory organs, and glands.

5. **Liquid tissue** carries food, waste products, and hormones by means of the blood and lymph.

◆ ◆ ORGANS

Organs are structures designed to accomplish a specific function. The most important organs of the body are described below.

The **brain** controls the body.

The **heart** circulates the blood.

The **lungs** supply oxygen to the blood.

The **liver** removes toxic products of digestion.

The **kidneys** excrete water and other waste products.

The **stomach** and **intestines** digest food.

◆ ◆ OVERVIEW OF SYSTEMS

Systems are groups of organs that cooperate for a common purpose, namely the welfare of the entire body. The human body is made up of ten important systems.

The **integumentary** (in-TEG-yoo-men-ta-ree) **system** is composed of two distinct layers, the dermis and epidermis. It provides a protective covering, contains sensory receptors that give us our sense of touch, and helps regulate the temperature of the body.

The **skeletal system** is the physical foundation or framework of the body. The bones of the skeletal system serve as a means of protection, support, and locomotion (movement).

The **muscular system** covers, shapes, and supports the skeleton. Its function is to produce all the movements of the body.

The **nervous system** controls and coordinates the functions of all the other systems of the body.

The **circulatory** (SUR-kyoo-lay-tohr-ee) **system** supplies blood throughout the body.

The **endocrine** (EN-doh-krin) **system** is made up of ductless glands that secrete hormones into the bloodstream.

The **excretory** (EK-skre-tohr-ee) **system** eliminates waste from the body.

The **respiratory** (RES-pi-rah-toh-ree) **system** supplies oxygen to the body.

The **digestive system** changes food into substances that can be used by the cells of the body.

The **reproductive system** enables human beings to reproduce.

◆ ◆ THE INTEGUMENTARY SYSTEM

The integumentary system is the largest system in the body and is the organ system in which the nail technician will be most closely involved. Most products used by the nail technician will have some direct or indirect effect on this organ system. The function of this system, which includes the

6

skin and its accessory organs such as the oil and sweat glands, sensory receptors, hair, and nails, is to provide a protective covering and sensory receptors for a sense of touch. This system also plays an important role in regulating the temperature of the body.

◆ ◆ ◆ THE SKELETAL SYSTEM

The **skeletal system** is the physical foundation of the body. The entire skeleton is composed of 206 bones. These bones have a variety of shapes and are connected by movable and immovable joints.

Bone, second to the tooth enamel, is the hardest tissue of the body. It is composed of connective tissues consisting of about one-third animal (organic) matter, such as cells and blood, and two-thirds mineral (inorganic) matter, mainly calcium carbonate and calcium phosphate. The scientific study of bones, their structure, and functions is called **osteology** (os-tee-OL-oh-jee). The technical term for bone is **os**.

The following are primary functions of the skeletal system.

1. Give shape and support to the body.

2. Protect various internal structures and organs.

3. Serve as attachments for muscles and act as levers to produce body movements.

4. Produce various blood cells in the red bone marrow.

5. Store various minerals, such as calcium, phosphorus, magnesium, and sodium.

Structure of Bone

Bone is a hard connective tissue consisting of bone cells called **osteocytes** (OS-tee-o-sitz). These cells are embedded within a hard substance primarily composed of calcium carbonate and calcium phosphate. By weight, bone is composed of 75 percent non-living substance and 25 percent living cells. Bones are covered by a specialized connective tissue called **periosteum** (pe-ree-OS-tee-um). The periosteum serves a number of functions. Cells within the periosteum aid in bone repair after injury. It also serves as a point of attachment to the bone for muscles and tendons. The bone immediately under the periosteum is hard and compact and is called *cortical bone.* Underlying the cortical bone is a spongy lattice-like layer of bone called *cancellous bone.* The center of long bones is hollow and filled with a connective tissue called marrow. Marrow also fills the spaces within cancellous bone and its primary function is to produce blood cells. Bone receives its nutrition from arteries that penetrate the periosteum and enter the bone structure through a series of microscopic canals or tunnels called Haversian canals. This system of canals is throughout the bone and allows the delivery of nutrients to all living tissue within the bone structure.

The structures attached to the bone include cartilage and ligaments. **Cartilage** (CAR-tih-ledj) is a tough elastic substance similar to bone but it has no mineral content. Cartilage cushions bones at the joints and gives shape to some external features such as the nose and ears. **Ligaments** (LIG-e-mentz) are bands or sheets of fibrous tissue that support and connect the bones at the joints.

Joints

The various bones of the body meet at junctions called **joints**. Bones are connected together at joints by **ligaments** and a bag-like structure called the **joint capsule**. The ligaments give the joint strength, while the capsule encloses and seals off the joint from the surrounding tissues. Within the joint each end of the bone is covered with cartilage, which helps to cushion the joint as well as to give a smooth surface on which the joint moves.

The joint is filled with **synovial** (sy-NOV-ee-al) **fluid**, which acts as a lubricant for the joint. Synovial fluid also helps to furnish nourishment to the cartilage of the joint. Although most joints move in many ways, there are some, like those that connect the various bones of the skull, that do not. The non-movable joints, therefore, generally do not have a joint capsule or synovial fluid, they may or may not be connected together by ligaments, and they do not have cartilage covering the ends of the bone.

At **pivot** (PIH-vut) **joints**, like the neck, one bone turns on another bone. At **hinge** (HINJ) **joints**, which are found in the elbow and knee, two or more bones connect like a door. At a **ball-and-socket joint**, such as the hip or shoulder, one bone is rounded and fits into the socket, or hollow part, of another bone. In **gliding joints**, which are found in the ankle and wrist, two bones glide over each other.

Bones of the Arm and Hand

The **scapula** (SKAP-yoo-lah) and the **clavicle** (KLAV-i-kul) form the shoulder. The clavicle is also known as the collar bone.

The **humerus** (HYOO-mo-rus) is the uppermost and largest bone of the arm.

The **ulna** (UL-nah) is the large bone on the small-finger side of the forearm.

The **radius** (RAY-dee-us) is the small bone in the forearm on the same side as your thumb (Figure 6–3).

The **carpus** (KAHR-pus) or wrist, is a flexible joint composed of eight small, irregular bones held together by ligaments.

The five **metacarpals** (met-a-KAHR-puls), the bones of the palm of the hand, are long and slender.

The **digits** or **fingers** consist of three **phalanges** (fl-LAN-jeez) in each finger and two in the thumb, totaling fourteen bones (Figure 6–4).

Bones of the Leg and Foot

The **femur** (FEE-mur) is a heavy, long bone that forms the leg above the knee.

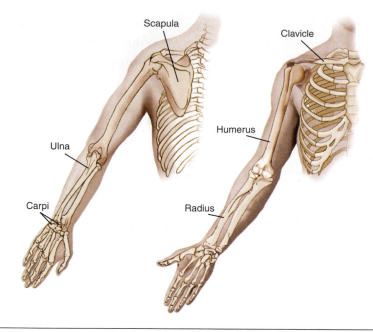

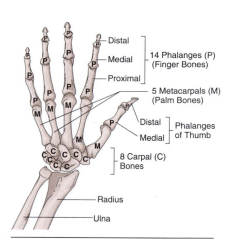

Figure 6-3 Bones of the arm

Figure 6-4 Bones of the hand and wrist

The **tibia** (TIB-ee-ah) is the larger of the two bones that form the leg below the knee. The tibia may be visualized as a "bump" on the big-toe side of the ankle.

The **fibula** (FIB-ya-lah) is the smaller of the two bones that form the leg below the knee. The fibula may be visualized as a "bump" on the little-toe side of the ankle.

The **patella** (pah-TEL-lah), also called the accessory bone, forms the knee cap joint (Figure 6–5).

The ankle joint is made up of three bones. The ankle joint is formed by the tibia, fibula, and the **talus** (TA-lus) or ankle bone of the foot.

The foot is made up of 26 bones. These can be subdivided into three general categories: seven **tarsal** (TAHR-sul) bones (talus, calcaneous, navicular, three cuneiform bones, and the cuboid), and five **metatarsal** (met-ah-TAHR-sul) bones, which are long and slender, like the metacarpal bones of the hand, and 14 bones called **phalanges**, which compose the toes. The phalanges are similar to the finger bones. There are three phalanges in each toe, except for the big toe, which has only two (Figure 6–6).

THE MUSCULAR SYSTEM

The **muscular** (MUS-kyoo-lahr) **system** covers, shapes, and supports the skeleton. Its function is to produce all movements of the body. **Myology** (meye-OL-oh-jee) is the study of the structure, functions, and diseases of the muscles.

The muscular system consists of over 500 muscles, large and small, comprising 40 to 50 percent of the weight of the human body.

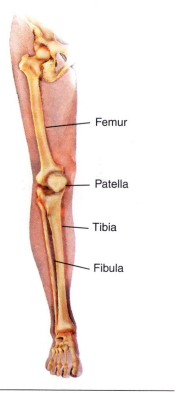

Figure 6-5 Bones of the leg

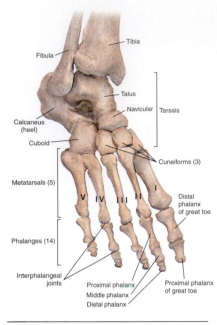

Figure 6-6 Bones of the foot and ankle

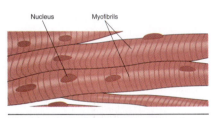

Figure 6-7 Striated muscle cells

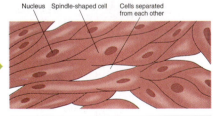

Figure 6-8 Non-striated muscle cells

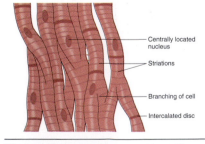

Figure 6-9 Cardiac muscle cells

Muscles are fibrous tissues that have the ability to stretch and contract according to our movements. Different types of movement—for example, stretching and bending—depend on muscles performing in specific ways.

There are three kinds of muscular tissue.

1. **Striated** (STRY-ate-id) **muscles** are voluntary muscles that you can move whenever you want. Muscles of the face, arm, and leg are striated muscles. The word striated means striped (Figure 6–7).

2. **Non-striated muscles** are involuntary. Muscles of the stomach and intestines are non-striated. These muscles function automatically. Non-striated means smooth or not striped (Figure 6–8).

3. **Cardiac** (CAR-dee-ak) **muscle** is heart muscle, which is not found anywhere else in the body (Figure 6–9).

Muscle Parts

A typical striated muscle is composed of a mass of muscle fibers, called the **belly** of the muscle. The belly is attached at each end to a bone or other structure by a **tendon** (TEN-dun). The more fixed or least movable attachment is called the **origin** of the muscle. The more movable attachment is called the **insertion** of the muscle. When the belly of the muscle contracts the muscle shortens, causing movement of the part into which it inserts. Tendons are composed of strong, fibrous tissues and may appear as a flat layer of tissue but are usually seen as a round rope-like cord. Tendons are smooth and have a white, glistening appearance.

Stimulation of Muscles

Muscle tissue can be stimulated in any of the following ways.

Nerve impulses—through the nervous system.

Massage—hand massage and electric vibrator.

Electric current—applied to the muscle area to produce visible muscle contractions.

Light rays—infrared rays and ultraviolet rays.

Heat rays—heating lamps and heating caps.

Moist heat—steamers or moderately warm steam towels.

Chemicals—certain acids and salts.

Muscles Affected by Massage

As a nail technician, you are concerned with the voluntary muscles of the hands, arms, legs, and feet. It is essential to know where these muscles are located and what they control. Pressure in massage is usually directed from the insertion to the origin.

The Consultation

A good consultation is the beginning of a successful client-professional relationship. Take time to talk with a new client about her nailcare goals—is she trying to grow her short nails long, to switch from extensions to natural nails, or simply to have better groomed hands? Understanding her goals helps you know how to proceed to meet her expectations. The initial consultation is also the time to look for an existing medical problem, such as a severe case of eczema, a fungal infection, or any other disorder. If you encounter such a problem, don't try to solve it yourself. Suggest that she see her physician who will give her the names of specialists who can help. Tell her that healthy nails sometimes require the help of a medical expert and that you look forward to working on her once the problem clears up. She'll be so impressed with your professional concern that she'll be sure to return once the condition is treated.

Muscles of the Shoulder and Upper Arm

The **deltoid** (DEL-toid) is a large, thick triangular muscle that covers the shoulder and lifts and turns the arm.

Biceps (BEYE-seps) is the muscle on the front of the upper arm that lifts the forearm, flexes the elbow and turns the palm up. It has two heads or points of attachment.

Triceps (TREYE-seps) are muscles that cover the entire back of the upper arm and extend the forearm forward. They have three heads or points of attachment.

Muscles of the Forearm

The **forearm** contains a series of muscles and strong tendons.

The **pronator** (PRO-nay-tor) turns the hand inward, so the palm faces downward.

Supinator (SUE-pi-nay-tor) turns the hand outward so the palm faces upward.

Flexors (FLEKS-ors) bend to the wrist, draw the hand upward, and close the fingers toward the forearm.

Extensor (eck-STEN-sur) straightens the wrist, hand, and fingers to form a straight line (Figure 6–10).

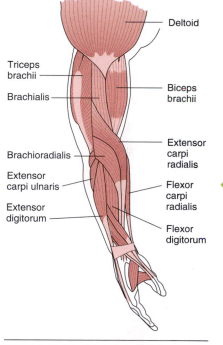

Figure 6–10 Muscles of the arm

Muscles of the Hand

The hand has many small muscles that overlap from joint to joint, giving flexibility and strength. When the hands are properly cared for, these muscles will remain supple and graceful. They close and open the hands and fingers.

Abductors (ab-DUK-tohrs) separate the fingers and **adductors** (a-DUK-tohrs) draw the fingers together. Both of these muscles are located at the base of the thumbs and fingers (Figure 6–11).

Opponent muscles are located in the palm of the hand and act to bring the thumb toward the fingers, allowing the grasping action of the hands.

Muscles of the Lower Leg and Foot

As a nail technician, you will use your knowledge of the muscles of the foot and leg during a pedicure. The muscles of the foot are small and provide proper support and cushioning for the foot and leg (Figure 6–12).

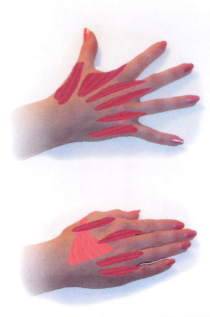

Figure 6–11 Muscles of the hand

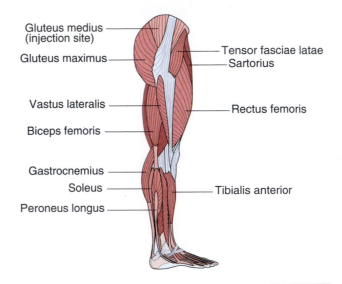

Figure 6–12 Muscles of the lower leg and foot

The **extensor digitorum longus** (eck-STEN-sur dij-it-TOHR-um LONG-us) bends the foot up and extends the toes.

The **tibialis anterior** (tib-ee-AHL-is an-TEHR-ee-ohr) covers the front of the shin. It bends the foot upward and inward.

The **peroneus longus** (per-oh-NEE-us LONG-us) covers the outer side of the calf and inverts the foot and turns it outward.

The **peroneus brevis** (BREV-us) originates on the lower surface of the fibula. It bends the foot down and out.

The **gastrocnemius** (gas-truc-NEEM-e-us) is attached to the lower rear surface of the heel and pulls the foot down.

The **soleus** (SO-lee-us) originates at the upper portion of the fibula and bends the foot down.

The muscles of the feet include the **extensor digitorum brevis** (ek-STEN-sur dij-it-TOHR-um BREV-us), **abductor hallucis** (ab-DUK-tohr ha-LU-sis), **flexor digitorum brevis** (FLEKS-or dij-it-TOHR-um BREV-us) and the **abductor**. The foot muscles move the toes and help maintain balance while walking and standing (Figure 6–13).

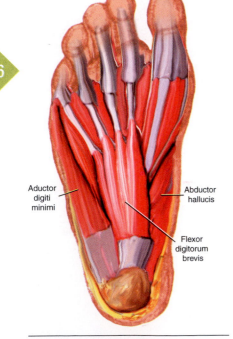

Figure 6–13 Muscles of the foot (bottom)

◆ ◆ ◆ THE NERVOUS SYSTEM

Neurology is the branch of medicine that deals with the nervous system and its disorders. The **nervous system** is one of the most important systems of the body because it controls and coordinates the functions of all the other systems and makes them work in harmony. Every square inch of the human body is supplied with fine fibers called **nerves**. As a nail technician, you should study the nervous system in order to understand the effect massage has on the nerves of the feet, legs, hands, arms, and the whole body.

The nervous system is composed of three divisions: the central nervous system, the peripheral system, and the autonomic nervous system.

1. The **cerebro-spinal** (ser-EE-broh SPEYE-nahl) or **central nervous system** consists of the brain and spinal cord and has the following functions.
   a. controls consciousness and all mental activities
   b. controls functions of the five senses: seeing, smelling, tasting, feeling, and hearing
   c. controls voluntary muscle actions, such as all body movements and facial expression

2. The **peripheral** (pe-RIF-er-al) **system** is made up of the sensory and motor nerve fibers that extend from the brain and spinal cord and are distributed to all parts of the body. Its function is to carry messages to and from the central nervous system.

3. The **autonomic** (aw-toh-NAHM-ik) **nervous system** is the portion of the nervous system that functions without conscious effort and regulates the activities of the smooth muscles, glands, blood vessels, and heart. The system has two divisions, the **sympathetic** and **parasympathetic systems**, which act in direct opposition to each other. They regulate such things as heart rate, blood pressure, breathing rate, and body temperature to aid the body in the maintenance of homeostasis, or normal internal stability. The sympathetic division is primarily activated during stressful, energy-demanding, or emergency situations; the parasympathetic division is most active in ordinary restful energy-conserving situations.

The Brain and the Spinal Cord

The brain is the largest mass of nerve tissue in the body and is contained in the cranium. The weight of the average brain is 44–48 ounces (1232–1344 g). It is considered to be the central processing unit of the body, sending and receiving digital messages. Twelve pairs of cranial nerves originate in the brain and reach various parts of the head, face, and neck.

The spinal cord is composed of masses of nerve cells, with fibers running upward and downward. It originates in the brain, extends the length of the trunk, and is enclosed and protected by the spinal column. Thirty-one pairs of spinal nerves, extending from the spinal cord, are distributed to the muscles and skin of the trunk and limbs. Some of the spinal nerves supply the internal organs controlled by the sympathetic nervous system.

Nerve Cells and Nerves

A **neuron** (NOOR-on) or **nerve cell** is the primary structural unit of the nervous system. It is composed of a cell body, **dendrites** (DEN-dreyets), which receive messages from other neurons, and an **axon** (AK-son) and axon terminal, which send messages to other neurons, glands, or muscles (Figure 6–14).

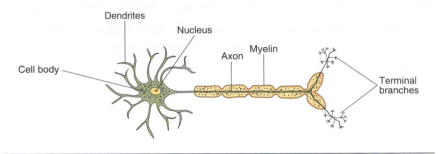

Figure 6–14 A neuron or nerve cell

Nerves are long, white cords made up of masses of neurons that carry messages to and from various parts of the body. Nerves have their origin in the brain and spinal cord, and distribute branches to all parts of the body.

Types of Nerves

Sensory nerves, also called **afferent** (AF-fer-ent) **nerves**, carry impulses or messages from sense organs to the brain, where sensations of touch, cold, heat, sight, hearing, taste, smell, pain, and pressure are experienced.

Motor nerves, also called **efferent** (EF-fer-ent) **nerves**, carry impulses from the brain to the muscles. The transmitted impulses produce movement.

Mixed nerves contain both sensory and motor fibers and have the ability to both send and receive messages.

Sensory nerve endings, called **receptors**, are located near the surface of the skin. Impulses pass from the sensory nerves to the brain and back over the motor nerves to the muscles. A complete circuit is established and movements of the muscles result.

A **reflex** is an automatic, involuntary response to a stimulus that involves the transmission of an impulse from a sensory receptor along an afferent nerve to the spinal cord, and a responsive impulse along an efferent neuron to a muscle, causing a reaction. An example of a reflex is the quick removal of the hand from a hot object. A reflex action does not have to be learned.

Nerves of the Arm and Hand

The **ulnar** (UL-ner) **nerve** and its branches supply the small finger side of the arm and the palm of the hand.

The **radial** (RAY-dee-al) **nerve** and its branches supply the thumb side of the arm and the back of the hand.

The **median** (MEE-di-an) **nerve** is a smaller nerve than the ulnar and radial nerves. With its branches, it supplies the arm and hand.

The **digital** (DIJ-it-al) **nerve** and its branches supply all fingers of the hand (Figure 6–15).

Nerves of the Lower Leg and Foot

The **tibial** (TIB-ee-al) **nerve**, a division of the sciatic nerve, passes behind the knee. It subdivides and supplies impulses to the knee, the muscles of the calf, the skin of the leg, and the sole, heel, and underside of the toes.

The **common peroneal** (per-oh-NEE-al) **nerve**, also a division of the sciatic nerve, extends from behind the knee to wind around the head of the fibula to the front of the leg where it divides into two branches. The **deep peroneal nerve**, also known as the **anterior tibial nerve**, extends down the front of the leg, behind the muscles. It supplies impulses to these muscles and also to the muscles and skin on the top of the foot and adjacent sides of the first and second toes. The **superficial peroneal nerve**, also known as the **musculo-cutaneous nerve**, extends down the leg, just under the skin, supplying impulses to the muscles and the skin of the leg, as well as to the skin and toes on the top of the foot, where it is called the **dorsal** (DOOR-sal) or **dorsal cutaneous nerve**.

The **saphenous** (sa-FEEN-us) **nerve** supplies impulses to the skin of the inner side of the leg and foot.

The **sural nerve** supplies impulses to the skin on the outer side and back of the foot and leg.

The **dorsal** (DOOR-sal) **nerve** supplies impulses to the skin on top of the foot (Figure 6–16).

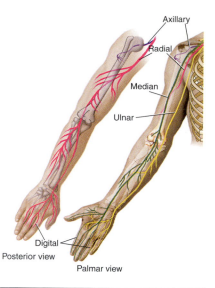

Figure 6–15 Nerves of the arm and hand

◆◆◆ THE CIRCULATORY SYSTEM

The **circulatory** (SUR-kyoo-lah-tohr-ee), or **vascular** (VAS-kyoo-lahr) **system** is vital to the maintenance of good health. It controls the steady circulation of the blood through the body by means of the heart and the blood vessels (the arteries, veins, and capillaries).

The **blood-vascular system** consists of the heart and blood vessels and circulates the blood. The **lymph** (LIMF)**-vascular** or **lymphatic** (lim-FAT-ik) **system** consists of lymph glands and vessels through which a slightly yellow fluid, called lymph, circulates. These two systems are intimately linked with each other. Lymph is derived from the blood and flows gradually back into the bloodstream.

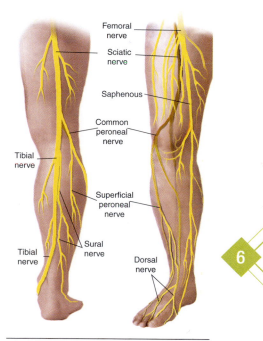

Figure 6–16 Nerves of the lower leg and foot

The Heart

The heart is a muscular, cone-shaped organ about the size of a closed fist. It is located in the chest cavity, and is enclosed in a membrane, the

pericardium (per-i-KAHR-dee-um). It is an efficient pump that keeps the blood moving within the circulatory system. At the normal resting rate, the heart beats about 72–80 times a minute. The **vagus** (VAY-gus) (tenth cranial nerve) and nerves from the autonomic nervous system regulate the heartbeat (Figure 6–17).

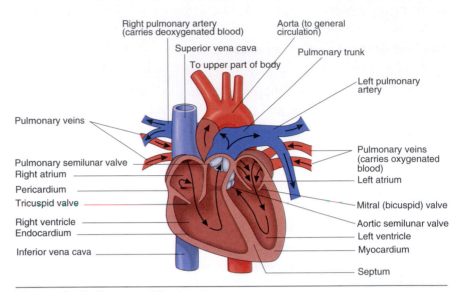

Figure 6–17 Diagram of the heart

The interior of the heart contains four chambers. The upper, thin-walled chambers are the **right atrium** (AY-tree-um) and **left atrium**. The lower, thick-walled chambers are the **right ventricle** (VEN-tri-kel) and **left ventricle**. **Valves** allow the blood to flow in only one direction. With each contraction and relaxation of the heart, the blood flows in, travels from the **atria** (both right atrium and left atrium) to the ventricles, and is then driven out, to be distributed all over the body. Another name for the atrium is **auricle** (OR-ik-kel).

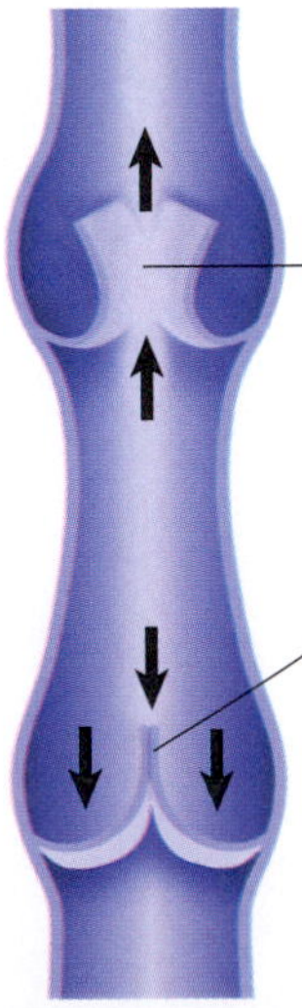

Blood Vessels

Blood vessels, which include arteries, capillaries, and veins, are tubelike in construction. They transport blood to and from the heart and to various tissues of the body.

Arteries are thick-walled muscular and elastic tubes that carry oxygen-filled blood from the heart to the capillaries throughout the body.

Capillaries are tiny, thin-walled blood vessels that connect the smaller arteries to the veins. Through their walls, the tissues receive nourishment and eliminate waste products.

Veins carry blood that lacks oxygen from the capillaries back to the heart. They are thin-walled blood vessels that are less elastic than arteries. They contain cuplike valves to prevent backflow. Veins are located closer to the outer surface of the body than arteries are (Figure 6–18).

Valve open to allow for venous blood flow

Valve closed to prevent venous back flow

Figure 6–18 Cross section of a vein

The Blood

Blood is a nutritive fluid that moves throughout the circulatory system. It is a red, salty fluid with a consistency similar to that of tomato juice. Blood has a normal temperature of 98.6°F (37°C), and it makes up about one-twentieth of the weight of the body. Approximately 8–10 pints of blood fill the blood vessels of an adult. Blood is bright red in color in the arteries, except for in the pulmonary artery, and dark red in the veins (except for in the pulmonary vein). This change in color is due to the exchange of carbon dioxide for oxygen as the blood passes through the lungs and the exchange of oxygen for carbon dioxide as the blood circulates throughout the body.

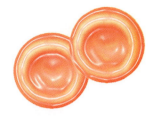

Figure 6-19 Red corpuscles

Circulation of the Blood

Blood is in constant circulation from the moment it leaves the heart until it returns. There are two systems that control this circulation.

The **pulmonary** (PUL-mo-ner-ee) **circulation** is the blood circulation that goes from the heart to the lungs to be purified.

The **systemic**, or **general**, **circulation** is the blood circulation from the heart throughout the body and back again to the heart.

Composition of the Blood

Blood is composed of red and white corpuscles, platelets, and plasma (Figures 6–19 and 6–20).

The function of **red corpuscles** (KOR-pus-els) (red blood cells), or **erythrocytes** (ih-RITH-ruh-syts) is to carry oxygen to the cells. **White corpuscles** (white blood cells), or **leucocytes** (LOO-ko-seyets), perform the function of destroying disease-causing germs.

Blood platelets (PLAY-tel-lets), or **thrombocytes** (throm-BOH-syts) are much smaller than the red blood cells. They play an important part in the clotting of the blood (Figure 6–21).

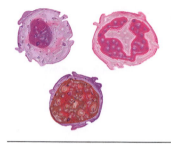

Figure 6-20 White corpuscles

Plasma is the fluid part of the blood, in which the red and white blood cells and blood platelets flow. It is straw-like in color and is about nine-tenths water. It carries food and secretions to the cells and carbon dioxide from the cells.

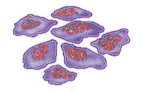

Figure 6-21 Platelets

Chief Functions of the Blood

The primary functions of the blood are described below.

1. carries water, oxygen, food, and secretions to all cells of the body

2. carries away carbon dioxide and waste products to be eliminated through the lungs, skin, kidneys, and large intestine

3. helps to equalize the body temperature, thus protecting the body from extreme heat and cold

4. aids in protecting the body from harmful bacteria and infections through the action of the white blood cells

5. clots, thereby closing tiny, injured blood vessels and preventing the loss of blood

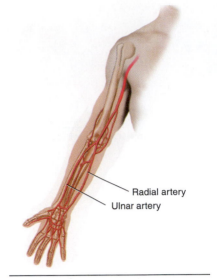

Figure 6-22 Arteries of the hand and arm

Blood Supply for the Arm and Hand

The **ulnar** (UL-ner) and **radial** (RAY-dee-ul) **arteries** are the main blood supply for the arm and hand.

The ulnar artery and its numerous branches supply the little-finger side of the arm and the palm of the hand. The radial artery and its branches supply the thumb side of the arm and the back of the hand.

The important veins are located almost parallel with the arteries and take the same names as the arteries. While the arteries are found deep in the tissues, the veins lie nearer to the surface of the arms, hands, legs, and feet (Figure 6–22).

Blood Supply to the Lower Leg and Foot

There are several major arteries that supply blood to the lower leg and foot. The **popliteal** (pop-lih-TEE-ul) **artery** divides into two separate arteries known as the **anterior tibial** (TIB-ee-al) and the **posterior tibial**. The anterior tibial goes to the foot and becomes the **dorsalis pedis** which supplies the foot with blood.

As in the arm and hand, the important veins of the lower leg and foot are almost parallel with the arteries and take the same names (Figure 6–23).

The Lymph-Vascular System

The **lymph-vascular system**, also called the **lymphatic system**, acts as an aid to the blood system, and consists of lymph spaces, lymph vessels, and lymph glands.

Lymph is a slightly yellow, watery fluid that is made from the plasma of blood. It is created when the plasma filters through the capillary walls into the tissue spaces. The tissue found in the tissue spaces bathes all cells and trades its nutritive materials to the cells in return for the waste products of metabolism. This fluid is absorbed into the lymphatics or lymph capillaries to become lymph and is then filtered and detoxified as it passes through the lymph nodes. It is eventually reintroduced into the blood circulation.

The following are the primary functions of lymph.

1. reaches parts of the body not reached by blood and carries on an interchange with the blood
2. carries nourishment from the blood to the body cells
3. acts as a bodily defense against invading bacteria and toxins
4. removes waste material from the body cells to the blood
5. provides a suitable fluid environment for the cells

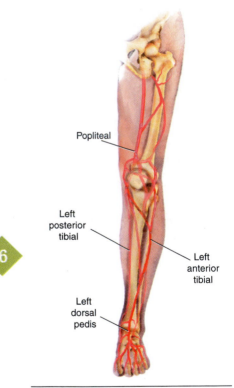

Figure 6-23 Arteries of the lower leg and foot

◆ ◆ ◆ THE ENDOCRINE SYSTEM

The **endocrine** (EN-doh-krin) **system** is made up of ductless glands that secrete substances into the bloodstream. A **gland** is a specialized organ that

6

secretes substances. Glands convert certain elements from the blood into new compounds that the body needs. The **endocrine glands** secrete **hormones**, chemicals that affect metabolism and other body processes, directly into the bloodstream. The endocrine system works with the nervous system to regulate and integrate the various organs and systems of the body. Examples of endocrine glands are the pituitary gland, thyroid gland, and ovaries.

THE EXCRETORY SYSTEM

The excretory (EK-skr-tohr-ee) system, including the kidneys, liver, skin, intestines, and lungs, purifies the body by eliminating waste matter. Metabolism of the cells of the body forms various toxic substances which, if retained, might poison the body.

Each of the following plays a part in the excretory system.

1. **Kidneys** excrete urine.
2. The **liver** discharges bile.
3. The **skin** eliminates perspiration.
4. The **large intestine** evacuates decomposed and undigested food.
5. The **lungs** exhale carbon dioxide.

THE RESPIRATORY SYSTEM

The respiratory system is situated within the chest cavity, which is protected on both sides by the ribs. The **diaphragm** is a muscular partition that controls breathing, and separates the chest from the **abdominal** region.

The **lungs** are spongy tissues composed of microscopic cells that take in air. These tiny air cells are enclosed in a skin-like tissue. Behind this, the fine capillaries of the vascular system are found.

When we breathe, an exchange of gases takes place. When we **inhale**, oxygen is absorbed into the blood. Carbon dioxide is expelled when we **exhale**. Oxygen is more essential than either food or water. Although a person may live more than 60 days without food, and a few days without water, if deprived of oxygen, he or she will die in a few minutes.

Breathing through your nose is healthier than breathing through your mouth because the air is warmed by the surface capillaries and the bacteria in the air are caught by the hairs that line the mucous membranes of the nasal passages.

Your rate of breathing depends on your level of activity. Muscular activities and energy expenditures increase the body's demands for oxygen. As a result, the rate of breathing is increased. You require about three times more oxygen when walking than when standing.

◆ ◆ ◆ THE DIGESTIVE SYSTEM

Digestion is the process of converting food into a form that can be used by the body. The **digestive system** changes food into soluble form, suitable for use by the cells of the body. Digestion begins in the mouth and is completed in the small intestine. From the mouth, the food passes down the **pharynx** (FAR-ingks) and **esophagus** (i-SOF-a-gus), or food pipe, and into the stomach. Food is completely digested in the stomach and small intestine and is assimilated or absorbed into the bloodstream. The large intestine (colon) stores the refuse for elimination through the rectum. The complete digestive process of food takes about nine hours.

   Enzymes are catalysts that are present in the digestive secretions and responsible for helping to speed up the chemical changes in food. **Digestive enzymes** are chemicals that assist in changing certain kinds of food into a form capable of being used by the body. Intense emotions, excitement, and fatigue seriously disturb digestion. On the other hand, happiness and relaxation promote good digestion.

6

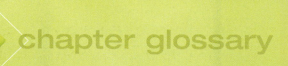

blood	The nutritive fluid that flows through the circulatory system to supply oxygen and nutrients to cells and tissues, and to remove carbon dioxide and waste from them.
blood-vascular system	The group of structures, including the heart, arteries, veins, and capillaries, that distribute blood throughout the body.
cells	Basic units of all living things; tiny masses of protoplasm capable of performing all the fundamental functions of life.
circulatory (vascular) system	The system that controls the steady circulation of blood through the body by means of the heart and blood vessels.
digestive system	Organs, including the mouth, stomach, intestines, salivary, and gastric glands, that change food into nutrients, for use by body cells, and wastes.
endocrine system	Group of specialized glands that affect the growth, development, sexual activity, and health of the entire body.
excretory system	Group of organs, including the kidneys, liver, skin, intestines, and lungs that purify the body by the elimination of waste.
integumentary system	Group of organs that make up the skin and its various accessory organs, such as oil and sweat glands, hair, and nails.
lymph	A slightly yellow, watery fluid that is made from the plasma of blood.
lymph-vascular (lymphatic) system	A bodily system, including the lymph vessels, lacteals, and lymph nodes, that allows lymph to flow through and circulate back into the bloodstream.
metabolism	The complex chemical process that takes place in living organisms whereby the cells are nourished and supplied with the energy needed to carry on their activities.
muscular system	The parts of the body that cover, shape, and support the skeletal system.
myology	The study of the structure, functions, and diseases of the muscles.
nerves	Long, white cords made up of masses of neurons and held together by connective tissue that carry messages to various parts of the body from the central nervous system.
nervous system	The bodily system that controls and coordinates the functions of all other systems of the body.
neurology	The branch of medicine that deals with the nervous system and its disorders.
neuron (nerve cell)	The basic structural unit of the nervous system, consisting of a cell body, dendrites, an axon, and an axon terminal. The neuron receives and sends messages to other neurons, glands, and muscles.
organs	Structures in the body, composed of specialized tissues, that perform specific functions.
osteology	The scientific study of bones, their structure, and function.
pulmonary circulation	Blood circulation from the heart to the lungs, to be purified, and back to the heart.

6

reflex	An automatic, involuntary response to a stimulus that involves the transmission of an impulse from a sensory receptor along an afferent nerve to the spinal cord, and a responsive impulse along an efferent neuron to a muscle, causing a reaction.
respiratory system	The system situated within the chest cavity, consisting of the nose, pharynx, larynx, trachea, bronchi, and lungs, that enables breathing.
skeletal system	The physical foundation or framework for the body
systemic (general) circulation	Blood circulation from the heart throughout the body and then back to the heart.
systems	Groups of bodily organs acting together to perform one or more functions, namely for the welfare of the entire body.
tissues	Collections of similar cells within the body, characterized by appearance, that perform particular functions.

1. How can an understanding of anatomy and physiology help you become a better nail technician?

2. What is the purpose of cells within the human body?

3. What is cell metabolism?

4. Name the five types of body tissue and explain the function of each.

5. What are the five most important organs of the body? Explain the function of each.

6. List the ten systems that make up the human body. What is the function of each system?

7. What are four ways in which muscles are stimulated?

8. What are four types of muscles that are affected by massage?

9. What are the three divisions of the nervous system? What is the function of each division?

10. What are the chief functions of the blood?

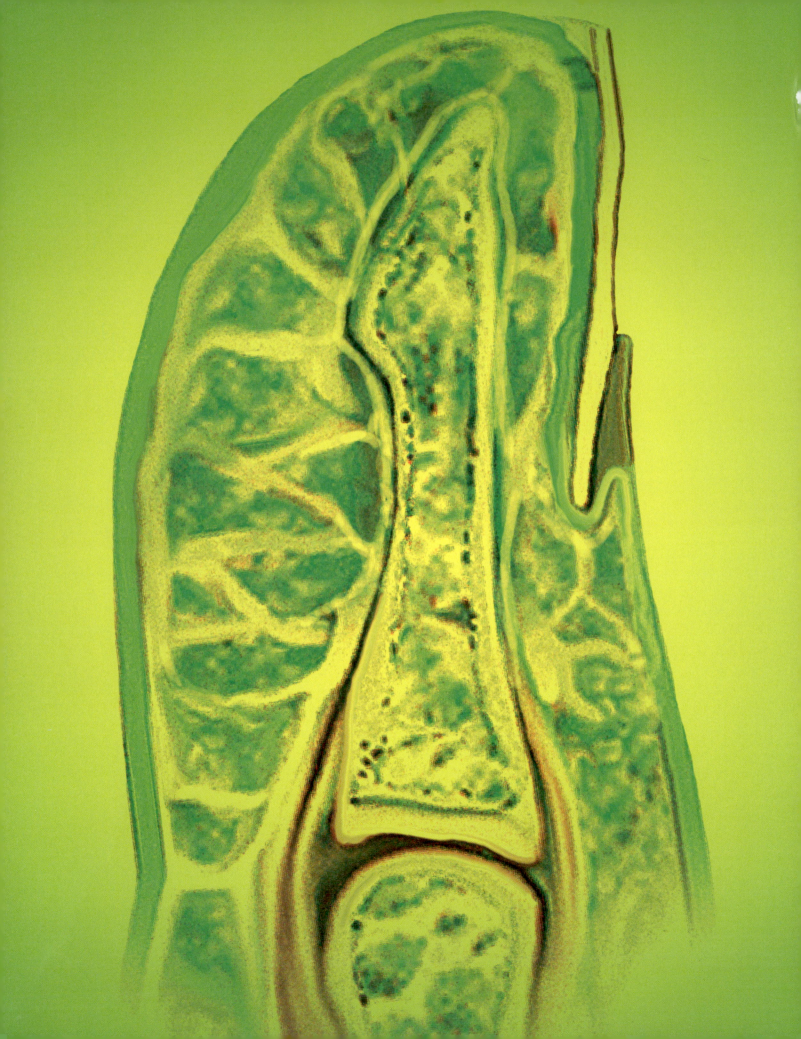

7

THE NAIL AND ITS DISORDERS

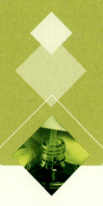

Author: Godfrey Mix, DPM

CHAPTER OUTLINE

Normal Nail Anatomy

Nail Disorders

Common Nail Disorders and Their Symptoms

Learning Objectives

After you have completed this chapter, you should be able to:

1. **Identify the basic parts of the nail unit.**

2. **Identify the part of the nail unit that produces the nail plate.**

3. **Define the term nail disorder.**

4. **Cite the golden rule for dealing with nail disorders.**

5. **Identify the term pterygium and describe how it relates to a nail disorder.**

6. **Determine if the terms cuticle and pterygium are interchangeable.**

7. **Determine why the nail technician should not aggressively push back or cut cuticles during a nail service.**

8. **Identify the nail disorders that can be serviced by a nail technician.**

9. **Identify the nail disorders that should not be serviced by a nail technician.**

Key Terms

Page number indicates where in the chapter the term is used.

bed epithelium
pg. 114

bruised nails
pg. 118

cuticle (eponychium)
pg. 114

discolored nails
pg. 118

eggshell nails
pg. 119

eponychium (cuticle)
pg. 114

furrows (corrugations)
pg. 119

hangnails (agnails)
pg. 119

hyponychium
pg. 114

infection
pg. 117

inflammation
pg. 117

keratin
pg. 113

leukonychia
pg. 119

lunula
pg. 114

matrix bed
pg. 114

melanonychia
pg. 119

mold (fungus)
pg. 123

nail bed
pg. 114

nail disorder
pg. 116

nail folds
pg. 115

nail plate
pg. 114

onychatrophia (atrophy)
pg. 119

onychauxis (hypertrophy)
pg. 120

onychia
pg. 123

onychocryptosis (ingrown nails)
pg. 121

onychodermal band (solehorn)
pg. 114

onychogryphosis (ram's horn nail)
pg. 121

onycholysis
pg. 125

onychomadesis
pg. 125

onychomycosis (tinea unguium)
pg. 124

onychophagy
pg. 121

onychophosis
pg. 121

onychophyma
pg. 121

onychoptosis
pg. 125

onychorrhexis
pg. 121

onychosis (onychopathy)
pg. 122

onyx
pg. 113

paronychia
pg. 126

plicatured nail
pg. 120

pterygium
pg. 122

pyogenic granuloma
pg. 126

specialized ligaments
pg. 115

tile-shaped nails
pg. 120

trumpet (pincer) nail
pg. 120

The technical term for nail is **onyx** (ON-iks). Nails are a part of the skin, or integumentary system, and are made of the same protein, **keratin** (KER-a-tin), as skin and hair. Nails are composed of the hardest keratin; hair is made of a hard keratin, but not as hard as the keratin in nails; and skin is made of soft keratin. To give clients professional and responsible service and care, you need to learn about the structure and function of the nails. You must know when it is safe to work on a client and when they need to see a dermatologist (a medical doctor who is a skin specialist) or a podiatrist (a foot specialist). Nails are an interesting and surprising part of the human body. They are small mirrors of the general health of the body. Healthy nails are smooth, shiny, and translucent pink. Systemic problems in the body can show in the nails as nail disorders or poor nail growth.

The normal nail has several different functions. In humans and primates it is adapted to enhance the use of the fingers for handling small objects. It is also used for scratching and grooming purposes, as well as having a protective function for the tips of the fingers and toes. In humans alone, nails are used to produce esthetic, as well as cosmetic, functions. You will become aware of the many manipulations and modifications that may be applied to the nails to enhance their beauty or appearance. The normal growth rate of fingernails is 0.1mm per day or approximately 3mm per month. Toenails grow at about one half to one third that rate. To completely replace a fingernail it takes about six months, while to replace a toenail it takes between 12 to 18 months. The growth rate of nails varies with age, gender, disease states, and temperature. Between ages 10 to 14 the growth rate peaks and gradually decreases with the aging process. Men's nails generally grow faster than women's. Certain diseases, such as psoriasis, causes the growth rate to increase. Other disease states such as arteriosclerosis, severe infections, high fevers, and paralysis or inactivity all decrease the growth rate of the nail. Cold temperatures decrease the growth rate while warm temperatures increase it. These are generalities and there are variations between individuals. In general, under normal conditions, members of the same family will have similar growth rates of their nails, indicating that we may inherit a factor which determines how fast our nails will grow.

It is important to remember that the nail plate is only the visible structure of a complex group of microscopic structures that actually produce the plate. Too many times when a deformity or abnormality of the plate is observed we fail to look to those deeper structures for answers to a particular problem. By caring for the visible abnormality it is mistakenly thought that the condition will be corrected. You, as a nail technician, must always understand this and look under the surface of the nail plate for the source of the abnormal condition of the nail. The cause or origin of the problem then, in most instances, will be easily understood or identified. You will then be better equipped to recommend those services, products, or referrals to other nail specialists that will benefit your client. For these reasons it is imperative for the nail technician to understand the anatomy and growth patterns of the normal nail.

◆ ◆ ◆ NORMAL NAIL ANATOMY

The normal *nail unit* is composed of six basic parts: **matrix** (MAY-triks) **bed**, **nail plate**, **cuticular** (KYOO-ti-u-lar) **system** consisting of the **cuticle** (KOOti-kel), the **eponychium** (ep-o-NIK-ee-um), and the **hyponychium** (heye-poh-NIK-ee-um), **nail bed**, **specialized ligaments**, and **nail folds** (Figures 7–1 and 7–2). The nail unit is the same in both fingernails and toenails.

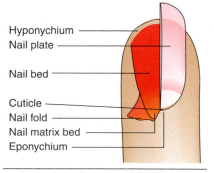

Hyponychium
Nail plate
Nail bed
Cuticle
Nail fold
Nail matrix bed
Eponychium

Figure 7–1 Diagram of the nail

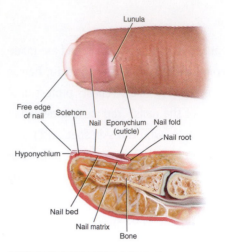

Figure 7-2 Cross section of the nail

1. The **matrix bed** is composed of matrix cells that produce the nail plate. It extends from under the proximal nail groove, where it can be seen as a whitish, moon-shaped area under the nail plate. This visible portion of the matrix bed is called the **lunula**.

2. The **nail plate**, formed by the matrix cells, is the most visible and functional part if the nail module. The free edge is the end of the nail plate that extends beyond the fingertip.

3. **The Cuticular System.** The proximal nail fold is the fold of skin at the **base** or proximal portion of the nail. The top of this fold appears to be normal skin. This skin then folds back under itself, onto the surface of the nail, extending proximally to where the matrix bed begins nail formation. The skin on the under surface of the proximal nail fold adheres to the top of the nail plate and as the nail plate is formed extends out onto the nail as a thin, translucent band of the stratum corneum of the skin's epidermal layer. This is called the **cuticle** or **eponychium**. The "true cuticle," which is living tissue, extends under the proximal nail fold and back to the point where nail plate originates at the base, or proximal portion, of the matrix bed. The "true cuticle," by its strong attachment to the nail, acts to seal the area against foreign material and microorganisms, thus helping to prevent injury and infection. For this reason the nail technician should not be too aggressive in removing cuticle during a pedicure or manicure service. The counterpart to the proximal nail fold and eponychium is the **hyponychium** that is found at the distal, or free, edge of the nail. The hyponychium lies under the nail plate where the free edge of the nail attaches to the underlying tissues. It seals the nail's free edge to the normal skin, thus preventing external moisture, bacteria, or fungi from getting under the nail. The nail technician should be careful here also not to break this seal when removing dead cuticle from under the free edge of the nail plate.

4. The **nail bed** lies under the nail plate and on top of the distal phalanx (the end of the finger or toe). Because it is richly supplied with blood vessels, it is observed under the nail plate as a reddish area extending from the lunula to the area just before the free edge of the nail. The nail is attached to the nail bed by a thin layer of tissue called the **bed epithelium** (ep-ih-THEE-lee-um) which originates at the junction of the matrix bed and the nail bed.

At the distal end of the nail bed the bed epithelium meets the hyponychium, where it becomes cornified and thicker. Here it forms a grayish band that is called the **onychodermal** (ahn-ih-koh-DERM-ul) **band** or **solehorn** of the nail. The onychodermal band is a combination build up of bed epithelium and hyponychial tissue. It plays a major role in attaching the nail plate to the underlying tissues. It serves a similar function as the "true cuticle" of the proximal nail fold helping to seal the free edge of the nail to the skin. (Remember, the free edge of the nail plate begins immediately beyond the onychodermal band and hyponychium.)

5. **Specialized ligaments** anchor the nail bed and matrix bed to the underlying bone. These ligaments are located at the proximal aspect of the matrix bed and around the edges of the nail bed, corresponding to the areas under the nail grooves.

6. **Nail folds** are those folds of normal skin that surround the nail plate. These folds of skin form the nail grooves and also serve a minor role in determining the shape of the nail plate.

The nail plate originates at the matrix bed. The shape and thickness of the nail is determined by the shape and length of the matrix bed, as well as how fast it produces nail plate. The matrix bed can be roughly divided into thirds. These are the proximal matrix bed, the intermediate or middle matrix bed, and the distal matrix bed. The nail plate grows from the proximal matrix, the central area of the matrix, as well as from the distal aspect of the matrix. The distal aspect of the matrix is generally seen as that area where the lunula stops and nail bed begins. The length of the matrix bed in an individual will determine his or her normal nail thickness (approximately 0.5mm in women and 0.6mm in men). This is because more matrix, or nail, will be formed in a longer matrix bed making a thicker nail plate than a nail that would be produced by a short matrix bed.

The cells at the base or proximal part of the matrix bed form the top of the plate, while those produced at the distal matrix bed form the bottom of the plate. The intermediate matrix bed forms the middle portion of the nail plate. The nail plate, therefore, is a multi-layered structure. It has been shown that the matrix cells at the base of the matrix bed form nail plate faster than those at the distal part of the bed. Thus the underlying, or deep, layers of the nail plate move forward on the nail bed at a slower rate than the surface layers of the nail. As long as the rate of nail plate production remains constant the nail will have a normal thickness. When abnormal conditions in the matrix occur because of infections, disease, or injury, the shape or thickness of the nail plate will change (Figure 7–3).

The nail plate, as previously discussed, is attached to the nail bed by a layer of tissue called the *bed epithelium*. The bed epithelium originates at the junction of the matrix bed and the nail bed. By attaching the nail plate to the nail bed it forces the plate to grow toward the end of the digit instead of growing straight up, off the matrix bed. The bed epithelium is tightly attached to the nail plate and loosely attached to the nail bed. The top of the nail bed has microscopic grooves extending from the distal end of the matrix bed (lunula) to the solehorn, or onychodermal band. The bed epithelium has ridges that correspond to the grooves in the nail bed. As the nail plate grows the bed epithelium glides over the nail bed rather than the nail moving over the bed epithelium. It is thought that the grooves and ridges function to keep the nail plate growing along a straight path from the matrix bed to its free edge. They also make a larger surface area for the bed epithelium to attach to the nail bed (Figure 7–4).

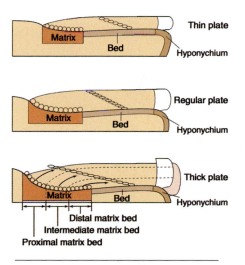

Figure 7–3 The length of the matrix bed determines the thickness of the nail plate. Notice that the cells of the proximal matrix end up on top of the plate while those of the distal matrix are on the bottom and the intermediate matrix cells are in the middle.

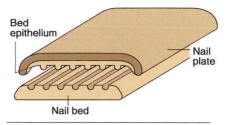

Figure 7–4 The bed epithelium is tightly attached to the nail plate. Notice the grooves in the nail bed which correspond to the ridges in the bed epithelium.

The free edge begins where the nail plate passes over the onychodermal band. Remnants of the bed epithelium and the onychodermal band remain attached to the under surface of the nail as a cuticle or part of the hyponychium.

Chemical Content of the Nail

What is the normal nail plate actually composed of? This is a much-studied topic with little universal agreement. Scientific literature seems to agree that the calcium content of nails is over rated. It is present but does not function to make the nail plate stronger or harder. In all probability its presence is not necessary for a healthy nail plate. Other inorganic elements also found in the nail plate include magnesium, sodium, potassium, iron, copper, zinc, sulfur, and nitrogen. Sulfur and nitrogen are usually found as chemical parts of organic compounds (amino acids) found in the nail. Many other amino acids are also present, and combine to form the main compounds of the nail plate that are fibrous proteins called keratin. Keratin is also found in hair and skin.

The nail is quite porous and water will pass through it much easier than through normal skin. The water content of the nail is related to the relative humidity of the surrounding environment. Nails, though they seem to be a dry, hard plate, have between 10 percent and 30 percent water content. The water content of the nail is directly related to its flexibility. The lower the water content in the nail, the more brittle it becomes. The application of nail enamel or an ointment-based nail conditioner on the nail plate will reduce the loss of water from the nail.

◆ ◆ ▶ NAIL DISORDERS

A **nail disorder** is a condition caused by injury to the nail or disease or imbalance in the body. Most, if not all, of your clients have had some type of common nail disorder and may have one when they are scheduled for a manicure. As a nail technician, you learn to recognize the symptoms of nail disorders so you can make a responsible decision about whether you should perform a service on your client.

You may be able to help your clients with nail disorders in one of two ways. You can tell clients that they may have a disorder and refer them to a physician. In other cases you can cosmetically improve a nail disorder and improve the overall beauty of your clients' nails.

It is your responsibility to know when it is safe to work on your clients' nails. You must learn to recognize the symptoms of nail disorders that cannot be worked on. In addition, you must know when to treat nails with extra care and when you can perform a service to cosmetically improve a disorder. Use the golden rule to make a responsible decision about the health of your clients' nails.

The **golden rule** is that, if the nail or skin to be worked on is infected, inflamed, broken, or swollen, a nail technician should not service the client. Instead refer the client to a doctor. An **inflammation** (in-flam-MAY-shun) is red and sore. An **infection** (in-FEK-shun) will have evidence of pus. Inflammation and infection are not the same thing, although they often occur at the same time. **Broken** skin or nail tissue is a cut or tear that exposes deeper layers of these structures. **Raised** or **swollen** skin will appear as fatter than normal skin and rise above the normal level.

To understand nail disorders, toenails or fingernails, it is necessary to understand what constitutes a normal nail. The exact cause of a particular disorder, in many cases, cannot be determined; however, in most instances the probable or possible cause may be. By understanding the previous section of this chapter with regard to how the nail plate is formed and grows from the matrix bed to its free edge, you are now better able to understand why particular nail disorders may be occurring.

Nail plate disorders can be roughly classified into four individual problem areas.

1. problems that affect the matrix bed

2. problems that affect the nail bed and bed epithelium

3. problems affecting the eponychium and hyponychium

4. problems that affect the structures surrounding the nail plate, such as the nail folds or the underlying bone

The previous section of this chapter discussed how each of these nail parts is related to the nail plate itself. The appearance of the nail plate will give an idea about which structures within the nail module are contributing to a particular disorder.

❖ **Matrix bed problems** are generally associated with nail thickness as well as some surface irregularities of the plate. As we have already learned, the proximal matrix bed cells form the surface of the nail plate, the middle portion of the matrix bed forms the middle layers of the nail, while the distal portion of the matrix forms the bottom layers of the nail plate. Therefore, if a disorder of the plate is on the surface it can generally be determined that there is a problem in the proximal matrix bed. A disorder affecting only the intermediate matrix bed will cause distortions within the nail plate such as the small white spots (leuconychia) often seen under the surface of the nail plate. If the entire plate is overly thick, the disorder is affecting the whole matrix bed. This is also true for an abnormally thin nail plate. Grooves or ridges across the nails, from one side to the other, are rate-of-growth disturbances within the entire matrix bed. These are called *Beau's Lines* and may be seen in all of the nail plates after severe illness, high fevers, or massive injuries such as those seen in automobile accidents. If only a single nail plate is involved, the cause is generally a local injury to the nail such as trauma or infection.

❖ **Nail bed disorders** are generally the cause of the nail being loosened (detached) from the onycholysis (on-i-KOL-I-sis), which is the underlying tissue. A build up of debris and callus under the plate is also generally a nail bed problem. Distortional or misalignment abnormalities of the nail plate, in most instances, can be traced to bed epithelium injuries or disorders. Bed epithelial problems may also cause onycholysis.

❖ **Eponychial** and **hyponychial disorders** are associated with pterygium (te-RIJ-ee-um) (abnormal adherence of the skin to the nail plate) formation. Some surface disorders on the nail plate or under the free edge are also associated with eponychial and hyponychial problems.

❖ **Injuries** or **chronic infections of the nail folds** may affect the shape and texture of the nail plate. Problems affecting the shape of the underlying bone, such as those associated with rheumatoid arthritis, will also affect the shape of the nail plate.

Fingernails and toenails have the same basic elements that form the nail plate. Because we walk on our feet the forces exerted through the toes, and thus through the toenails, are tremendous. These forces magnify any disorders of the toenails as compared to a similar disorder in the fingernails. Foot gear adds extra stress and creates a warm, moist environment that complicates, as well as creates, many nail disorders not seen in the hands. When looking at the toenails of a client always keep these facts in mind when trying to decide what may be causing or contributing to a nail disorder that you are observing.

The list below contains the names of nail disorders and a short description of each. The list contains the names of some nail disorders that nail technicians can work on if there is not evidence of infection, inflammation, broken tissue, or swelling. The list also suggests services you might perform and contains descriptions of nail disorders that are too serious for a nail technician to work on and that must be referred to a physician.

◆ ◆ COMMON NAIL DISORDERS AND THEIR SYMPTOMS

There are many nail conditions that will not be affected by providing nail services, as long as the nail technician takes proper safety precautions and does nothing to contribute to the condition. Following are examples of nail disorders that can generally be serviced by nail technicians.

Bruised nails are a condition in which a clot of blood forms under the nail plate. The clot is caused by injury to the matrix bed or nail bed. It can vary in color from maroon to black. In some cases, a bruised nail will fall off during the healing process. Applying artificial nail services to a bruised nail is not recommended (Figure 7–5).

Discolored nails are a condition in which the nails turn a variety of colors including yellow, blue, blue-grey, green, red, and purple. Discoloration can be caused by poor blood circulation, a heart condition, or topical or oral medications. It may also indicate the presence of a systemic disorder. Artificial tips, wraps, or an application of colored nail polish can hide this condition.

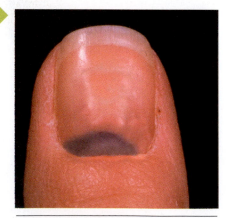

Figure 7–5 Bruised nail

Eggshell nails are thin, white, and curved over the free edge. The condition is caused by improper diet, internal disease, medication, or nervous disorders. Be very careful when manicuring these nails because they are fragile and can break easily. Use the fine side of an emery board to file gently and do not use pressure with a metal pusher at the base of the nail (Figure 7–6).

Furrows, also known as corrugations, are long ridges that run either lengthwise or across the nail. Some lengthwise ridges are normal in adult nails, and they increase with age. Lengthwise ridges can also be caused by conditions such as psoriasis, poor circulation, and frostbite. Ridges or grooves that run across the nail can be caused by conditions such as injury or a high fever, pregnancy, measles in childhood, and a zinc deficiency in the body. If ridges are not deep and the nail is not broken, you can correct the appearance of this disorder. Since these nails are exceedingly fragile, great care must be exercised when giving a manicure. Avoid the use of the metal pusher; use a cotton-tipped orange-wood stick around the cuticle. Carefully buff the nails with a fine grit buffer to remove or shorten the ridges. The remaining ridges can be filled with ridge filler and covered with colored polish to give a smooth, healthy look to the nail (Figure 7–7).

Hangnails, also known as agnails, is a common condition in which the cuticle around the nail splits. Hangnails are caused by dry cuticles or cuticles that have been cut too close to the nail. This disorder can be improved by softening the cuticles with oil and trimming the hangnail with nippers. Though this is a simple and common disorder, hangnails can become infected if not serviced properly (Figure 7–8).

Leukonychia (loo-ko-NIK-ee-ah) is a condition in which white spots appear on the nails. It is caused by air bubbles, a bruise, or other injury to the nail. Leukonychia cannot be corrected, but it will grow out (Figure 7–9).

Melanonychia (mel-ah-no-NIK-e-ah) may be seen as a black band under or within the nail plate, extending from the proximal nail fold to the free edge. In some cases it may affect the entire nail plate. This condition is caused by a localized area of increased **melanocytes** (pigment cells) usually within the proximal matrix bed. As matrix cells form nail plate, melanin is laid down within the plate by the melanocytes. As the plate grows toward the free edge a dark band of melanin becomes visible. This condition is present in all dark-skinned races. Nearly 100 percent of Afro-Americans over the age of 50 exhibit this condition. This condition is seen in approximately 12 to 25 percent of the Japanese. In Caucasians melanonychia is extremely rare. If seen, a malignant melanoma must be suspected, and melononychia medically ruled out as the cause. Nail services can be given to clients who have melanonychia (Figure 7–10).

Onychatrophia (on-i-kah-TROH-fee-ah), also known as **atrophy**, describes the wasting away of the nail. The nail loses its shine, shrinks, and falls off. Onychatrophia can be caused by injury to the nail matrix or by internal disease. Handle this condition with extreme care. File the nail with the fine side of the emery board and do not use a metal pusher or strong soaps or washing powders. If the condition is caused by internal disease and the disease is cured, new nails may grow back.

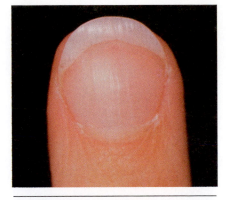

Figure 7–6 Eggshell nail

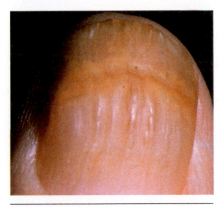

Figure 7–7 Furrows or corrugations

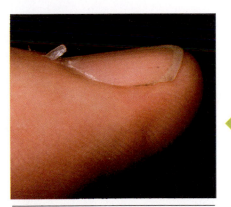

Figure 7–8 Hangnail

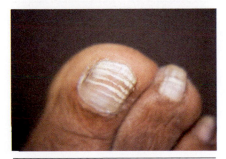

Figure 7–9 Leukonychia

7

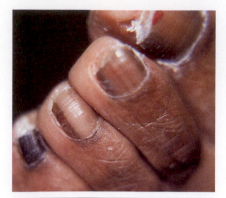

Figure 7–10 Melanonychia

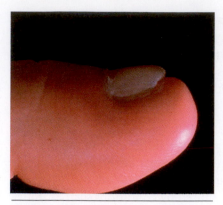

Figure 7–11 Onychauxis – side

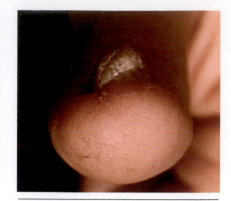

Figure 7–12 Onychauxis – end view

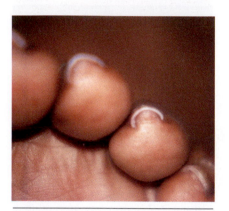

Figure 7–13 Tile-shaped nails

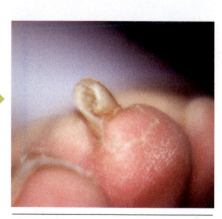

Figure 7–14 Trumpet nails

Onychauxis (on-i-KAWK-sis) or **hypertrophy** (hy-PER-troh-fee) shows the opposite symptoms of onychatrophia. Onychauxis is the overgrowth of nails. Nails with this disorder have abnormally thick hypertrophy or thickening of the nail plate. The condition is usually caused by internal imbalance, local infection, injury, or heredity. File the nail smooth and buff it with pumice powder (Figures 7–11 and 7–12).

Tile-shaped nails have an increased transverse curvature throughout the nail plate. The curve is caused by an increased curvature of the matrix bed. The borders of the nail are parallel with each other. This nail condition usually will not cause discomfort to the individual. Nail services can be given to a client with tile-shaped nails (Figure 7–13).

Trumpet or **pincer nail** deformities begin as a normal nail configuration in the matrix area. As the nail grows toward the end of the digit the edges of the plate begin to curl inward. When the nail reaches the end of the digit, depending on the severity of the deformity, it may curl completely in on itself and appear as a trumpet or cone formation. The underlying nail bed and distal skin are constricted within this curl and may become painful. This condition is seen more often on toes than on fingers. Causes of this deformity may be a bone spur on the top of the underlying bone; however, the most likely cause is an inherited disorder. On rare occasions, improperly fit shoes may produce the deformity. In most instances, the nail technician can carefully trim the margins of the nail to make the client comfortable. If the nail plate is adherent to the underlying tissues along the margins, this client must be sent to the physician or podiatrist (Figure 7–14).

Plicatured (plik-a-CHOOR-ed) **nail** deformity figuratively means folded nail. The surface of the nail is generally flat, while one or both of the edges of the plate are folded at a 90° or more angle down into the soft tissue nail margins. This deformity, like the tile-shaped deformity, also originates with a "folded" matrix bed, causing the plate to be formed in the plicatured fashion, and is more common in the toes than in fingers. This condition is most often seen as the cause of ingrown nails. It may result from an injury that deforms the matrix bed or it can be inherited. Shoe pressure over a period of time may result in a remolding and folding of the matrix bed in this manner. The nail technician can carefully round the corners of a plicatured nail (Figure 7–15).

Onychocryptosis (on-i-koh-krip-TOH-sis) or **ingrown nails** is a familiar condition of the fingers and toes in which the nail grows into the sides of the tissue around the nail. This disorder is the result of the matrix bed being folded or involuted deep into the soft tissues. Plicatured nails and some tile-shaped nails are most commonly associated with this problem. The mechanical forces of walking press the soft tissues against the nail margin, adding to the problem in toenails. As the nail grows toward its free edge it encounters a soft tissue wall at the end of the deepened nail groove. At this point it continues growing toward the end of the toe or finger, penetrating the soft tissue and creating a "portal of entry" for bacteria. This results in an acute infection (paronychia) usually caused by *Staphylococcus*. The distal end of the digit becomes red, acutely painful, and a small abscess or pus pocket forms. If the infection persists for any length of time a reddish hamburger-like mass of tissue forms along the edge of the nail. This is called granulation tissue, which forms as the result of the body's attempt to heal the infected area. Relief from this condition is obtained *only* by trimming away the offending nail margin and draining the abscess. The nail technician must not work on an infected ingrown nail. Refer the client to a physician or podiatrist. If the tissue around the nail is not infected or if the nail is not too deeply imbedded in the flesh, you can trim the corner of the nail in a curved shape to relieve the pressure on the nail groove (Figure 7–16).

Onychophagy (on-i-KOH-fa-jee) is the medical term for nails that have been bitten enough to become deformed. This condition can be improved greatly by professional manicuring techniques. Give frequent manicures, using the techniques described in the manicuring chapters of this book. As those chapters suggest, any of the artificial tips and wraps can hide and beautify deformed nails (Figure 7–17).

Onychophosis (on-ih-KOH-foh-sis) refers to a growth of horny epithelium in the nail bed.

Onychophyma (on-ih-koh-FEE-mah), more commonly referred to as onychauxis, denotes a swelling of the nail.

Onychorrhexis (on-i-kohr-REK-sis) refers to split or brittle nails that also have a series of lengthwise ridges. It can be caused by injury to the fingers, excessive use of cuticle solvents, nail polish removers, and careless, rough filing. Nail services can be performed only if the nail is not split below the free edge. This condition may be corrected by softening the nails with a reconditioning treatment and discontinuing the use of harsh soaps, polish removers, or improper filing (Figure 7–18).

Onychogryphosis (on-i-kho-greye-PHO-sis) is also called **ram's horn nail**. This disorder is usually the result of injury to the matrix bed. It may also be hereditary and can occur as the result of long-term neglect of nails. It is most commonly seen in the great toe but may be seen in other toes,

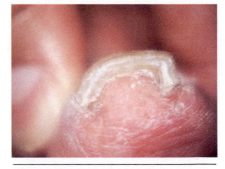

Figure 7–15 Plicatured nail

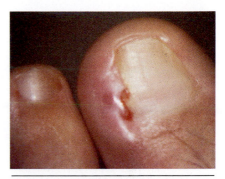

Figure 7–16 Onychocryptosis

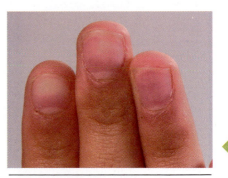

Figure 7–17 Bitten nails

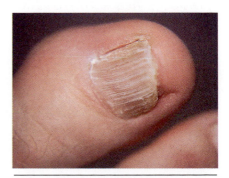

Figure 7–18 Onychorrhexis

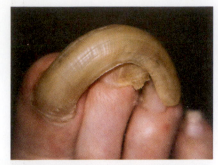

Figure 7–19 Onychogryphosis (1)

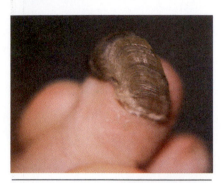

Figure 7–20 Onychogryphosis (2)

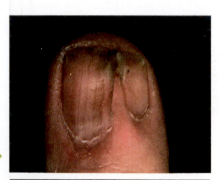

Figure 7–21 Pterygium

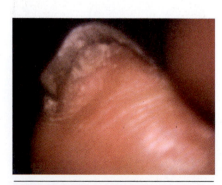

Figure 7–22 Ventral pterygium

as well as in fingernails. The nail usually has many transverse grooves and ridges, is brownish in color, and one side of the nail grows faster than the other, curving the nail plate and giving it the typical ram's horn configuration. This results in a thick, curved, hard-to-cut nail that remains untrimmed, adding to the severity of the disorder. There is no treatment for this disorder other than keeping the nail trimmed back and thinned. In the absence of an infection this may be carefully done by the nail technician with proper nail nippers and a file. Each of the grooves is a weak area of the nail plate. Trim the nail across the plate at a groove taking only small bites. The nail will break off through the groove when it has been trimmed about half way across (Figures 7–19 and 7–20).

Onychosis (on-ih-KOH-sis), also called onychopathy (on-ee-KOP-ah-thee), is a technical term applied to nail disease.

Pterygium (te-RIJ-ee-um) is defined in the medical dictionary as "a wing-like structure." The words "cuticle" and "pterygium" are not interchangeable. The term "pterygium" relates to the nail when there is an abnormal scarring of the proximal nail fold (eponychium) or the distal nail fold (hyponychium). *Dorsal pterygium* occurs on the top of the plate when the skin of the eponychium and the true cuticle abnormally attach to the nail plate. As the nail grows the proximal nail fold is stretched over the nail, forming the wing-like extension of skin. In severe cases, the cuticle may adhere to the matrix, stopping plate formation in that area that results in a split in the nail. If the process continues, the entire matrix bed can adhere to the cuticle, causing the loss of the nail plate (Figure 7–21).

The opposite of dorsal pterygium is *ventral pterygium.* This process involves the free edge of the nail. The hyponychium remains adherent to the underlying portion of the plate. In this disorder the distal nail groove is eliminated, and the hyponychium will appear thickened because of this. Ventral pterygium is common in toenails. When trimming nails, (fingernails or toenails) the underside of the free edge should be visualized and if a ventral pterygium is present care must be taken not to trim it off along with the nail (Figure 7–22).

The most common causes of dorsal pterygium are lichen planus (a skin disease) and trauma. Underlying bone diseases, such as those seen in rheumatoid arthritis, may also cause the formation of a dorsal pterygium. Ventral pterygium is most often associated with Raynaud's disease, as seen with scleroderma, and also arteriosclerosis. Dorsal or ventral pterygium associated with disease processes, generally affects more than one nail. Traumatic pterygium formation generally involves only the injured nail. There are also congenital forms of dorsal and ventral pterygium.

The nail technician cannot treat pterygium by pushing the extension of skin back with an instrument. To do so will cause more injury to the tissues and make the condition worse. Gentle massage, with cuticle creams and conditioners, into the affected area by the nail technician and the client may be beneficial; however, once the disorder has occurred it is most usually not reversible.

7

BUSINESS TIP

The Power of Diversity

Just as a successful hairstylist must offer a spectrum of hair services to be successful, so must a nail professional. Although many technicians may rely on only one system — natural, acrylic, fiberglass, or gel wraps — it's important to learn as many systems as possible. This way you'll be covered if someone develops an allergy or a client insists on a specific type of service. For help, visit nail trade shows, read nail magazines and enroll regularly in continuing education classes. Avoid the mind set of believing any technique is too difficult or that your business is going so well, you don't need to learn more.

There are also many nail conditions that should not be serviced by a nail technician. In some of the following examples, the client should be referred to a doctor before the nail technician performs any services.

Mold (fungus) is an infection of the nail usually caused when moisture seeps between an artificial nail and the free edge of the nail, but can also affect a natural nail. Mold starts with a yellow-green color and darkens to black. Many clinicians believe that the small green areas often seen under nail enhancements are not mold (fungus), but a limited growth of a bacteria called *Pseudomonas aeruginosa*. This bacteria is found in soil and water and often contaminates open wounds. If an enhancement is hit straight on or is not applied properly, small air pockets are created between the nail plate and the enhancement. *Pseudomonas* bacteria will infiltrate these areas as the client gets her hands wet or works in a garden. The waste products from the bacterial growth are then seen as the green patches in these pockets under the enhancement.

If the mold or bacteria is between the artificial nail and nail plate the nail technician must remove the enhancement. The nail plate should, at that time, be sanitized. It then must be disinfected with a disinfectant made for use on the natural nail. Do not reapply another enhancement for at least one week or until there are no visible signs of a mold or bacteria being present. If the discoloration persists or if it is under the nail plate the client should be referred to a physician for treatment. By maintaining proper sanitizing *and* disinfecting procedures of instruments and equipment, the nail technician will not pass the infection to other clients (Figure 7–23).

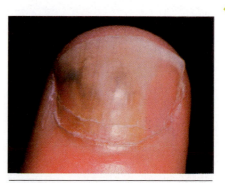

Figure 7–23 Mold

Onychia (on-NIK-ee-ah) is an inflammation of the entire nail unit or a portion of the unit. The tissues may be red and swollen; pus may or may not be present. Any opening of the skin or the seals of the eponychium or hyponychium to the nail plate will allow entry of bacteria, fungi, or foreign materials, which may result in an onychia of the nail unit. For this reason, the nail technician must be careful not to cause an abrasion or opening in the tissues around the nail plate while performing a nail service. If an onychia is present prior to the service, the nail technician should not perform a nail service. Refer the client to a dermatologist or podiatrist for treatment.

Onychomycosis (oni-koh-meye-KOH-sis), **tinea unguium** (TIN-ee-ah UN-gwee-um), of the nails, is an infectious disease caused by a fungus (vegetable parasite). There are over 100,000 species of fungi. Less than 50 cause infections in humans. Fungi are quite opportunistic in that they take advantage of any deficiency of the organism they infect. Fungi are everywhere in the environment. In theory they may be transmitted from one person to another; however, in practicality, and with the practice of proper sanitation and disinfection procedures, the risk of doing so is minimal. The nail technician should always be aware of this when performing nail services for clients.

Fungal infections of the nails usually occur because of some weakness in the nail unit. Injuries, even minor ones, which produce a portal of entry for the fungi, are taken advantage of. Multiple micro injuries or a single severe injury to the nail unit can create an unhealthy nail that is less resistant to disease and will allow access for fungi to infect the area. For this reason the cuticles should not be aggressively reduced when providing a nail service. Any small injuries to the eponychium or hyponychium that break the seal between these structures and the nail plate create openings for a fungus to enter the nail unit. If the individual is debilitated from a disease such as diabetes or arteriosclerosis the nail unit will not be as healthy as it should be and fungi will have an easy time invading it. Prolonged illnesses of any type will have the same affect on the nail unit. Localized disease processes, such as psoriasis and or chronic infections of the nail unit, also allow a fungi to begin growing within the nail unit.

Toenails are much more susceptible to fungal infections than are fingernails. Small injuries from shoes over a period of time produce an unhealthy nail unit. Add to this the warm, moist, dark environment within the shoe and perfect conditions are created for the growth of fungus. Few individuals over the age of 65 do not have some evidence of nail fungus. The nail technician should not cut the cuticles around toenails, because this is the easiest way to create an injury, which will lead to a fungal nail infection. Also, be extremely careful when removing the dead cuticle on the top or under the free edge of the nail plate so that no break in the seal is created between the nail plate and the eponychium or hyponychium.

Fungus infects the nail unit in many different ways. One form is often seen as whitish patches that may be scraped from the surface of the nail (Figure 7–24). This is called *Leukonychia Mycotica* (loo-ko-NIK-e-ah mi-KOT-i-ca).

Other species of fungus infect the nail bed, matrix bed, or tissues surrounding the nail unit. They are seen in many colors depending on the individual species of fungi. The most common is yellow but black, brown,

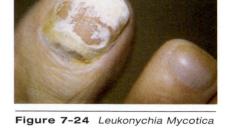

Figure 7-24 *Leukonychia Mycotica*

orange, or green forms are also seen. The infection usually starts along the nail margin or under the hyponychium at the free edge of the nail.

Onycholysis (on-i-KOL-i-sis) is a condition in which the nail loosens from the nail bed, beginning usually at the free edge and continuing to the lunula, but does not come off. It is caused by an internal disorder, trauma, infection, or certain drug treatments. It can also be caused by an allergic reaction to certain nail products. An infection may be the only sign of this disorder in its early stages. Onycholysis can occur on the nails of the hands or feet. As the disorder progresses, color changes are seen, the nail bed becomes thickened and as the infection progresses further, the nail plate becomes crumbly and malformed. The nail technician should refer the client to a dermatologist or podiatrist for an evaluation and treatment if the fungal infection becomes severe. As long as the fungal infection is not moist or draining, natural manicures and pedicures may be given to these clients when sanitation and disinfection practices are strictly adhered to within the salon (Figures 7–25 and 7–26).

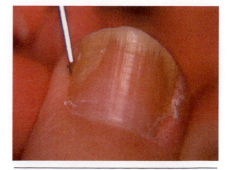
Figure 7-25 Onycholysis

Onychomadesis (on-i-ko-MAH-de-sis) is shedding of the nail plate. This nail disorder is characterized by a separation of the nail plate from the matrix bed. It can occur on fingernails and toenails. In most cases the cause can be traced to a localized infection, minor injuries to the matrix bed, or a severe systemic illness. Some chemotherapy or x-ray treatments for cancer may also cause this condition. Localized causes involve individual nails, while in systemic problems all the nails are usually involved. This disorder occurs when the matrix bed stops producing nail plate for a period of at least one to two weeks. When the matrix bed stops producing nail plate for only a short period of time, Beau's lines occur, so a groove is formed rather than the complete separation of the plate from the matrix as seen in this disorder. In cases of onychomadesis, when the causative factors are removed a new nail plate will form (Figure 7–27).

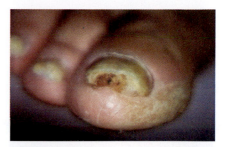
Figure 7-26 Fungal infection

The nail technician may cause this condition by aggressively pushing back the cuticle or by the improper use of the drill during manicures or fills. Care must always be taken not to injure or break the natural seal between the nail plate and the "true cuticle" that may result in an infection. Excessive heat caused by the drill bit can cause a thermal injury to the matrix bed, and as a result, this disorder may occur. If onychomadesis is present the nail technician should not apply enhancements to the nail. If there is no active infection present a natural manicure or a pedicure service may be given. Do not apply polish over the defect in the plate as this will seal in any infective organisms that may be present, thus enhancing the possibility of further infection and injury to the matrix. Care must be taken to avoid further injury to the nail unit during these services.

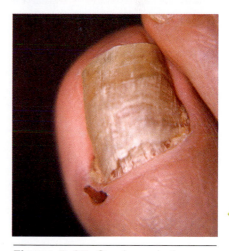
Figure 7-27 Onychomadesis

Onychoptosis (on-i-kop-TOH-sis) is a condition in which part or all of the nail sheds periodically and falls off the finger and can affect one or more nails. It can occur during or after certain diseases of the body, such as syphilis, as a result of a fever and system upsets, as a reaction to prescription drugs, or as a result of trauma.

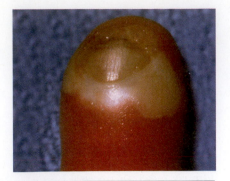

Figure 7-28 Paronychia runaround

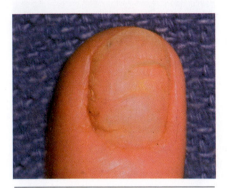

Figure 7-29 Chronic paronychia

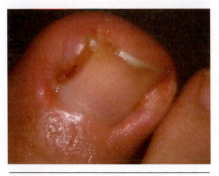

Figure 7-30 Chronic paronychia—toe nail

Paronychia (par-oh-NIK-ee-ah) is an infection of the tissue around the nail. It is most commonly caused by bacteria (*streptococcus* or *staphylococcus*) or fungi, including yeast. These organisms enter the tissues around or under the nail through an opening (portal of entry) in the skin. Refer to onychia. The symptoms are redness, swelling, and tenderness of the tissue surrounding the nail. Pus is usually present (Figure 7–28).

Paronychia can occur at the base of the nail, around the entire nail plate, or on the fingertip. Paronychia around the entire nail is sometimes referred to as runaround. Chronic paronychia occurs continually over a long period of time and may cause damage to the nail plate.

Chronic paronychia is most often caused by a yeast infection (candida) of the soft tissues around the nail (Figure 7–29). Individuals who work with their hands in water (dishwashers, bartenders) or must wash their hands continually (health care workers, food processors) are prone to this type of infection. Toenails, because of perspiration and footgear, quite often will exhibit chronic paronychia infections caused by yeast (Figure 7–30).

Nail technicians should never aggressively push or cut the cuticles of their clients. This is the easiest way to create an opening for bacteria or fungi to invade the tissues around the nail and cause a paronychia. Do not cut the cuticles around toenails and only gently remove the dead cuticle from the top of the toenail in order not to break the normal seal between the nail plate and the true cuticle. There are products available that will safely remove and soften excess cuticle formations.

Proper sanitation and disinfection of all instruments is important in helping to prevent infections, should the nail technician accidentally cause an opening through the skin. These procedures also help to stop cross-contamination of infections from one client to another. If a client has a paronychia, chronic or acute, the nail technician must not give a nail service to that client. Refer them to a dermatologist or podiatrist for treatment.

Pyogenic granuloma is a severe inflammation of the nail in which a lump of red tissue grows up from the nail bed to the nail plate. It is an overgrowth of vascular tissue most commonly caused by injury or infection (Figure 7–31).

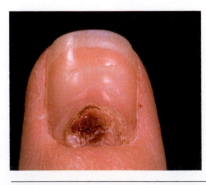 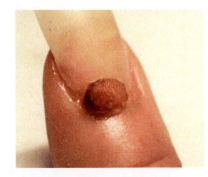

Figure 7-31 Pyogenic granuloma

bed epithelium	The thin layer of tissue that attaches the nail to the nail bed.
bruised nails	A condition in which a clot of blood forms under the nail plate, usually due to an injury, characterized by a dark maroon or black spot.
cuticle (eponychium)	The crescent of toughened skin, around the base of the fingernails and toenails, that partially overlaps the lunula.
discolored nails	A condition in which the nails turn a variety of colors, including yellow, blue, blue-grey, green, red, and purple. Discoloration can be caused by poor blood circulation, a heart condition, or topical or oral medications.
eggshell nails	A condition, caused by improper diet, internal disease, medication, or nervous disorders, in which the nails become thin, white, and curved over the free edge.
eponychium (cuticle)	The crescent of toughened skin, around the base of the fingernails and toenails, that partially overlaps the lunula.
furrows (corrugations)	Long ridges that run either lengthwise or across the nail that create ridges or grooves in the nail. Furrows are caused by psoriasis, poor circulation, and frostbite.
hangnails (agnails)	A common condition, caused by dry cuticles or cuticles that have been cut too close to the nail, in which the cuticle around the nail splits.
hyponychium	The toughened skin that lies underneath the distal edge of the nail, where it seals the nail's free edge to the normal skin.
infection	The result of germs or disease-causing bacteria entering the body, characterized by pus.
inflammation	A condition responding to body injury, irritation, or infection, characterized by redness, heat, pain, and swelling.
keratin	The principal fiber protein found in hair and nails.
leukonychia	A condition, caused by air bubbles, a bruise, or other injury to the nail, in which white spots appear on the nail.
lunula	The white, half-moon-shaped area of the matrix bed, found at the root of the nail.
matrix bed	The part of the nail extending from under the proximal nail groove, where it can be seen as a white, moon-shaped area under the nail plate.
melanonychia	A condition, present in all dark-skinned races and extremely rare in caucasians, in which a black band of pigment cells grows from the proximal matrix bed toward the free edge of the nail.
mold (fungus)	A growth that starts with a yellowish-green color and darkens to black. It is usually caused by moisture that has seeped under the edge of an artificial nail, but can also affect a natural nail.
nail bed	The portion of skin on which the body of the nail rests.
nail disorder	Any condition of the nail caused by injury to the nail or disease or imbalance in the body.
nail folds	Folds of normal skin that surround the nail plate, forming grooves and a wall to help determine the shape of the nail plate.
nail plate	Formed by the matrix cells, it is the visible and functional body of the nail module.
onychatrophia (atrophy)	A condition, caused by injury to the nail matrix or by internal disease, in which the nail wastes away, loses its shine, shrinks, and falls off.
onychauxis (hypertrophy)	A condition, caused by internal imbalance, local infection, injury, or heredity, is the abnormal overgrowth of nails and thickening of the nail plate.

7

onychia	An inflammation of the entire nail unit or a portion of the nail, characterized by red and swollen tissue, and possibly pus. The condition is usually caused by the entry of bacteria, fungi, or foreign materials through an opening in the skin.
onychocryptosis (ingrown nails)	A common disorder in which the nail grows into the sides of the tissue around the nail. It can be a result of the matrix bed being folded or involuted deep into the soft tissues, penetrating the tissue, and creating a portal of entry for bacteria.
onychodermal band (solehorn)	A combination build up of bed epithelium and hyponychial tissue found at the distal end of the nail. The grayish band of tissue helps attach the nail plate to the underlying tissues.
onychogryphosis (ram's horn nail)	This disorder is characterized by a brownish, thick, hard-to-cut nail plate that is curved into the shape of a ram's horn because one side of the nail grew faster than the other. This condition is the result of an injury to the matrix bed, long-term neglect of the nails, or can be inherited.
onycholysis	A condition in which the nail loosens from the nail bed, usually beginning at the free edge and continuing to the lunula, but does not come off. It can be caused by an internal disorder, trauma, infection, certain drug treatments, or an allergic reaction to certain nail products.
onychomadesis	A condition, characterized by a shedding of the nail plate from the matrix bed, that occurs when the matrix bed stops producing nail plate for one to two weeks. It is caused by a localized infection, minor injury to the matrix bed, severe systemic illness, and, in some cases, chemotherapy or x-ray treatments for cancer.
onychomycosis (tinea unguium)	An infectious disease of the nails caused by a fungus.
onychophagy	Medical term for nails that have been bitten enough to become deformed.
onychophosis	Growth of horny epithelium in the nail bed.
onychophyma	Swelling of the nail.
onychoptosis	A condition in which part or all of the nail sheds periodically and falls off the finger. It can be caused by syphilis, high fever, system upsets, a reaction to prescription drugs, or trauma.
onychorrhexis	A condition, caused by injury to the fingers; excessive use of cuticle solvents and nail polish removers; or careless, rough filing, in which split or brittle nails have a series of lengthwise ridges.
onychosis (onychopathy)	The technical term applied to nail disease.
onyx	The technical term for nail of the fingers or toes.
paronychia	An infection of the tissue around the nail. Characteristics include redness, swelling, and tenderness of that tissue. In the later stages of this condition, the nail bed will thicken and discolor, and the nail plate will become crumbly and malformed.
plicatured nail	A deformity caused by an injury to the matrix bed or can be inherited in which the surface of the nail is flat, while the edge(s) of the plate are folded at a 90° or more angle. This condition is most often seen as the cause of ingrown nails.
pterygium	Forward growth of the cuticle, abnormally adhering the skin to the nail plate.
pyogenic granuloma	A severe inflammation of the nail in which a lump of red vascular tissue grows up from the nail bed to the nail plate. It is commonly caused by injury or infection.
specialized ligaments	Ligaments located at the proximal portion of the matrix bed and around the edges of the nail bed that anchor the matrix and the nail bed to the underlying bone.

7

tile-shaped nails	A condition, caused by abnormal curvature of the matrix bed, in which there is an increased transverse curvature throughout the nail plate.
trumpet (pincer) nail	A condition, seen more often on toes than on fingers, caused by a bone spur on the top of the underlying bone or has been inherited. As the nail grows toward the end of the toe or finger, the edges of the nail plate curl inward, eventually forming the shape of a trumpet or cone.

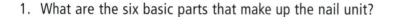

review questions

1. What are the six basic parts that make up the nail unit?

2. What is the only part of the nail unit that produces the nail plate?

3. Define nail disorder.

4. What is the golden rule for dealing with nail disorders?

5. What does the term "pterygium" mean as it relates to a nail disorder?

6. Are the terms "cuticle" and "pterygium" interchangeable?

7. Why should the nail technician not aggressively push back or cut cuticles during a nail service?

8. List five nail disorders that can be serviced by a nail technician.

9. List five nail disorders that cannot be serviced by a nail technician.

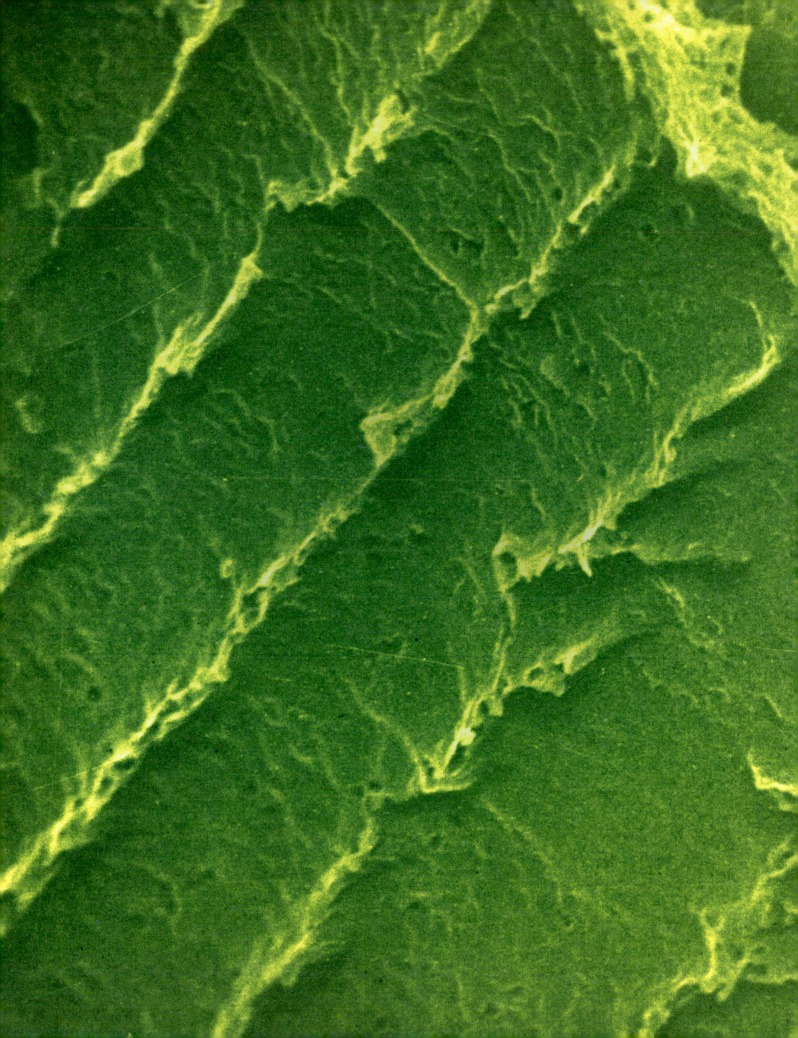

8

THE SKIN AND ITS DISORDERS

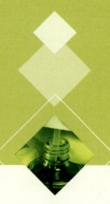

Author: Godfrey Mix, DPM

CHAPTER OUTLINE

Healthy Skin

Skin Disorders

Pigmentation of the Skin

Learning Objectives

After you have completed this chapter, you should be able to:

1 Describe the characteristics of healthy skin.

2 List the functions of the skin.

3 Describe the epidermis and dermis.

4 Explain how the skin is nourished.

5 Describe the function of sweat glands.

6 Define lesion.

7 Describe the characteristics of eczema and psoriasis.

Key Terms

Page number indicates where in the chapter the term is used.

adipose
pg. 136

albinism
pg. 145

arrector pili muscles
pg. 136

Basal layer
pg. 135
pg. 145

bulla
pg. 138

calluses (Tyloma)
pg. 141

chloasma
pg. 145

crust
pg. 138

cyst
pg. 138

dermatology
pg. 133

dermis
pg. 136

eczema
pg. 140

elasticity
pg. 133

elastic tissue
pg. 138

epidermis (cuticle)
pg. 134

excoriation
pg. 139

fissure
pg. 139

friction blisters
pg. 141

fungi
pg. 143

herpes simplex
pg. 145

hypodermis (fatty layer)
pg. 136

keratinization
pg. 135

lentigines (freckles)
pg. 145

leucoderma
pg. 145

macule
pg. 139

melanin
pg. 135

melanoma
pg. 144

molds
pg. 143

motor nerves
pg. 136

nerve
pg. 136

objective symptoms
pg. 138

papillae
pg. 136

papillary layer
pg. 136

papule
pg. 139

pigmented nevus (mole)
pg. 144

psoriasis
pg. 140

pustule
pg. 139

reticular layer
pg. 136

scales
pg. 139

scar
pg. 139

sebaceous glands (oil glands)
pg. 137

secretory nerves
pg. 137

sensory nerves
pg. 136

stain
pg. 139

stratum corneum (horny layer)
pg. 135

stratum granulosum
pg. 135

stratum lucidum
pg. 135

subcutaneous tissue
pg. 136

subjective symptoms
pg. 138

sudoriferous glands (sweat glands)
pg. 137

tactile corpuscles
pg. 136

tan
pg. 145

tubercule
pg. 140

tumor
pg. 140

ulcer
pg. 140

vesicle
pg. 140

vitiligo
pg. 145

warts (papilloma, verruca, and plantar wart)
pg. 142

wheals (hives)
pg. 140

yeasts
pg. 143

As a nail technician you must have a basic understanding of the skin and its disorders in order to serve your clients responsibly and professionally. You will have the opportunity to improve the appearance of the skin on the hands and feet and, therefore, to enhance your client's appearance. The finished nails will look their best when set off by beautiful, healthy skin. In addition, it is your responsibility to know when you cannot work on a client or must not use certain products on your client due to a skin condition. Knowledge of the skin will help you avoid the spread of infectious disease and aggravation of skin conditions or sensitivities. Before you can judge whether a particular service or product is appropriate for your client's skin, you must have a general understanding of what the skin is and how it functions. Because the nails are an appendage of the skin, problems with the skin can cause nail problems.

◆ ◆ HEALTHY SKIN

To be a nail technician, you must learn about **dermatology** (der-mah-TOL-o-jee), the study of healthy skin and skin disorders. Healthy skin is slightly moist and acid, soft, and flexible. Unless the skin is aged, healthy skin has **elasticity** that allows it to regain its shape immediately after being pulled away from the bone. Healthy skin is free of blemishes and disease and its texture is smooth and fine-grained. The skin on the human body varies in thickness. It is thinnest on the eyelids and thickest on the palms of the hands and soles of the feet. It is the largest organ system of the body, covering an area almost the size of a 10' x 12' rug.

Function of the Skin

The skin performs eight jobs for the body. They include protection, the prevention of fluid loss, response to external stimuli, heat regulation, secretion, excretion, absorption, and respiration.

1. **Protection.** The skin covers every part of the body acting as a physical barrier protecting it from injury and invasion by bacteria.

2. **Prevention of fluid loss.** The skin seals blood and other bodily fluids inside the body.

3. **Response to external stimuli.** The skin contains nerve endings that respond to stimuli from outside the body, such as heat, cold, touch, pressure, and pain. This sensitivity helps the body find the most comfortable environment while acting as a protection against injury from these stimuli.

4. **Heat regulation.** The skin keeps the body's internal temperature at 98.6 degrees Fahrenheit (37 degrees Celsius). When the temperature outside the body changes, the blood and sweat glands of the skin heat or cool the body to maintain its temperature.

5. **Secretion.** The oil (sebaceous) glands secrete **sebum**, a fatty, oily substance that maintains the skin's moisture level by slowing the evaporation of moisture from the skin and preventing excess water from penetrating the skin.

6. **Excretion.** The sweat (sudoriferous) glands excrete salt and other waste chemicals from the body through the pores of the skin (perspiration).

7. **Absorption.** The skin absorbs small amounts of chemicals, drugs, and cosmetics through the pores.

8. **Respiration.** The skin breathes through the pores. Oxygen is absorbed and carbon dioxide is discharged.

◆ ◆ STRUCTURE OF THE SKIN

The skin has three layers or parts. The outer layer is called the epidermis; the deep layer under the epidermis is called the dermis. The deepest layer is the hypodermis, or subcutaneous layer (Figures 8–1 and 8–2).

Epidermis

The **epidermis** (ep-i-DUR-mis), also called the **cuticle**, is the outermost protective covering of the skin. It contains no blood vessels, but contains many small nerve endings. The epidermis is made of the following four layers.

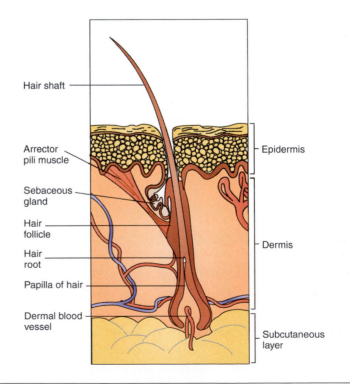

Hair shaft
Arrector pili muscle
Sebaceous gland
Hair follicle
Hair root
Papilla of hair
Dermal blood vessel
Epidermis
Dermis
Subcutaneous layer

Figure 8–1 A microscopic section of the skin

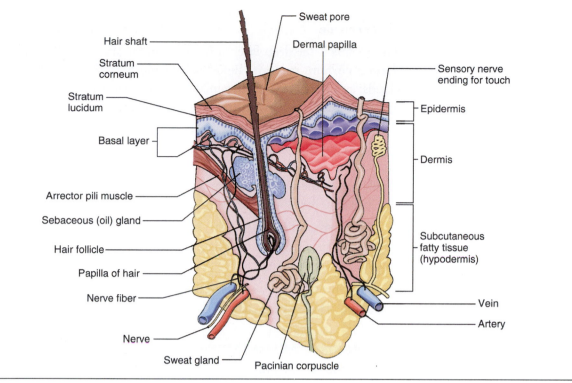

Figure 8-2 Diagram of the skin

The **stratum corneum** (STRAT-um KOHR-nee-um), also called the **horny layer**, which consists of tightly packed, scalelike cells that are continually shed and replaced. This layer is composed of dead epithelial cells that have become horney or keratinized.

The **stratum lucidum** (STRAT-um LOO-si-dum) is a small layer of clear cells. It is most prominent on the palms of the hands and soles of the feet.

The **stratum granulosum** (STRAT-um gran-yoo-LOH-sum) consists of cells that look like granules. This layer is where the process of keratinization is most active. (**Keratinization** describes the microscopically visible changes, as well as the biochemical changes, that occur within the cells of the skin as they progress upward from the stratum germinativum to the stratum corneum.)

The **Basal layer**, formerly known as the *stratum germinativum* (STRAT-um jur-mi-nah-TIV-um), is composed of several layers of differently shaped cells. The deepest layer is responsible for supplying new cells to make up for the ones that are continually worn away. From this layer, all other cells of the epidermis arise. It also contains a dark skin pigment, called **melanin** (MEL-a-nin), which determines skin color and protects the sensitive cells below from the destructive effects of excessive ultraviolet rays from the sun or an ultraviolet lamp.

The Dermis

The **dermis** is the deep layer of the skin and is also called the "true skin," **derma**, **corium**, or **cutis**. Blood vessels and lymph vessels, nerves, sweat glands, and oil glands are contained in this layer in an elastic network made up of collagen. The dermis contains three separate layers.

The **papillary** (PA-pil-ah-ry) **layer** lies directly under the epidermis and contains the **papillae** (pa-PIL-e), little cone-like projections that extend upward into the epidermis. Some of the papillae contain looped capillaries, and small blood vessels; others contain nerve endings, called tactile corpuscles. This layer also contains some of the melanin pigment.

The **reticular** (re-TIK-u-lar) **layer** contains fat cells, blood and lymph vessels, sweat and oil glands, hair follicles, and the arrector pili muscles attached to the hair follicles.

The **hypodermis**, also called the **subcutis** or **fatty layer**, is the deepest skin layer. This layer is characterized by closely packed fat cells.

The **subcutaneous** (sub-kyoo-TAY-nee-us) **tissue** is made up of fatty tissue known as **adipose** (AD-i-pohs). This tissue gives smoothness and shape to the body, contains stored fat to be burned for energy, and acts as a protective cushion for the outer skin. It varies in thickness according to the age, sex, and general health of the individual.

Nourishment of the Skin

The skin is nourished by blood and lymph. See Chapter 6 for more information about blood and lymph. One-half to two-thirds of the total blood supply of the body is distributed to the skin. Blood and lymph supply essential nourishment for growth and repair of skin, hair, and nails. The subcutaneous layer of the skin contains arteries and lymphatic vessels that send small branches to provide nourishment to hair papillae, hair follicles, and skin glands. The skin also contains numerous capillaries.

Nerves of the Skin

A **nerve** is made of cordlike fibers and sends messages from body organs to the central nervous system, which consists of the brain and spinal cord. The skin contains the surface endings of many nerve fibers.

These nerve endings are called **tactile corpuscles** (TAK-til KOR-puh-sils) and they perform the following functions.

Motor nerves cause the blood vessels to constrict or expand and the **arrector pili** (a-REK-tohr PIGH-ligh) **muscles** that are attached to the hair follicles to contract. These muscles can cause goose bumps.

Sensory nerves, which are found in the papillary layer of the dermis, give the skin a sense of touch. They allow you to react to heat, cold, touch, pressure, and pain. Sensory nerve endings are most abundant in the fingertips and on the soles of the feet. Complex sensations, such as vibrations, seem to depend on the sensitivity of a combination of these nerve endings (Figure 8–3).

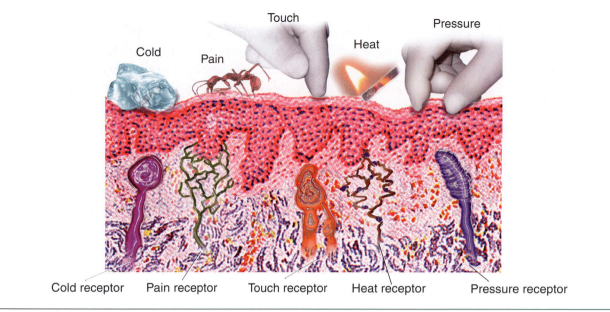

Cold Pain Touch Heat Pressure

Cold receptor   Pain receptor   Touch receptor   Heat receptor   Pressure receptor

Figure 8-3 Sensory nerves of the skin

Secretory (se-KREET-e-ree) **nerves** are the nerves of the sweat and oil glands. They cause the glands to secrete their products (sweat or sebum).

Glands of the Skin

The skin contains two types of duct glands that extract materials from the blood and turn them into different substances. These new substances are secreted for use by the body or excreted from the body.

The **sudoriferous** (su-dohr-IF-er-us) **glands**, or **sweat glands**, regulate body temperature and eliminate waste products through perspiration. Though the nervous system controls the excretion of sweat, activity is greatly increased by heat, exercise, emotions, and certain drugs. One to two pints of liquids containing salts are normally eliminated daily through the sweat pores in the skin (Figure 8–4).

Sweat glands consist of a coiled base, called a **fundus** (FUN-dus) and a tubelike duct that ends at the skin surface to form a **sweat pore**. A sweat pore is a small opening in the skin surface from which the sweat gland eliminates waste. Most parts of the body have sweat glands. The palms of the hands, soles of the feet, forehead, and armpits have the greatest number of sweat glands.

The **sebaceous** (si-BAY-shus) or **oil glands** secrete an oily substance, called sebum, as you learned earlier in this chapter. Sebum lubricates the skin and softens the hair. All parts of the body, except the palms of the hands and soles of the feet, have oil glands. The oil glands consist of little sacs with ducts that open into the other follicles. When the oil gland produces sebum in the sac, it flows through the oil duct into the hair follicle. If the sebum hardens and the duct becomes clogged, a blackhead, or comedone, forms. Cleansing skin regularly will prevent the oil ducts from clogging (Figure 8–5).

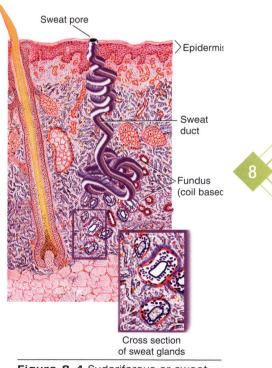

Sweat pore
Epidermis
Sweat duct
Fundus (coil based)
Cross section of sweat glands

Figure 8-4 Sudoriferous or sweat glands

8

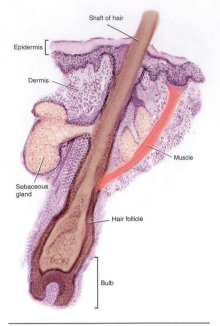

Figure 8–5 Sebaceous or oil glands

Elasticity of the Skin

The **elastic tissue** composed primarily of elastin which is similiar to collagen, is found in the papillary layer of the dermis. It gives the skin the ability to return to its original shape after it has been stretched. As a person ages, the papillary tissue begins to lose its elastic nature. The skin begins to sag or wrinkle because it no longer can return to its original shape.

◆ ◆ SKIN DISORDERS

As a nail technician, you need to learn about skin disorders to decide when it is safe and appropriate to work on a client. Your goal is to prevent the spread of an infectious disease and to avoid worsening a condition your client already has. You will observe the skin of a client during the consultation and use your special knowledge to make an informed decision about servicing your client. While only a medical doctor is qualified to make a diagnosis, you should learn to recognize the symptoms that indicate a disorder is present. It is difficult to recognize some skin disorders in practice, so you must use the following "golden rule" when making your decision.

The **golden rule** of skin disorders is that if the area of skin to be worked on is infected, inflamed, broken, or raised, a nail technician should not service the client. The client should be referred to a dermatologist. Inflamed skin is red, sore, and swollen. **Inflamed skin** is not the same as infected skin. **Infected skin** will have evidence of pus. **Broken skin** occurs when the epidermis is cut or torn, exposing the deeper layers of skin. **Raised skin** is a symptom of a variety of skin conditions, some of which are lesions, and will be described next.

Lesions of the Skin

A **lesion** (LEE-zhun) is a structural change in tissue caused by injury and disease. There are two main types: primary and secondary. Primary lesions are the original lesions manifesting a disease. Secondary lesions are those that develop in the later stages of the disease. While studying the different skin lesions, remember that you will always use your "golden rule" to decide whether or not it is safe to work on your client. The symptoms or signs of diseases of the skin are divided into two groups:

1. **Subjective symptoms** are those that can be felt by the client, such as itching, burning, or pain.
2. **Objective symptoms** are those that are visible to the nail technician, such as pimples, pustules, or inflammation (Figure 8–6).

A **bulla** (BYOO-lah) is a blister containing watery fluid.

A **crust** is an accumulation of serum and pus mixed with epidermal flakes. An example of crust is a scab on a sore.

A **cyst** (SIST) is a semisolid or fluid lump above and below the skin surface.

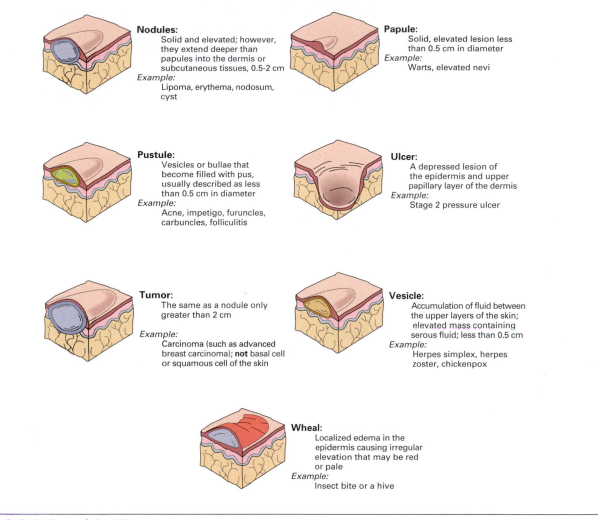

Nodules:
Solid and elevated; however, they extend deeper than papules into the dermis or subcutaneous tissues, 0.5-2 cm
Example:
Lipoma, erythema, nodosum, cyst

Papule:
Solid, elevated lesion less than 0.5 cm in diameter
Example:
Warts, elevated nevi

Pustule:
Vesicles or bullae that become filled with pus, usually described as less than 0.5 cm in diameter
Example:
Acne, impetigo, furuncles, carbuncles, folliculitis

Ulcer:
A depressed lesion of the epidermis and upper papillary layer of the dermis
Example:
Stage 2 pressure ulcer

Tumor:
The same as a nodule only greater than 2 cm
Example:
Carcinoma (such as advanced breast carcinoma); **not** basal cell or squamous cell of the skin

Vesicle:
Accumulation of fluid between the upper layers of the skin; elevated mass containing serous fluid; less than 0.5 cm
Example:
Herpes simplex, herpes zoster, chickenpox

Wheal:
Localized edema in the epidermis causing irregular elevation that may be red or pale
Example:
Insect bite or a hive

Figure 8-6 Lesions of the skin

Excoriation (ed-skohr-i-AY-shun) is a sore or abrasion caused by scratching or scraping off the superficial layer of the skin.

A **fissure** (FISH-ur) is a crack in the skin that penetrates the dermis. Chapped hands or lips are an example.

A **macule** (MAK-ul) is a small, discolored spot or patch on the surface of the skin. Some macules are safe and some are not.

A **papule** (PAP-yool) is a small elevation above the skin surface. It has a solid center that can be felt.

A **pustule** (PUS-chool) is a lump on the skin with an inflamed base and a head containing pus.

Scales are produced during the shedding of the epidermis. Severe dandruff is an example of scales.

A **scar** is a light-colored, slightly raised mark on the skin formed after an injury or lesion of the skin has healed.

A **stain** is an abnormal discoloration that remains after moles, freckles, or liver spots disappear, or after certain diseases.

8

A **tubercle** (Too-ber-kul) is a solid lump larger than a papule. It varies in size from a pea to a hickory nut.

A **tumor** is an abnormal cell mass that varies in size, shape, and color. Nodules are small tumors.

An **ulcer** (UL-ser) is an open lesion on the skin or mucous membrane of the body. Ulcers are accompanied by pus and loss of skin depth.

A **vesicle** (VES-i-kell) is a blister containing clear fluid. Poison ivy is an example of a condition that produces vesicles.

Wheals (HWEELS) or **hives** are swollen, itchy bumps on the skin that last for several hours. They are often caused by insect bites or by allergic reactions.

Inflammatory and Infectious Disorders of the Skin

There are several types of **inflammations** of the skin, also known as dermatitis. If inflammation, infection, or raised or broken skin is present, do not work on the inflamed area. Be very cautious when working on a client who suffers from these disorders because the skin is sensitive and the condition can be aggravated by the use of chemicals.

Eczema (EK-se-mah) is a generic term used to describe a chronic, long-lasting, inflammatory skin disorder of unknown cause (Figure 8–7). In the adult and in some juvenile stages it is characterized by itching, burning, and the formation of scales and oozing blisters. In the chronic, long-lasting stages it may even affect the nail plates, causing growth disturbances (Beaus Lines) and pitting on the surface of the nail. The nail technician should not give services to a client with this condition if any cracking, oozing, or open areas of skin are visible. Follow the "golden rule" for these clients.

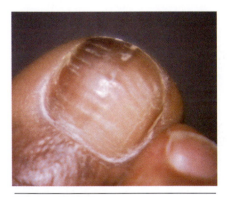
Figure 8-7 Eczema

8

Psoriasis (so-REYE-a-sis) is a generalized disease that produces mild to severe effects on the skin (Figure 8–8). The actual cause of psoriasis is unknown. In affected individuals, the time required for the basal cells to reach the epithelial layer of the skin (epidermal turnover time, keratinization) is extremely short. Normally it takes 28 to 30 days for this process, while in the psoriatic individual this time is reduced to 3 or 4 days. This extremely active turnover time of the skin cells produces the typical silvery, scaly plaques of skin seen with this disease. On removal of the scale the underlying skin will appear red and inflamed because of the dilated capillaries underlying the area. There may also be some pinpoint bleeding from the capillaries in the area after the scale is removed. Psoriasis can affect any area of the skin.

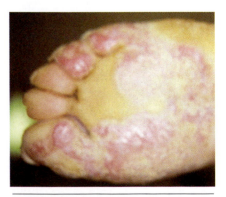
Figure 8-8 Psoriasis

There are many forms of psoriasis. Those seen most commonly are silvery plaque, like lesions on the elbows. **Pustular psoriasis** and **psoriatic keratoderma** of the sole of the foot may also affect the palm of the hand. **Interdigital psoriasis**, also known as white psoriasis (rare), **psoriasis of the nails** (to be discussed in another chapter), and **psoriatic arthritis** are also seen in the hands and feet. All of these forms may vary from mild to severe. The plaque form is the type generally seen on other areas of the body. The pustular form is first seen on the soles as small sterile blisters of pus that dry as dark brown crusts before peeling off. As this form progresses, the entire sole may be involved, with the skin between the blisters having the silvery, scaly appearance of psoriasis. In the keratoderma form, massive amounts of yellow or gray callus-like tissues are formed. Deep, painful fissures are generally present. This and the pustular forms may be so severe as to cause the individual great pain during walking. The interdigital or white form appears as white, macerated tissue in the web spaces between the toes. It is hard to distinguish this form from a fungal infection and a surgical biopsy of the tissue, in most cases, is the only way to arrive at a definitive diagnosis.

As a nail professional, you will see some forms of psoriasis during your career. It is recommended that you consult with the client's dermatologist or podiatrist before providing a service. The skin of a person with psoriasis is quite fragile and any injury, no matter how slight, may cause an extension of the psoriatic lesions.

Friction blisters are a localized reaction of the skin to friction from an external source. They are the most common reaction of the skin to injury and are classified as a bulla. They are really only seen in the human species. Friction blisters are filled with a straw-colored, tissue fluid. This fluid collects in the space created by the injury to the skin just below the stratum granulosum, or middle layer, of the skin. It is best not to break the blister but rather to let it heal itself. If the blister does break before it is healed, a topical antibiotic ointment and a dressing should be applied until it is healed. An open blister is easily infected and what may have been only a minor discomfort may become a major problem. All blisters should be treated with care. Services in the presence of friction blisters should not be provided. Provide foot services only after the blister is totally healed. If the blister is infected or appears too severe for the client to care for themselves, refer them to their physician.

Burns, chemical irritants, fungal infections, bacterial infections, and many other internal or external causes can also produce skin blisters. Some pressure sores start as a simple blister appearing on the skin. It is, therefore, important to be able to determine the cause of the blister in order to give it proper care. If there is the slightest suspicion that a blister you observe is anything other than a simple, non-infected friction blister, refer the client to their physician for care. Without treatment of the primary cause, the condition may become more severe.

Calluses (Tyloma) are caused by friction on the skin from an external force (Figure 8–9). They occur where excessive, intermittent friction and rubbing occur with any regularity. The callus usually is an enlarged area of irritated skin and its edges blend into the normal, surrounding skin. The classical friction callus is seen under the ball of the foot. Calluses are the result of long-term, abnormal stresses on the skin. This is in contrast

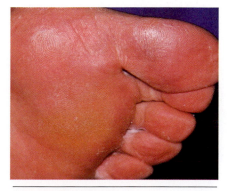

Figure 8-9 Callus

to blisters which form after short-term, excessive stress to the affected area of skin. The skin does not have time to produce the extra keratin to protect itself and, as a result, a blister forms instead of a callus.

The formation of callus is the skin's attempt to protect itself from excessive irritation or mechanical stresses. An abnormal gait pattern will result in extra shearing, or friction forces, being applied to the bottom of the foot. The intermittent force of this abnormal walking causes the basal cell layer of the skin to produce extra keratin. This results in the thickening of the skin in the irritated area. The yellow discoloration of the callus is due to the extra keratin within the tissue. The same mechanism causes calluses in other areas of the body. The nail technician can give services if a client has calluses. Soften and smooth calluses, but do not remove them.

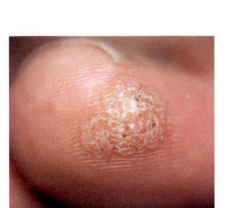

Figure 8-10 Wart

Common names for **warts** are **papilloma**, and **plantar wart verruca** Figure 8–10. Warts are viral infections of the skin caused by a specific human papillomavirus (HPV). The virus multiplies within the nuclei of the cells that produce the skin. They cause papillary growth structures, which are elongated nipple-like projections that are seen as the wart. A wart is one of the very few true tumors of the skin. It is not a cancer, but is the result of the body trying to protect itself from the virus by forming a growth, or barrier, around the virus. Incubation periods have ranged experimentally from one to twenty months. Viral particles invade the skin through direct introduction that may be caused by occupational injuries, friction, nail biting, and scratching. An open sore or cut that creates a portal of entry may be the opening through the skin that allows the virus to produce the infection.

Since only about 10 percent of the population ever has a wart, there is no rule stating that everyone exposed to the HPV virus will subsequently become infected. The long incubation periods and differences in resistance seen within individuals make it impossible for clear-cut epidemiological patterns to be determined. Warts are rare in children under 5 and in the elderly. They are seen most commonly in the age groups between 5 to 20 years with the peak incidence being from 12 to 15 years of age. Warts however may occur at any age. From these statistics it appears that we are born with immunity to the virus. About 10 percent lose the immunity, and as they become infected the immunity is regained. This may explain why warts spontaneously regress in 30 percent of the infected people in 3 to 6 months and in 50 percent of the cases within 24 months. It is believed that this is because the body redevelops the antibodies against HPV during the course of the infection. A few individuals never develop antibodies against the virus and these are the people who seem to have warts all their lives.

Warts may occur on any area of the body, but seem to be found more commonly on the hands and feet. On the palmar surface of the hands and the plantar surfaces of the feet they appear as flat or slightly elevated circular callused areas, which generally have small black dots or sliver-like areas within them. These black dots or sliver-like areas are really dried blood within a capillary that is located in the center of one of the wart's papillary structures. Warts on non-weight-bearing surfaces appear as small, elevated cauliflower-like lesions with black dots, or dried areas of blood, at the tips of the easily visible papillary structures that make up the wart. A wart on the weight-bearing surface of the foot, plantar aspect or sole, is harder to identify. This is because the pressure of walking on the wart flattens it slightly, but more importantly, the wart is a foreign growth to the bottom of the foot. The skin in the area of the wart tries to protect itself from this foreign body by building callus over and around the wart. This callus, the body's natural protection from added pressure or friction on the bottom of the foot, covers the wart. The callus makes the wart appear totally different from the cauliflower look of a wart on a non-weight-bearing area of the body. The callus may build up to such an extent that it totally hides the underlying wart.

As a nail professional you should not be afraid to provide a service to a client with a wart. The probability of the nail professional contracting the wart virus, based on statistics, is less than 10 percent. The probability is further reduced to near zero if the service does not cause the wart to bleed, and the nail professional does not have an open cut or sore on his or her hands. Using proper sanitation/disinfection procedures in the salon before and after client services also makes it nearly impossible for other clients to become infected after services have been provided to a client with a wart.

Fungal Infections of the Skin

As discussed in Chapter 7, there are more than 100,000 known species of **fungi** present in nature! Of this vast group of fungi only about 175 of these live on or in the human body. Of these 175, under normal conditions, approximately 20 will cause systemic disease to develop within the body. **Yeasts** and **molds** also fall within the classification of fungi. Some of the infections caused by these fungi are referred to as **Tinea** infections. This word comes from the Latin word for worm and is used because of the worm-like appearance of the advancing edges of the infection. From this comes the common term **Ringworm** used to describe many fungal infections of the skin.

Fungi form **spores**. Spores have a hard outer coating like an egg. Under proper circumstances when a spore comes in contact with the skin it will **germinate** within four to six hours and cause an infection. Intact, healthy skin is a good barrier against fungal infections. In addition, the normal dryness of the skin inhibits the growth of fungi, particularly the candidia (yeast, monilia) species, which is always with us.

Fungal infections of the skin can be acquired from contact with an infected person or from their clothes, the soil, or an infected pet. Others that normally live on the human body may cause infection when our resistance is lowered because of injuries or other disease processes. Fungi are very opportunistic and will take advantage of any weakness that allows them to grow. An excoriation, or open cut in the skin, is a prime area for a fungi to start growing. Candidia is a good example of this process. It is always present on and within our body, and is quick to overgrow and cause infection when our resistance is reduced or the skin is injured.

Fungal infections are generally seen as two distinct types. One is a dry, scaly form called **chronic hyperkeratotic** (Figure 8–11). The second is a more acute form called **acute inflammatory**. The hyperkeratotic form is characterized by a dry, scaly formation on the skin. The edges of the scaly areas are usually slightly inflamed and red. Itching may or may not be present. It is not unusual for an individual to have this type of tinea only on one foot. On occasion, if the hand is also infected, only one may be involved. This condition may persist in this pattern for years. There is no explanation for why this happens. Using proper sanitation and disinfection procedures, the nail technician may give services to a client with this form of fungus.

The acute inflammatory form is characterized by blisters (large or small) which may break and ooze. Itching is present, the skin may crack and become soft in the infected area. With openings in the skin, it is not uncommon for a secondary bacterial infection to start. This type of infection occurs on any area of the skin. One of the first areas in which this form of fungus usually occurs is between the fourth and fifth toes. The skin becomes whitish and a painful fissure (crack) occurs deep between the toes. This is the typical form of tinea pedis that we refer to as **athletes foot** (Figure 8–12). The nail technician should not give services to a client with the acute inflammatory form of a fungal infection.

Pigmented nevus (mole) is the most common tumor of the skin (Figure 8–13). They appear in childhood and also in adulthood. In the early stages they appear as non-raised tan or brown areas on the skin. As they mature they may become raised and will exhibit many varying sizes, shapes, surfaces, and colors ranging from tan to dark brown. Generally speaking they will have a well-defined margin and in some cases will have hair growing out of them. Most pigmented nevi do not cause a problem and there is no need for them to be removed. Nevi on the palms of the hands and the soles of the feet seem to have a higher incidence of becoming malignant than those in other areas of the body.

As a nail professional you will have occasion to observe nevi on the extremities. The main thing is to discuss the presence of the nevus with the client. You should advise your client to seek a medical opinion if a change in color or size in the nevus is noticed. Also, medical attention should be sought for nevi that have not been injured but bleed, ooze, or ulcerate. If you, as the nail professional, have any question or suspicion about a nevus you should strongly recommend a consultation with a dermatologist. Early detection of malignant changes within a nevus can save a life.

Melanoma is cancer of the pigment-producing cells of the skin (Figure 8–14). It is the most serious malignancy of the skin and, if left untreated, will spread throughout the body and cause death. A complete cure of this disease depends on early detection and subsequent surgical excision. This condition may arise from a non-malignant pigmented nevus

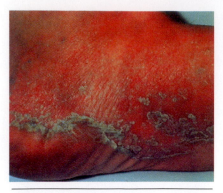

Figure 8–11 Chronic hyperkeratotic

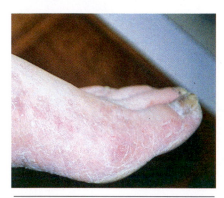

Figure 8–12 Tinea pedis (athlete's foot)

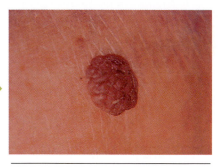

Figure 8–13 Mole (nevus)

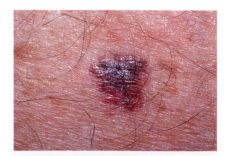

Figure 8–14 Melanoma

or from pigment cells within skin that appear normal. Its cause is unknown; however, an association with the exposure to ultraviolet light may be a contributing factor.

Approximately 1 percent of the cancers diagnosed in the United States are melanomas. Of those diagnosed melanomas, some 30 to 40 percent occur on the lower extremities. Melanomas are usually quite dark in color but can range from brownish to reddish colors. The **amelanotic melanoma** appears as a red, moist tumor-like structure on the skin. The margins of the melanoma are uneven and tend to blend into the surrounding tissues. In some cases on the palms and soles they mimic the appearance of a wart. As a nail professional, you must be on the look-out for any suspicious pigmented lesions of the skin. Know what to watch for based on what we have discussed in the pigmented nevus section and here. Advise your clients about the subject of melanomas and refer any questionable or suspicious lesions to a dermatologist for evaluation.

Herpes simplex is a skin infection common in dental staff and others involved with the care of the mouth. It may start as a painful paronychia (see Chapter 6). This is a serious viral infection that may recur periodically. Nail services should not be provided by the nail technician to a client with this condition.

◆ ◆ ◆ PIGMENTATION OF THE SKIN

The color of the skin is determined in part by the blood supply to the skin, but mostly by melanin, or coloring matter. Abnormal pigmentary conditions may be caused by internal or external factors. Certain medications are also known to cause pigmentary irregularities. Clients with these irregularities can receive nail services.

Albinism (AL-bi-niz-em) is a congenital absence of melanin pigment in the body, including the skin, hair, and eyes. The hair is silky white. The skin is pinkish white and does not tan. The eyes are pink and the skin ages early. Albinism is a form of **leucoderma** (loo-ko-DER-ma), a general term for the abnormal lack of pigmentation.

Chloasma (kloh-AZ-mah) are brown spots on the skin, especially the face and hands. Chloasma are also called "liver spots" or "moth patches."

Lentigines (len-ti-JEE-neez), or **freckles**, are small brown or yellow spots.

A **birthmark** or **nevus** (NEE-vus) is a malformation of the skin due to abnormal pigmentation or dilated capillaries. The condition may be inherited.

A **tan** is the darkening of the skin caused by exposure to the ultraviolet rays of the sun.

Vitiligo (vit-l-EYE-go) is an acquired form of leucoderma that affects the skin or hair. People with vitiligo must be protected from the sun.

chapter glossary

adipose	Fatty connective tissue that gives smoothness and shape to the body.
albinism	A congenital absence of melanin pigment in the body, including the skin, hair, and eyes.
arrector pili muscles	Minute involuntary muscle fibers in the skin inserted to the base of the hair follicles that cause goose bumps.
Basal layer	Formerly known as the stratum germinativum, it is the deepest layer of the epidermis, laying on the corneum. From this layer, all other cells of the epidermis arise.
birthmark (nevus)	A malformation of the skin due to abnormal pigmentation or dilated capillaries. This condition may be inherited.
bulla	A large blister containing watery fluid.
calluses (Tyloma)	Superficial, thickened patches of epidermis resulting from excessive friction to areas such as hands and feet.
chloasma	Brown spots on the skin, especially the face and hands; also called liver spots or moth patches.
crust	An accumulation of serum and pus mixed with epidermal flakes; e.g., a scab on a sore.
cyst	A semisolid or fluid lump above and below the skin's surface.
dermatology	The study of healthy skin and skin disorders.
dermis	The underlying or inner layer of the skin, located below the epidermis; also refers to the derma, corium, cutis, or "true skin."
eczema	The generic term used to describe a chronic, long-lasting, inflammatory skin disorder of unknown cause.
elasticity	The tissue's ability to return to normal and regain its original shape when a stress that is placed on it is removed.
elastic tissue	Tissue found in the papillary layer of the dermis, composed primarily of elastin, that gives skin its ability to return to its original shape after it has been stretched.
epidermis (cuticle)	The outermost protective covering of the skin. It contains no blood vessels, but does include many small nerve endings. It consists of four layers.
excoriation	A sore or abrasion caused by scratching or scraping off the superficial layer of the skin.
fissure	A crack in the skin that penetrates the dermis; e.g., chapped hands or lips.
friction blisters	Localized reactions of the skin to friction from an external source. The middle layer of skin fills with a straw-colored fluid, creating the blisters.
fungi	The general term used to describe plantlike parasites that can spread easily from nail to nail.
herpes simplex	A viral infection commonly seen as a fever blister or cold sore.
hypodermis (fatty layer)	Also known as the subcutis; the deepest layer of the skin, characterized by closely-packed fat cells.
keratinization	The microscopically visible changes, as well as the biochemical changes, that occur within the cells of the skin as they progress upward to the outer layer of the epidermis.

8

lentigines (freckles)	Small brown or yellow spots found on the skin.
lesion	A structural change in tissue; can be either primary (an original lesion manifesting a disease) or secondary (a lesion that develops in the later stages of a disease).
leucoderma	A general term for abnormal lack of pigmentation.
macule	Small, discolored spot or patch on the surface of the skin. Some macules are safe and some are not.
melanin	The tiny grain of pigment in the epidermis that determines natural skin color and protects the sensitive cells against strong light rays.
melanoma	Cancer of the pigment-producing cells of the skin. If left untreated, it will spread throughout the body and cause death.
molds	Fungus growth in dark, damp places, usually forming particular shapes.
motor nerves	Nerves that carry impulses from nerve centers to muscles.
nerve	A long, white cord made up of masses of neurons and held together by connective tissue that carries messages to various parts of the body from the central nervous system.
nodules	Small tumors.
objective symptoms	Symptoms that are visible to the nail technician, such a pimples, pustules, or inflammation.
papillae	Small, cone-shaped projections that extend upward into the epidermis from the dermis. Some contain looped capillaries, others contain small blood vessels, and yet others contain the melanin pigment.
papillary layer	The outer layer of the dermis, directly beneath the epidermis.
papule	Small elevation above the skin surface with a solid center.
pigmented nevus (mole)	Raised tan or brown tumor on the skin, varying in size, shape, and surface. Some may have hair growing from them.
psoriasis	A generalized disease, characterized by red patches and scales, that produces mild to severe effects on the skin.
pustule	Lump on the skin with an inflamed base and a head containing pus.
reticular layer	The deeper layer of the dermis, containing cells, vessels, glands, nerve endings, and follicles, that supplies the skin with oxygen and nutrients.
scales	Dead skin produced during the shedding of the epidermis; e.g., severe dandruff.
scar	A light-colored, slightly raised mark on the skin formed after an injury or lesion has healed.
sebaceous glands (oil glands)	Glands of the skin, connected to the hair follicles, that secrete sebum.

8

secretory nerves	Nerves of the sweat and oil glands that regulate perspiration and sebum excretion.
sensory nerves	Nerves that carry impulses from sense organs to the brain to experience sensations like touch, cold, heat, pain, and pressure.
stain	An abnormal discoloration that remains after moles, freckles, or liver spots disappear, or after certain diseases.
stratum corneum (horny layer)	The outer layer of the epidermis composed of dead epithelial cells that continually shed and replace themselves.
stratum granulosum	The granular layer of the epidermis where the process of keratinization is most active.
stratum lucidum	The clear, transparent layer of the epidermis under the stratum corneum. It is most prominent on the palms of the hands and the soles of the feet.
subcutaneous tissue	Fatty tissue known as adipose that gives smoothness and shape to the body. It contains stored fat to be burned for energy and acts as a protective cushion for the outer skin.
subjective symptoms	Symptoms that can be felt by the client, such as itching, burning, or pain.
sudoriferous glands (sweat glands)	Small, convoluted tubules that secrete sweat; found in the subcutaneous tissue and ending at the opening of the pores.
tactile corpuscles	Small epidermal structures with nerve endings that are sensitive to touch and pressure.
tan	Darkening of the skin caused by exposure to ultraviolet rays of the sun.
tubercle	A solid lump larger than a papule, varying in size from a pea to a hickory nut.
tumor	An abnormal cell mass that varies in size, shape, and color.
ulcer	An open lesion on the skin or mucous membrane of the body. Ulcers are accompanied by pus and loss of skin depth.
vesicle	A blister containing clear fluid. Poison ivy is an example of a condition that produces vesicles.
vitiligo	An acquired form of leucoderma that affects the skin or hair. People with vitiligo must be protected from the sun.
warts (papilloma, verruca, and plantar wart)	Non-cancerous viral infections of the skin, caused by a specific human papillomavirus (HPV), that multiply within the nuclei of skin-producing cells.
wheals (hives)	Swollen, itchy bumps on the skin that last for several hours; often caused by insect bites or by allergic reactions.
yeasts	Substances containing minute cells of fungi used to promote fermentation; a high source of vitamin B.

8

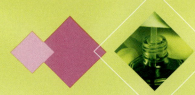

1. What are the characteristics of healthy skin?

2. What are five functions of the skin?

3. Describe the epidermis and dermis.

4. How is the skin nourished?

5. What are the functions of sweat glands?

6. Name five types of lesions.

7. What are the characteristics of eczema and psoriasis?

8

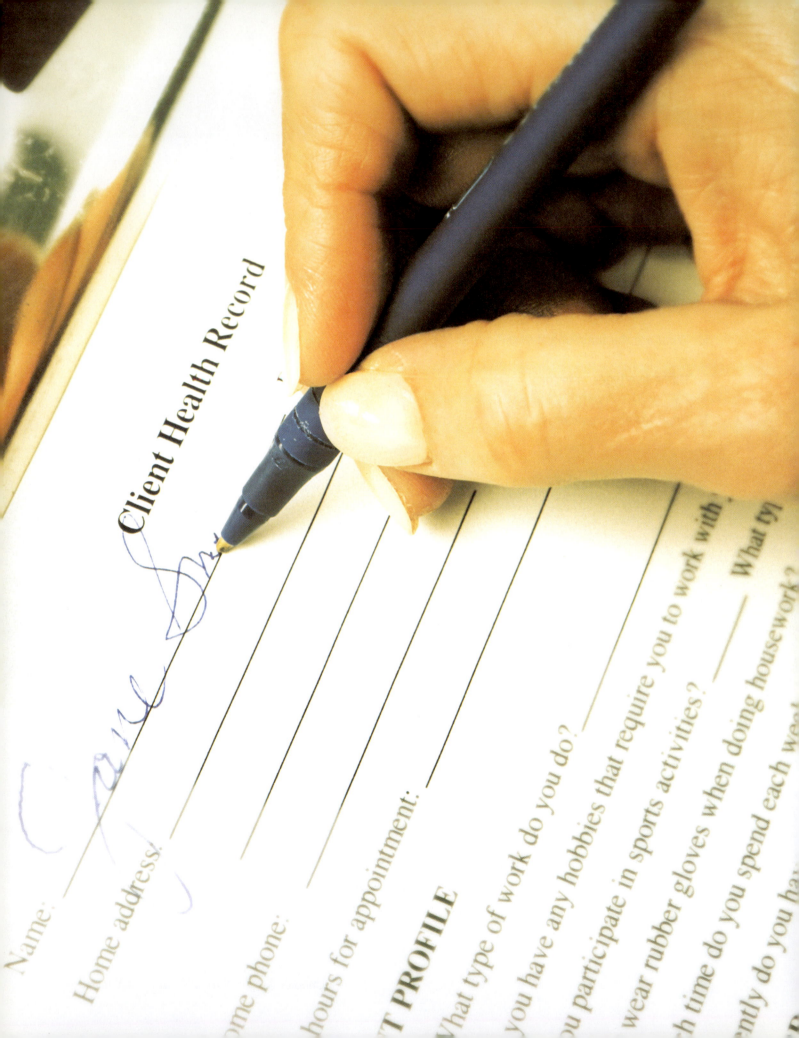

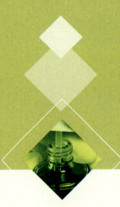

9

CLIENT CONSULTATION

Author: Janet McCormick

CHAPTER OUTLINE

Determining the Condition of Nails and Skin
Determining the Client's Needs • Meeting Your Client's Needs
Completing the Client Health/Record Form
Maintaining the Client Service and Product Record

Learning Objectives

After you have completed this chapter, you should be able to:

1 **Explain the purpose of a client consultation.**

2 **Explain the parts of a consultation.**

3 **Describe the consultative technique.**

4 **Describe the appearance of healthy nails.**

5 **Describe the symptoms of allergies.**

6 **Explain why knowing a client's lifestyle is helpful in making decisions about products and services.**

7 **Determine when it is necessary to refer a client to a physician.**

8 **Describe the information that should be gathered on the client health/record form.**

9 **Name the reasons for maintaining a client health/ record form.**

10 **Name the reasons for maintaining a client service and product record.**

Key Terms

Page number indicates where in the chapter the term is used.

analysis
pg. 153

client consultation
pg. 153

recommendations
pg. 153

Before you perform a service on a client, you should take time to talk with that client and complete a client health/record form and a client service and product record. During this conversation, called the **client consultation**, you will discuss the client's general health, the health of his or her nails and skin, the client's lifestyle and needs, and the nail services that you can perform. You will use your knowledge of skin, nails, and each type of nail service to help your client select the most appropriate service. If the client has a nail or skin disorder that prevents you from performing a service, you should refer that client to his or her physician and offer to perform a service as soon as the disorder has been treated.

A **client consultation** has two parts, the **analysis** and the **recommendations**. For best results, you will perform them as separate and distinct parts. The **analysis** is the first section of the process, the information-gathering portion. You ask questions in this section, looking closely at the client's skin and nails. Touch them, define their texture, moisture content, coloration, and condition in verbal observations to the client. Always point out what you see and ask more questions concerning lifestyle and home care. Ask the client what her goal is for you in the care of her skin and nails. Then, after all the information is gathered and her goals are known, **recommendations** are made for the appropriate service that will aid her in achieving them. The benefits and results of the recommended service are explained in full. Supportive home care products are recommended to aid clients in reaching their goals, and instructions are provided on how and when they are to be used.

A professional, consultative technique should be used to make a good first impression. The consultation is your first opportunity to portray yourself as a professional to your client. It should be performed in a straightforward and confident manner. You will need to

❖ focus on the client.

❖ look directly at your client while speaking, in a tone that demonstrates integrity and confidence.

❖ support your recommendations with facts and information.

❖ be friendly and helpful.

A well-done consultation can place you solidly as a professional in the eyes of a client. It is the difference between being a professional and just "doing nails."

DETERMINING THE CONDITION OF NAILS AND SKIN

Are your client's nails and skin healthy? Look at the nails and skin of the hands or feet (depending on the service). Examine them for disorders. Generally, if there is no inflammation, infection, swelling, or broken skin it is okay to work on that client. It may be necessary to refer a client to his or her physician if you find a problem. It is important to handle this situation very delicately (Figure 9–1).

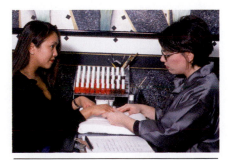

Figure 9-1 Are your client's nails and skin healthy?

If you need to refer a client to a physician, you must act responsibly and tactfully. Explain to your client that you think there may be a problem and to be safe you will not perform a service until the client has visited a doctor. Never attempt to diagnose the problem because you could cause unnecessary stress for your client. While it may be difficult to turn a client away, you must do so. Performing a service on an infected nail could cause great pain to your client, for which you could be blamed. In addition, your client will be impressed with your professionalism and concern for health and safety.

The consultation should include a discussion of the client's general health. The safety of your client can depend upon your knowledge obtained from questions or observations concerning her general health. Always read the completed health/record form to gain awareness of appropriate precautions you must take during services. For example, be particularly careful while filing the nails or pushing back the pterygium of a diabetic client, and *never* nip the cuticles. A pedicure for this client should be in warm, not hot, water as a diabetic client's skin is particularly sensitive to heat. Diabetics get infections easily and heal slowly, sometimes not at all. The potentials can be deadly if the skin is cut or scraped. Clients with arthritis should be held gently during the service and clients who have a circulatory disease, such as varicose veins, should be massaged very gently, if at all. It is the responsibility of the technician to seek out information that will ensure the health of the clients (Figure 9–2).

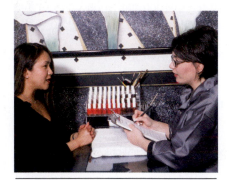

Figure 9-2 Always fill out a client health form prior to beginning any service

Does your client have allergies? You should always try to avoid using products that can cause an allergic reaction. As a professional, you must be alert to any change or discomfort on the client's skin or nails, and thoroughly investigate the causes. Some of the symptoms of allergies are severe dryness and cracking of the cuticles, onycholysis, throbbing nail beds after a fill, itching of the cuticles, and swelling around the nails. Any one, or a combination of these and other symptoms, may indicate a need for a change or a cessation of the service or a product. If your client does have a reaction to a product, be sure to make a note on his or her client health/record form that includes both the product and the type of reaction.

DETERMINING YOUR CLIENT'S NEEDS

What nail service does the client want? If your client asks for a specific nail service, discuss the procedure used to create that service, the benefits, and proper maintenance. Make sure that your client's expectations are realistic. Keep this desired service in mind as you discuss the client's lifestyle. You may know of a nail service that is better suited to the client's needs. Keep your client's goals in mind at all times.

What kind of lifestyle does the client have? What kind of job does your client have? What hobbies? Are your client's hands often in water? Does your client walk a lot? By learning the answers to these types of questions, you will be able to decide such things as the best length for your client's nails or how much callus to remove from the feet. Is the client a gardener, model, guitar player, or runner? A gardener might need short nails because it would be difficult to remove dirt from under a long nail. Dirt that cannot be removed can lead to infection or a painful break. A guitar player may need short nails on the left hand and want longer nails on the right hand. He or she also needs calluses on the fingertips of the left hand. A model needs beautiful nails and skin (Figure 9–3). A runner may have calluses on the feet that protect the feet during running. You must always consider your client's personality styles and activities when choosing a nail service (Figure 9–4). In each of these cases the wrong service could make a client unhappy and even cause pain. You're the professional; it's your job to make the client happy. If your client gets a service and is not happy with it, he or she may not return. If you offer a different service than originally requested and explain why you feel that service is better suited for the client, you will have that client for life.

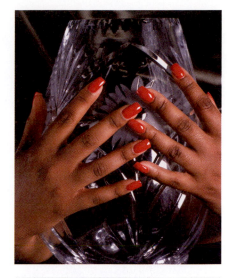

Figure 9-3 A model needs beautiful nails.

◆◆ MEETING YOUR CLIENT'S NEEDS

What is the client's final decision about nail services? After talking with your client about his or her needs, expectations, and nail health you will either confirm the client's service choice or recommend another service. Think of your recommendations as "educating your client." Clients like to learn about their skin and nails and will respond positively to recommendations made in this manner. Explain why a service is best for the client, what you will do during the procedure, and fully explain the results the client can expect. For example, you would not want your client to believe that nail wraps stayed on forever and needed no maintenance. The client would be very disappointed, despite having a very professional service, when the wrap began to grow out. This is the appropriate time to explain any safety precautions you will take during the procedure. For example, if you are going to apply acrylic nails, you should explain why you will wear safety goggles while applying primer. It is also a good idea to offer your client the same protection (Figure 9–5).

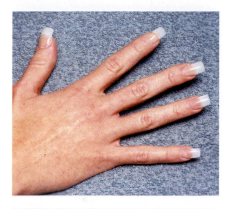

Figure 9-4 Many people prefer natural looking nails.

After you have completed this process with your client you will start the procedure. You and your client can be sure that it is the appropriate service. Time and money are being spent wisely. The nail service will not conflict with the client's lifestyle and should meet all expectations; your client will also know that you are concerned about health and safety. Your client will leave your salon satisfied, and will also return to you again and again as a steady client!

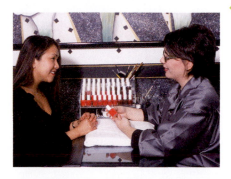

Figure 9-5 Explain why you think a particular service is best for your client.

BUSINESS ◆ TIP

Thank you for coming...

In today's competitive business climate, it is important to win your client's loyalty immediately. For that reason, it is crucial to perform your duties professionally during the client's first exposure to your services, and to follow up with a reminder of your professional care. A "thank you for visiting me at (salon name)" is a good way to cement your professional relationship and to win future loyalty. Cards of this type are available at shows and in beauty catalogues. With a note and signature by the professional who worked on them, they are very well received. Handwritten ones on commercial thank-you note stationery are also appreciated. Also, placing the new client on the mailing list for any salon communications, such as newsletters and promotional notices, will remind her of your service every time it comes to her home. New clients like to be reminded of how much you enjoyed doing their service and if the first service was top notch and professionally done, they will respond with reappointments.

COMPLETING THE CLIENT HEALTH/RECORD FORM

The form for client health/record information will vary from one salon to another. If cards are used, they should be kept in a convenient location where they can provide ready reference for every nail technician in the salon and may easily be retrieved for every client visit. If the salon is computerized, client health/record information can be kept in the computer and accessed, even printed out, by a few simple keystrokes.

Client health/record forms usually include three valuable types of information including

1. **General information** asks for the client's name, address, telephone number, the name of the person who referred her, and preferred appointment hours.

2. The **client profile** asks for information about the type of work and leisure activities in which the client participates.

3. The **medical record** asks for information about the client's general health. This information will help you determine whether it is safe to perform nail services or hand and foot massage on the client (Figures 9–6 and 9–7).

CLIENT HEALTH/RECORD FORM

Name: _____   Birthday: _____

Home address: _____   Work address: _____

_____   _____

_____   _____

Home telephone: _____   Work telephone: _____

Best hours for appointment are: _____

CLIENT PROFILE

1. What type of work do you do? _____

2. Do you have any hobbies that require you to work with your hands? _____ If so,

   what are they? _____

3. Do you participate in sports activities? If so, what type? _____

4. Do you wear rubber gloves when doing housework? _____

5. How much time do you spend each week caring for your own nails? _____

6. How frequently do you have professional nail services? _____

MEDICAL RECORD

Your health can be important to our professional care of your hands and feet. Please circle any of the following that are relevant to your health, and fill in the name where necessary.

Circulatory disease_____	Diabetes	Thyroid disease
Skin disease_____	Pregnancy	Acute Arthritis
Fungal infection (hands or feet)	Heart disease	Retinoid therapy
Reynaud's disease	Presently taking Chemo/Radiation	Stroke
Prominent varicose veins	Alpha Hydroxy Acid treatments/products	
Lupus	Photosensitive medications	

Are you currently on any medication on a regular basis?_____ If so, what?_____

_____

For an acrylic/gel/wrap service, please fill out the following also.

Have you worn nail enhancements prior to this time?_____ If so, what kind?_____

Are you allergic to any kind of enhancement?_____ If so, what kind?_____

Is your skin oily or dry?_____

Comments: _____

_____

Figure 9-6 Client health form

CLIENT SERVICE RECORD

Name: _____

Home address: _____   Work address: _____

_____   _____

_____   _____

Home telephone: _____   Work telephone: _____

Best hours for appointment are: _____

DATE	SERVICE PERFORMED	OBSERVATIONS	PRICE

DATE	RETAIL PRODUCTS SOLD	PRICE

What future nail services were discussed?

_____

_____

_____

Figure 9-7 Client service record

◆ ◆ MAINTAINING THE CLIENT SERVICE AND PRODUCT RECORD

Each time a client receives a service in the salon, an entry should be made in the client's service and product record. This record can be maintained manually on a client health/record form, in a file or binder, or in the client's computer file. It is retrieved for every visit because it includes information about services performed, retail products sold, future nail services discussed, and the client's goals. The client service and product record is a valuable asset for the salon to maintain. For example, a client comes in for a service when his or her usual nail technician is not available, or when a service or product problem occurs at a later time. The client's health/record form and service/product records are consultation tools. When used and maintained conscientiously, it shows your clients you are a professional, that you care about their health and safety, as well as the quality of the service they receive.

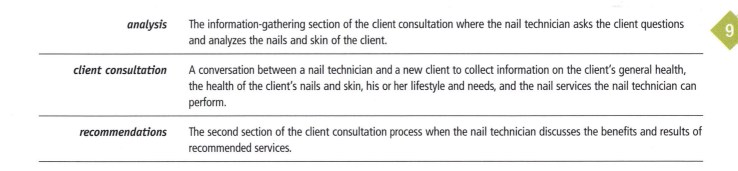

chapter glossary

analysis	The information-gathering section of the client consultation where the nail technician asks the client questions and analyzes the nails and skin of the client.
client consultation	A conversation between a nail technician and a new client to collect information on the client's general health, the health of the client's nails and skin, his or her lifestyle and needs, and the nail services the nail technician can perform.
recommendations	The second section of the client consultation process when the nail technician discusses the benefits and results of recommended services.

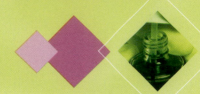
1. What is the purpose of a client consultation?

2. What are the parts of the consultation?

3. What are the characteristics of healthy nails?

4. How would your services differ for a runner and a guitar player?

5. Under what circumstances would you refer a client to a physician?

6. What are the three types of information on the client health/record form?

7. Why do you maintain a client health/record form and client service and product records?

part 3

BASIC PROCEDURES

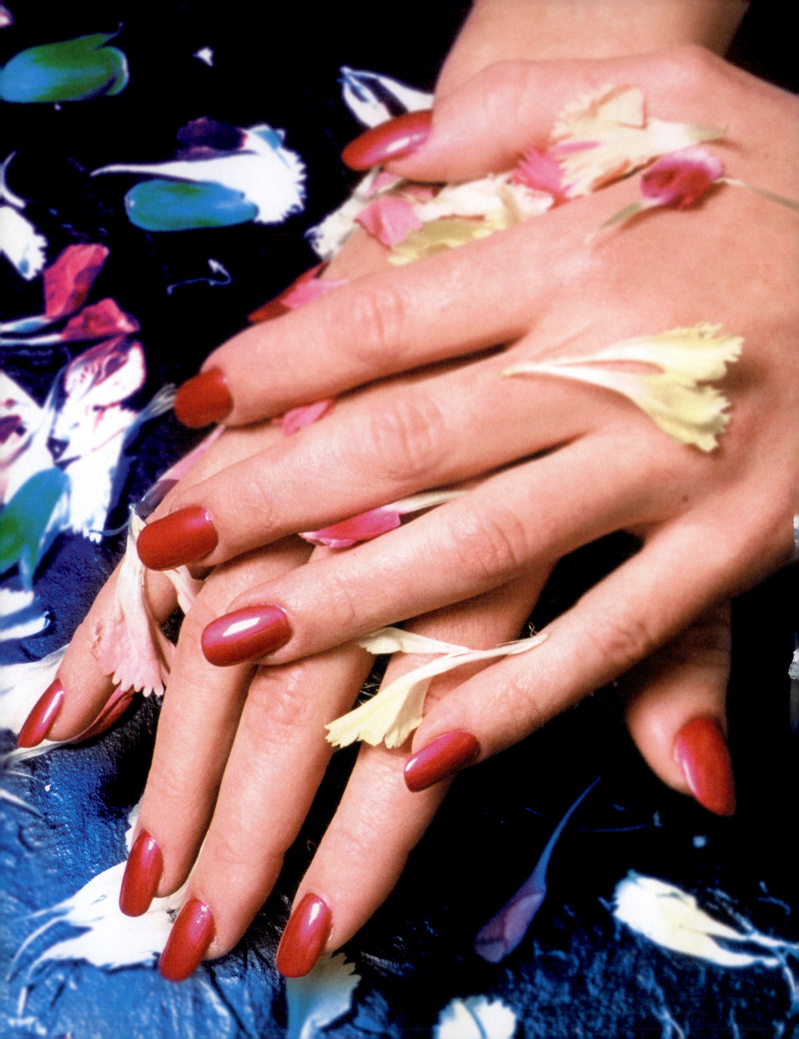

The importance of having well-manicured nails and hands has become a significant part of our culture for both men and women of today. It is among one of the fastest growing services requested in a salon. Once you have learned the basic knowledge and mastered the fundamental techniques in this chapter, you will be on your way to becoming a professional and providing the much-requested services of a professional nail technician. As a professional it is imperative that you learn to work with the tools required for your trade, and incorporate all safety and sanitation specifications during any procedure. The four types of nail technology tools you will incorporate into your services are

1. equipment.
2. implements.
3. materials.
4. nail cosmetics.

◆◆◆ NAIL TECHNOLOGY SUPPLIES

Equipment

Equipment includes all permanent tools used to perform nail services that do not require replacement until they are no longer in good repair or need replacement.

Manicure Table with Adjustable Lamp

Most standard manicuring tables include a drawer (for storing sanitized implements and cosmetics) and have an attached, adjustable lamp. The lamp should have a 40 watt bulb. The heat from a higher wattage bulb will interfere with manicuring and sculptured nail procedures. A lower wattage bulb will not adequately warm a client's nails in a room that is exceptionally cool. The warmth from the bulb will help you maintain product consistency.

Nail Technician's Chair and Client's Chair

The nail technician's chair should be selected for ergonomics, comfort, durability, and easy sanitizing. The client's chair should be durable, comfortable, and easy to sanitize. For sanitary purposes the client's set cushion can be covered with a clean, laundered terry towel or disposable towel before each client. Another option is to sanitize the cushion with a disinfectant spray before each client.

Fingerbowl

A fingerbowl is a bowl specifically designed for soaking the client's fingers in warm water with an antibacterial soap added. A fingerbowl can be designed from several materials such as plastic, metal, or glass, but should be durable and easy to sanitize after use on each client (Figure 10–1).

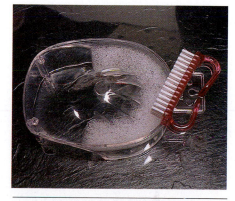

Figure 10–1 Fingerbowl filled with warm water and liquid soap, with nail brush

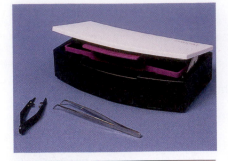

Figure 10-2 Disinfection container

Disinfection Container

A disinfection container is a receptacle that is large enough to hold a disinfectant solution in which the implements requiring sanitization can be completely immersed. Disinfectant containers come in a number of shapes, sizes, and material. They should have a lid, which is used to keep the disinfectant solution from becoming contaminated when not in use. Some containers have a lift tray that allows the implements to be removed from the solution by lifting the tray by a handle and removing the implements without contaminating the solution. After removing the implements from the disinfectant container they should be sprayed with water or alcohol thoroughly, as disinfectants should never be allowed to come in contact with the skin. If your disinfectant container does not have a lift tray, remove the implements using tongs or tweezers. Never allow your fingers to come in contact with the solutions, as this can cause contamination. Never place any used implements back into the disinfectant container until they have been properly cleaned (Figure 10–2).

Client's Arm Cushion

The cushion can be 8" x 12" and especially made for manicuring; a towel that is folded to cushion size can also be used. The cushion or folded towel should be covered with a clean or disposable towel before each appointment.

Sanitized Wipe Container

This container will hold clean, absorbent cotton or lint-free wipes.

Heater for a Reconditioning Hot Oil Manicure

A hot oil manicure heater warms the lotion that will be used when performing a reconditioning hot oil manicure.

Supply Tray

The tray holds cosmetics such as polishes, polish removers, and creams. It should be durable, balanced, and easy to clean and sanitize.

Electric Nail Dryer

A nail dryer is an optional item designed to shorten the length of time necessary for the client's nails to dry.

Electric File

An electric file can help speed up time and save energy while performing some nail services. Refer to Chapter 12 for more information.

Implements

Implements are tools that must be sanitized or disposed of after use with each client. They are small enough to be sanitized in a disinfection container.

Orangewood Stick

Use the orangewood stick to loosen cuticle around the base of a nail or to clean under the free edge. Hold the stick as you would a pencil. When you

10

SANITATION CAUTION

If you drop an orangewood stick on the floor, it must be discarded. It is a disposable implement that cannot be sanitized or reused.

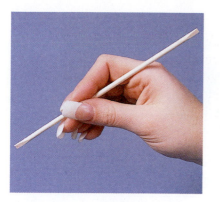

Figure 10-3 Orangewood stick

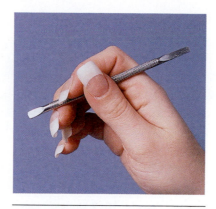

Figure 10-4 Steel pusher

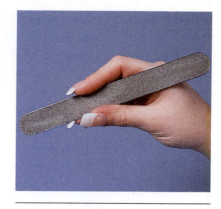

Figure 10-5 Metal nail file

use it to apply cosmetics, wrap a small piece of cotton around the end. An orangewood stick cannot be sanitized, so you must either give it to your client or break it in half and discard it after use (Figure 10–3).

Steel Pusher

The steel pusher, also called a cuticle pusher, is used to push back excess cuticle growth. Hold the steel pusher the way you hold a pencil. The spoon end is used to loosen and push back cuticle. If you have rough or sharp edges on your pusher, use an emery board to dull them. This prevents digging into the nail plate. They are reusable, so strict sanitation procedures are required before use on every client (Figure 10–4).

Metal Nail File

A metal nail file is used to shape the free edge of hard or sculptured nails. Most professional nail technicians use 7"–8" nail files because some states do not allow shorter files to be used. Since a nail file is metal and reusable, it must be disinfected after each use. When using a nail file, hold it with your thumb on one side and the handle and four fingers on the other side (Figure 10–5).

Emery Board

Many nail technicians prefer an emery board to a metal nail file. It is also a good choice for filing soft or fragile nails, because it is not as coarse as a nail file. An emery board can have two sides, a coarse-grained side and a fine-grained side. The coarse side is used to shape the free edge of the nail, and the fine side is used to **bevel** the nail or smooth the free edge. Hold the emery board the way you hold a nail file, with the wider end in your hand so you can file with the narrow end. To bevel, hold the emery board at a 45-degree angle and file, using light pressure, on the top or underside of the nail. Most professional nail technicians use 7"–8" emery boards because some states do not allow the use of smaller ones. The emery board cannot be sanitized, so you must either give it to your client or break it in half and discard it after use. It is not a good idea to save an emery board in a plastic bag for each client. Bacteria can grow on the unsanitized implement before your client's next appointment (Figure 10–6).

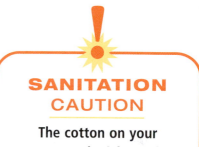

SANITATION CAUTION

The cotton on your orangewood stick needs to be changed after each use.

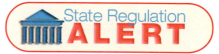

State Regulation **ALERT**

Some states do not permit nail technicians to use metal nail files. Be guided by your instructor.

10

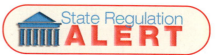

State Regulation **ALERT**

Some states do not permit nail technicians to clip cuticles. Be guided by your instructor.

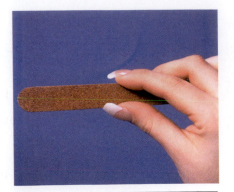

Figure 10-6 Emery board

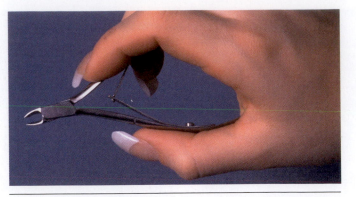

Figure 10-7 Cuticle nippers

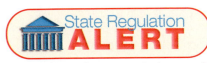

SANITATION CAUTION

If you drop an emery board on the floor during a procedure, it must be discarded. This is a disposable item and cannot be reused or sanitized.

State Regulation ALERT

Some states do not permit the use of a chamois buffer. Be guided by your instructor.

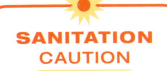

SANITATION CAUTION

Your chamois buffer must be designed so the chamois can be changed for each client. Be sure to discard the used chamois after each use.

Cuticle Nipper

A cuticle nipper is used to trim away excess cuticle at the base of the nail. To use the nippers, hold them in the palm of your hand with the blades facing the cuticle. Place your thumb on one handle and three fingers on the other handle, with your index finger on the screw to help guide the blade around the cuticle. They are reusable so strict sanitation procedures are required before use on every client (Figure 10–7).

Tweezers

Tweezers can be used to lift small bits of cuticle from the nail. They are reusable, so strict sanitation procedures are required before use on every client.

Nail Brush

A nail brush is used to clean fingernails and remove bits of cuticle with warm soapy water. Hold the nail brush with the bristles turned down and away from you. Place your thumb on the handle side of the brush that is facing you and your fingers on the other side. They are reusable, so strict sanitation procedures are required before use on every client.

Chamois Buffer

The **chamois** (SHAM-ee) **buffer** is used to add shine to the nail and to smooth out corrugations or wavy ridges on nails. There are two types of chamois buffer. The first has an open handle; the second has a closed handle on the top. To use the open-handled buffer, place your fingers around the handle with your thumb on the side of the handle to help guide it. To use the closed-handled type, rest your thumb along the edge of the buffer to guide and support your use of this implement. Another way to hold a closed-handled chamois buffer is to place the middle and ring fingers through the closed-handled buffer if it has an open slot. Be guided by your instructor on how to hold the chamois buffer. The chamois buffer must be designed so the chamois can be changed for use on each client. The used chamois must be disposed of after use on every client (Figures 10–8 and 10–9).

10

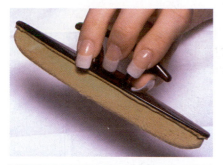

Figure 10-8 Holding a nail buffer

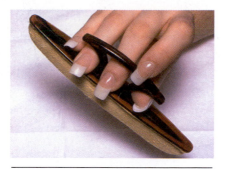

Figure 10-9 Alternative way to hold a nail buffer

Fingernail Clippers

Fingernail clippers are used to shorten nails. If your client's nails are very long, clipping cuts filing time. They are reusable, so strict sanitation procedures are required before use on every client.

Sanitation for Implements

It is a good idea to have two complete sets of metal implements, so you will always have a completely sanitized set for each client, with no waiting between appointments. If you have only one set of implements, remember that it takes approximately twenty minutes to sanitize implements after each use. A few sanitation hints follow. For a complete discussion of sanitation, see page 36.

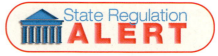

In some states, it is a violation of sanitary codes to have metal implements on your table when not in use. Be guided by your instructor about proper storage.

* Wash all implements thoroughly with soap and warm water and rinse off all traces of soap with plain water. Dry thoroughly with a clean or disposable towel.
* Metal implements should be immersed in a disinfection container that is filled with an approved disinfectant. Follow manufacturer's instructions for the required sanitation time. Rinse the implements, then dry them with a clean or disposable towel when you remove them from the disinfection container.
* Follow your state regulations for storage of sanitized manicuring implements. The regulations will tell you to store them in sealed containers, sealed plastic bags, or in a cabinet sanitizer until they are ready for use.

Materials

Materials are supplies that are used during a manicure and must be replaced for each client.

Disposable Towels or Terry Cloth Towels

A fresh, clean terry cloth towel or a disposable towel is used to cover the client's cushion before each manicure. Another fresh towel should be used to dry the client's hands after soaking in the fingerbowl. Other terry cloth or lint-free disposable towels are used to wipe spills that may occur around the fingerbowl.

Cotton/Cotton Balls or Pledgets

Cotton can be used for removing nail polish from the nails or wrapped around the end of an orangewood stick and used for removing nail polish from areas that are hard to reach. It can also be used for applying nail cosmetics. Small fiber-free squares known as pledgets are often used and preferred by nail technicians to remove polish because the cotton fibers from the squares do not adhere to the nails, which can interfere with the polish application.

Plastic Spatula

A plastic or wooden spatula is used for removing any nail cosmetics from their container. If a spatula comes in contact with your skin or the client's skin it must be disposed of immediately and a new one used to remove more product from the container if needed. Never use the same spatula to remove unlike products from different containers. Never use your fingers to remove any cosmetics from a container as they can contaminate cosmetics. A closed, contaminated container of nail cosmetics is a perfect place for bacteria from fingers to grow. All containers should be closed when not in use to avoid contamination.

Plastic Bags

Tape or clip a bag to the side of the manicuring table to hold the used materials you discard during a service. Be sure to have a generous supply of bags so you can change them regularly during the day.

Trash Containers

A trash container with a lid that can be operated by a foot pedal can be located at your work station. The trash container should be lined and closed when not in use. It should be emptied at the end of every day.

Powdered Alum or Styptic Powder

Powdered alum, or **styptic** (STIP-tik) **powder**, is used to contract the skin to stop minor bleeding that may occur during a manicure. To use, blot cut with powdered alum on a cotton-tipped orangewood stick.

Nail Cosmetics

As a professional nail technician, you need to know how to use each nail cosmetic and what ingredients it contains. You must know how to apply each cosmetic and when to avoid using a product because of a client's allergies or sensitivities. This section discusses some of the basic nail cosmetics, what each product does, and the basic ingredients in each.

Soap

Soap is used to clean the nail technician's and client's hands before a service begins. It is also mixed with warm water and used in the finger bowl as a soak during a plain manicure. Soap comes in four forms: flaked, beaded, cake, and liquid. It is recommended to use the liquid form because bar soap harbors bacteria and is a breeding place for pathogens.

10

State Regulation ALERT

Styptic pencils are not permitted for use in most states because they are unsanitary.

Polish Remover

Polish remover is used to dissolve and remove nail polish. It usually contains organic solvents and acetone. Sometimes, oil is added to offset the drying effect of the acetone. Use non-acetone polish remover for clients who have artificial nails, because acetone will weaken or dissolve tips, wrap glues, and sculptured nail compound.

Cuticle Cream

Cuticle cream is used to lubricate and soften dry cuticles and brittle nails. It contains fats and waxes, such as lanolin, cocoa butter, petroleum, and beeswax and is excellent for your client to use on a daily basis.

Cuticle Oil

Cuticle oil keeps the cuticle soft and helps to prevent hangnails or rough cuticles. It gives an added touch to the finish of a manicure. Cuticle oil contains ingredients such as vegetable oil, vitamin E, mineral oil, jojoba, and palm nut oil. Suggest that your clients use it at bedtime to keep their cuticles soft.

Cuticle Solvent or Cuticle Remover

Cuticle solvent makes cuticles easier to remove and minimizes clipping. It contains 2–5 percent sodium or potassium hydroxide plus glycerin.

Nail Bleach

Apply nail bleach to nail plate and under free edge to remove yellow stains. It contains hydrogen peroxide. If nail bleach cannot be purchased, use 20 volume (6 percent) hydrogen peroxide.

Nail Whitener

Nail whiteners are applied under the free edge of a nail to make the nail appear white. They contain zinc oxide or titanium dioxide. Nail whiteners are available in a paste, cream, coated string, and pencil form.

Dry Nail Polish

Dry nail polish, or **pumice** (PUM-is) **powder** is used with the chamois buffer to add shine to the nail. Some clients prefer it to liquid clear polish. Dry nail polish contains **mild abrasives** (ah-BRAY-sihvs), which are used for smoothing or sanding, such as tin oxide, talc, silica, and kaolin. Dry nail polish is available in powder and cream form.

Colored Polish, Liquid Enamel, or Lacquer (LAK-er)

Colored polish is used to add color and gloss to the nail. It is usually applied in two coats. Colored polish contains a solution of nitrocellulose in a volatile solvent, such as amyl acetate and evaporates easily. Manufacturers add castor oil to prevent the polish from drying too rapidly.

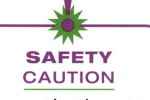

SAFETY CAUTION

Care must be taken not to get nail bleach on cuticles or skin because it can cause irritation.

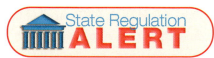

Nail white pencils are not permitted in most states because they are unsanitary.

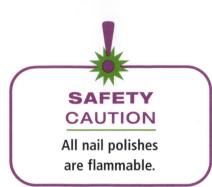

Base Coat

The base coat is colorless and is applied to the natural nail before the application of colored polish. It prevents red or dark polish from yellowing or staining the nail plate. Base coat is the first polish you apply in the polish procedure, unless you are using a nail strengthener. It is designed to provide a better intercoat adhesion. It contains ethyl acetate, a solvent, isopropyl alcohol, butyl acetate, nitrocellulose, and sometimes formaldehyde.

Nail Strengthener/Hardener

Nail strengthener is applied to the natural nail before the base coat. It prevents splitting and peeling of the nail. There are three types of nail strengthener:

Protein hardener is a combination of clear polish and protein, such as collagen.

Nylon fiber is a combination of clear polish with nylon fibers. It is applied first vertically and then horizontally on the nail plate. It can be hard to cover smoothly because the fibers on the nail are visible. It is sometimes referred to as a liquid wrap.

Formaldehyde strengthener contains 5 percent formaldehyde.

Top Coat or Sealer

The top coat, a colorless polish, is applied over colored polish to prevent chipping and to add a shine to the finished nail. It could contain acrylic- or cellulose-type film formers.

Liquid Nail Dry

Liquid "nail dry" is used to prevent smudging of the polish. It promotes rapid drying so that the polish is not tacky and prevents the polish from dulling. It has an alcohol base and is available in brush-on or spray.

Hand Cream and Hand Lotion

Hand lotion and hand cream add a finishing touch to a manicure. Since they soften and smooth the hands, they make the finished manicure look as beautiful as possible. Hand cream helps the skin retain moisture, so hands are not dry, cracked, and wrinkled. Hand cream is thicker than hand lotion and is made of emollients and humectants, such as glycerin, cocoa butter, lecithin, and gums. Hand lotion has a thinner consistency than hand cream because it contains more oil. In addition to oil, hand lotion can contain stearic acid, water, mucilage of quince seed as a healing agent, lanolin, glycerin, and gum. Hand cream or hand lotion can be used as oil in a reconditioning hot oil manicure.

Nail Conditioner

Nail conditioner contains moisturizers, and should be applied at night before bedtime to help prevent brittle nails and dry cuticles.

PROCEDURE

Basic Table Set-up

It is important that your manicure table is sanitary and properly equipped with implements, materials, and cosmetics. Anything you need during a service should be at your fingertips. Having an orderly table will give you and your client confidence during the manicure. The actual placement of supplies on the manicuring table is a suggestion. Since regulations regarding table set-up vary from state to state, be guided by your instructor. To set up your table, use the following procedure.

1. Wipe manicure table and drawer with approved sanitizer.

2. Wrap your client's arm cushion with a clean towel, either terry cloth or disposable. Put it in the middle of the table so the cushion is toward the client and the end of the towel is extended toward you.

3. Fill the disinfection container with an approved hospital-grade disinfectant 20 minutes before your first manicure of the day. Put all metal implements into the disinfection container after being washed and dried. Place the disinfection container to your right if you are right-handed, or to your left if you are left-handed.

4. Place the cosmetics (except polish) on the right side of the table behind your disinfection container (if left-handed, place on left).

5. Place emery boards and chamois buffer on the table to your right (if left-handed, to the left).

6. Place the fingerbowl and brush in the middle or to the left of the table, toward the client. The fingerbowl or hot oil heater should not be moved from side to side of the manicure table. It should stay where you place it for the duration of your manicure. If you're doing a reconditioning hot oil manicure, replace fingerbowl and brush with electric hot oil heater.

7. Tape or clip a plastic bag to right side of table (if left-handed, tape to left side). This is used for depositing used materials during your manicure.

8. Place polishes to the left (if left-handed, place on right).

9. Your drawer can be used to keep the following items: extra cotton or cotton balls in their original container or in a fresh plastic bag, pumice stone or powder, extra chamois for buffer, instant nail dry, or other supplies. Never place used materials in your drawer. Only completely sanitized implements (sealed in air-tight containers) and extra materials or cosmetics should be placed in this drawer. Always keep it clean and sanitary (Figure 10–10).

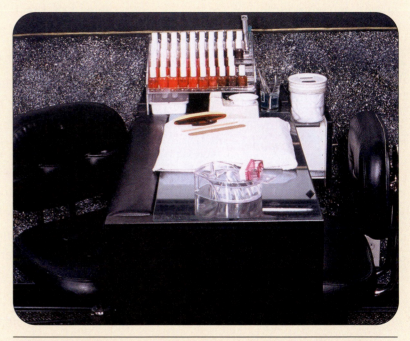

Figure 10–10 Basic table setup. Your instructor's table set-up is equally correct.

◆◆ CHOOSING A NAIL SHAPE

After the client consultation, you will discuss what shape and color nails your client prefers. Keep the following considerations in mind: the shape of the hands, length of fingers, shape of the cuticles, and the type of work clients do. It is a general thought that the nails should be shaped to mirror the shape of the cuticles (Figure 10–11). The following are five shapes from which to choose.

❖ The **square nail** is completely straight across with no rounding at the edges. The length depends on the client's preference.

❖ The **squoval nail** should extend only slightly past the tip of the finger with the free edge rounded off. This shape is sturdy because the full width of the nail remains at the free edge. Clients who work with their hands—on a typewriter, computer, or assembly line—will need shorter, square nails.

❖ The **round nail** should be slightly tapered and extend just a bit past the tip of the finger. Round nails are the most common choice for male clients because of their natural shape.

❖ The **oval nail** is an attractive nail shape for most women's hands. It is a square nail with slightly rounded corners. Professional clients who have their hands on display (professional business people, teachers, or salespeople, for example) may want longer oval nails.

❖ The **pointed nail** is suited to thin hands with narrow nail beds. The nail is tapered somewhat longer than usual to enhance the slender appearance of the hand; however, these nails are weak and break easily.

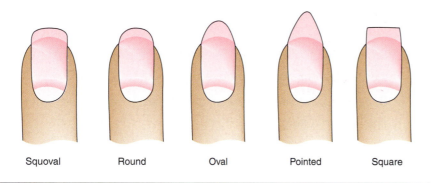

| Squoval | Round | Oval | Pointed | Square |

Figure 10-11 The five basic nail shapes: squoval, round, oval, pointed, and square.

PROCEDURE 10-2

Handling Blood During a Manicure

At times during a manicure blood may be visible from overzealous filing or other reasons. First and foremost, the safety and sanitation factors involved in an incident of this nature for both you and your client is of the utmost importance. You should incorporate the following procedure if this should happen.

1. Immediately put on gloves and inform your client of what has occurred. Apologize and proceed.

2. Apply slight pressure to the area with cotton and an antiseptic.

3. Apply alum or styptic powder (if needed) using the end of a cotton-wrapped orangewood stick. Never place the orangewood stick back into the container once it has been applied to an opened area on the skin. Styptic pencils should not be used, as they are unsanitary after they have been used on a client.

4. Complete the service if applicable.

5. Properly dispose of any blood contaminated materials and implements. Be guided by your instructor for proper disposal.

6. Properly and thoroughly disinfect all implements that require sanitization using an approved disinfectant.

7. Once you have removed your gloves, wash your hands using an antibacterial soap.

Always remember to use Universal Precautions when handling blood or bodily fluids. (Refer back to the chapter on sanitation and disinfection.) Be guided by your instructor for your state's mandatory and approved products and procedures for disinfecting any implements that have come in contact with blood or bodily fluids.

◆◆ PLAIN MANICURE

Three-part Procedure

As a professional nail technician you will follow a three-part procedure sequence for all services you perform. The sequence will include pre-service, actual performance, and post-service.

Pre-service

❖ Sanitize your table. (This procedure is described on pages 41–43.)

❖ Sanitize all additional equipment, tools, and implements and set up your standard manicuring table.

❖ Wash your hands with an antibacterial soap.

❖ Greet your client with a smile (Figure 10–12).

❖ Have your client remove jewelry and place it in a safe, secure place.

❖ Have your client wash his or her hands using an antibacterial soap and dry them thoroughly with a clean terry cloth or disposable towel.

❖ Perform a client consultation using a health and record form. This form will be used to record responses from clients and observations before and after the service. Before beginning always check the nails and skin area for any disorders or deviations from the normal. Decide if the service can be performed in a safe and appropriate manner. If there is a reason the service cannot be performed, explain the reason to the client, and suggest they seek medical attention; then record this information on their health and record form. If no deviation from the normal is noted, continue with the service.

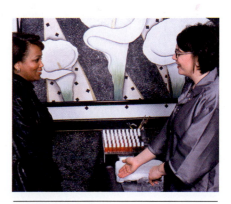

Figure 10-12 Greet your client with a smile.

Actual Procedure

❖ *During* the actual manicure, talk with your clients about the products you are using and suggest the products they need to purchase to maintain their nails and skin care between appointments.

❖ *Before* the polish application, ask your client to replace jewelry, locate necessary keys, pay for the service and retail products, and put on any outer clothing such as a sweater or jacket. By suggesting that your client complete these steps ahead of the polish application, chances of smudging the polish once the application is completed are decreased.

Post-service

❖ Schedule your client's next appointment. Set up the date, time, and services for your client's next appointment.

❖ Write down information on your business or appointment card.

❖ Clean up your work area and properly dispose of all used materials.

❖ Sanitize your table and any additional equipment, tools, and implements that need disinfecting. (It takes approximately 20 minutes to disinfect reusable implements.)

❖ Record service information on your client's heath and record form.

PROCEDURE 10-3

Performing a Plain Manicure

Begin Manicure

Begin working with the hand that is *not* the client's favored hand. The favored hand will need to soak longer, because it is used more often. If the client is left-handed, begin with the right hand and if the client is right-handed, begin with the left hand.

During the manicure, talk with your client about the products and procedures you are using. Suggest products the client will need to maintain the manicure between salon visits. These products might include polish, lotion, top coat, and emery boards.

❖ **NOTE:** This procedure is written for a right-handed client.

1. **Remove polish.** Begin with your client's left hand, little finger. Saturate cotton with polish remover. If your client is wearing artificial nails, use non-acetone remover to avoid damaging them. Hold saturated cotton on nail while you count to ten in your mind. Wipe the old polish off the nail with a stroking motion towards the free edge. If all polish is not removed, repeat this step until all traces of polish are gone. It may be necessary to put cotton around the tip of an orangewood stick and use it to clean polish away from the cuticle area. Repeat this procedure on each finger (Figure 10-13).

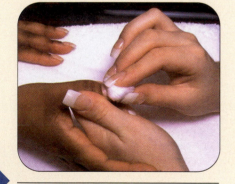

Figure 10-13 Remove polish.

10

Here's a Tip:

Roll a piece of cotton between your hands before you use it. This keeps loose cotton fibers from sticking to the nail or finger. An alternative way to remove nail polish is to moisten small pieces of cotton, called **pledgets** (**PLEJ**-ets), with nail polish remover and put them on all the nails at the same time. Pledgets absorb and do not leave a polish smear on the cuticles.

---

2. **Shape the nails.** Using your emery board or nail file, shape the nails as you and the client have agreed. Start with the left hand, little finger, holding it between your thumb and index

finger. Use the coarse side of an emery board to shape the nail. File from the right side to the center of the free edge and from the left side to the center of the free edge (Figure 10–14). Do not file into the corners of the nails (Figure 10–15). File each hand from the little finger to the thumb. Never use a sawing back and forth motion when filing the natural nail, as this can disrupt the nail platelayers and cause splitting and peeling. Never file nails that have been soaking. Soaking the nails makes them softer and easy to break or split when filed. If the nails need to be shortened, they can be cut with fingernail clippers. This will save time during the filing process.

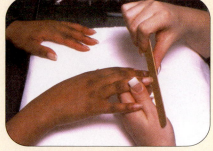

Figure 10–14 Shape nails.

3. **Soften the cuticles.** After filing the nails on the left hand place the fingertips in the fingerbowl to soak and soften the cuticles while you file the nails on the right hand.

4. **Clean nails.** Brushing the nails and hands with a sanitized nail brush cleans fingers and helps remove pieces of cuticle from the nails. Remove the left hand from the fingerbowl and brush the fingers with your nail brush. Use downward strokes, starting at the first knuckle and brushing toward the free edge (Figure 10–16).

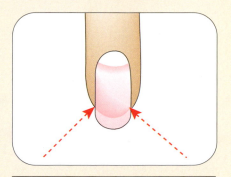

Figure 10–15 Do not file into the corners of the nail.

5. **Dry hand.** Dry the hand with the end of a fresh towel. Make sure you dry between the fingers. As you dry, gently push back the cuticle (Figure 10–17).

6. **Apply cuticle remover.** Use a cotton-tipped orangewood stick or cotton swab to apply cuticle remover to the cuticle on each nail of the left hand (Figure 10–18). Spread generously around cuticles and under the free edge of each finger. This softens and removes cuticle that remains after brushing. Now place the right hand into the fingerbowl to soak while you continue to work on your client's left hand (Figure 10–19).

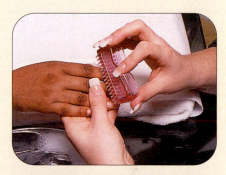

Figure 10–16 Clean nails.

7. **Loosen cuticles.** Use your orangewood stick and/or the spoon end of your steel pusher to gently push back and lift cuticle off the nails of the left hand. Use a circular movement to help lift

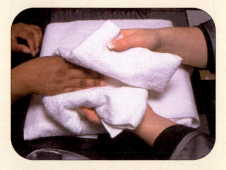

Figure 10–17 Dry hand.

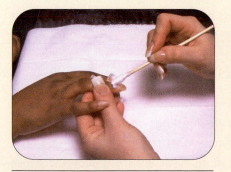

Figure 10–18 Apply cuticle remover.

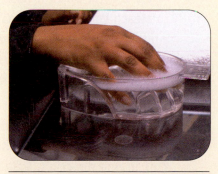

Figure 10–19 Soak hand.

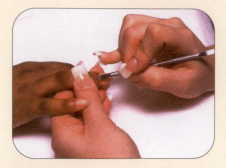

Figure 10-20 Loosen cuticle.

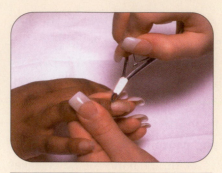

Figure 10-21 Nip cuticles.

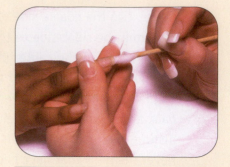

Figure 10-22 Clean under free edge.

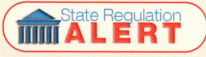

Some states do not permit nail technicians to nip cuticles or hangnails. Be guided by your instructor.

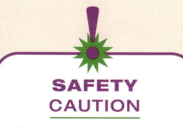

SAFETY CAUTION

When the cuticle is difficult to push back, be careful not to apply too much pressure at the base of the nail because it could damage the matrix.

10

cuticles that cling to the nail plate. The cuticle remover will probably remove enough cuticle so that you will not need to clip any. Light pressure should be used to avoid damaging the rest of the nail and the nail plate itself (Figure 10–20).

8. **Nip cuticles.** Use your cuticle nippers to nip any ragged excess cuticle or hangnails. Try to remove cuticle in one piece. You may need to wipe away excess cuticle remover to see the cuticle clearly. Be careful not to cut into the mantle, as this can cause damage and could hurt your client (Figure 10–21).

9. **Clean under free edge.** Clean under the free edge using a cotton swab or cotton-tipped orangewood stick. Remove right hand from the fingerbowl. Hold the left hand over the fingerbowl and brush a last time to remove bits of cuticle and traces of solvent. Then let client rest the left hand on the towel (Figure 10–22).

10. **Repeat steps 5–9 on right hand.**

11. **Bleach nails—optional.** After the filing and cleaning steps, if the client's nails are yellow, you can bleach them with a prepared nail bleach or apply 20 volume (6 percent) hydrogen peroxide. Apply the bleaching agent to the yellowed nail with a cotton-tipped orangewood stick. Be careful not to brush bleach on your client's skin or cuticle, because it will cause irritation. Apply several times if nails are extremely yellow. You may need to bleach certain clients' nails every time you manicure them for a period of time. Since all yellow may not fade after one service, you should plan to repeat the procedure when the client receives their next manicure.

12. **Buff with chamois buffer—optional.** To buff nails, apply dry nail polish to the nail with your orangewood stick. Buff on a diagonal from the base of the nail to its free edge (Figure 10–23). Buff in one direction, from left to right with a downward stroke

and then from right to left with a downward stroke, forming an "X" pattern (Figure 10–24). As you buff, lift the back of the buffer off the nail to prevent friction that can cause your client to experience a burning sensation. After buffing, the client should wash hands to remove any traces of abrasive or dry polish. A chamois buffer can also be used to smooth out wavy ridges or corrugated nails, but again, remember, these are not sanitizable and may not be appropriate for use in your state. A three-way buffer can be used here, then discarded.

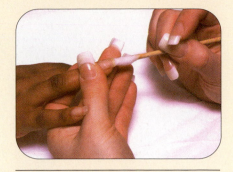
Figure 10-23 Buff nail.

Here's a Tip:

You may want to spray your client's nail with water before buffing to reduce the heat generated during buffing.

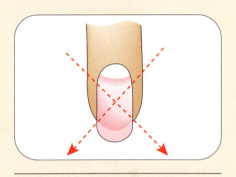
Figure 10-24 Buff nail in an "X" pattern with downward strokes.

13. **Apply cuticle oil.** Use a cotton-tipped orangewood stick or cotton swab to apply cuticle oil to each nail. Start with the little finger, left hand, and massage oil into each cuticle using a circular motion (Figure 10–25).

14. **Bevel nails.** To **bevel** (BEH-vel) the underside of the free edge, hold emery board at a 45-degree angle, and file with an upward stroke. This removes any rough edges or cuticle particles. A fine grit block buffer, which can be sanitized, may also be used (Figure 10–26).

15. **Apply hand lotion and massage hand and arm.** As a pleasant addition to your manicure before you apply polish, you can treat your client to a hand and arm massage. Apply lotion or cream to the hand and arm with a sanitary spatula. (Follow the procedure for hand and arm massage on pages 192–194.)

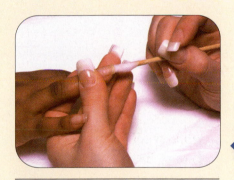
Figure 10-25 Apply cuticle oil.

16. **Remove traces of oil.** You must remove all traces of oil from the nail so the polish will adhere better. Use a small piece of cotton saturated with alcohol or polish remover, and clean the nail thoroughly.

17. **Choose a color.** If your client is undecided about the color of the nail polish, help her choose one. Suggest a shade that complements the skin tone. If the manicure and polish are for a special occasion, pick a color that matches the client's clothing. Generally, darker shades are appropriate for fall and winter and lighter shades are better for spring and summer. Always have a variety of nail polish colors available. Before

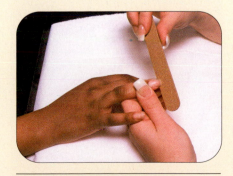
Figure 10-26 Bevel nail.

applying polish, you may ask your client to pay for the service, put on any jewelry, sweater, or jacket, and get out car keys. This will avoid smudges to the fresh polish.

18. **Apply polish.** Polish is generally applied in four coats. The first, the base coat, is followed by two coats of color and one application of top coat. The technique for polish application is used for all polishes including base coat, colored polish, and top coat. Never shake your polish bottles. Shaking will cause air bubbles to form and make the polish application rough and appear irregular. Gently roll the polish bottles between your palms to mix.

When applying the polish, remove the brush from the bottle and wipe the side away from you on the neck of the bottle. You should have a bead of polish on the end of the brush. There should be enough polish on the brush to complete the polish application for one nail without having to dip the brush back into the polish bottle, unless the nail is unusually long.

Hold the brush at approximately a 30–35-degree angle. Place it 1/16 inch away from the cuticle, starting in the center of the nail. Brush toward the free edge of the nail. Use the same technique for the entire nail. If you go back and dab at any spots you missed, the polish might appear uneven on the nail. When applying the colored polish, if you miss a small area on your client's nail you can cover this area before you apply the second coat, but definitely practice covering the entire nail each time especially near the cuticle to avoid a shadow of the polish. In addition to the finished nail appearance, the purpose of the polish application is to build layers allowing for adhesion and staying power. It is not necessary to put thick heavy coats of polish on the nail with each application. Use thin, even coats to allow for smoothness, drying, and building. On completion of the polish application the polish should appear smooth and even on the nails.

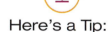

Here's a Tip:

When applying an iridescent or frosted polish, it is imperative to make sure the strokes are parallel to the sides of the nail.

Finishing the Nails

The following points provide guidelines for the proper application of nail finishes.

- ❖ **Nail strengthener/hardener—optional.** Apply this before the base coat if one is warranted.
- ❖ **Base coat.** Apply the base coat to keep polish from staining the nails and to help colored polish adhere to the nail.
- ❖ **Colored polish.** Apply two coats of colored polish. Complete your first color coat on both hands before starting the second coat. If you get polish on the cuticle, use a cotton-tipped orangewood stick saturated with polish remover to clean it off. Never use a polish corrector pen because it is unsanitary.

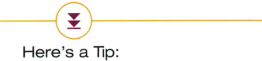

Here's a Tip:

A flat nylon bristle brush, size 6 or 8, can be used to remove polish around the cuticle area and the sides of the nail. Dip it into acetone, touch it to the towel to release excess acetone, and clean around the perimeter of the nail. Never leave this brush sitting in the acetone, as it will loosen the bristles from the ferrule. This brush can be sanitized.

- ❖ **Top coat.** Apply one coat of top coat to prevent chipping and to give nails a glossy, finished appearance.
- ❖ **Instant nail dry—optional.** Apply instant nail dry on each nail to prevent smudging and dulling, and decrease drying time.

Here's a Tip:

If you use an electric nail dryer, put one of your client's hands in the dryer while you polish the other. Put setting on cool; this helps to dry polish surface and make it less likely to smudge. Another option is to apply a UV top coat and place both hands under the UV dryer.

Five Types of Polish Application

Once you have mastered the techniques necessary to apply polish correctly and expertly, you can create the following five types of polish applications (Figure 10–27).

1. **Full coverage.** Entire nail plate is polished.
2. **Free edge.** The free edge of the nail is unpolished. This helps to prevent polish from chipping.

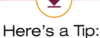

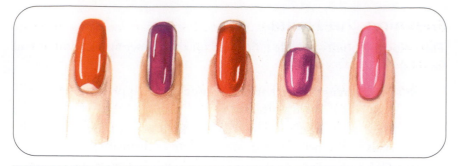

Figure 10-27 Five polish options: half moon or lunula, slimline or free walls, hairline tip, free edge, or full coverage.

3. **Hairline tip.** The nail plate is polished and 1/16 inch is removed from the free edge. This prevents polish from chipping.

4. **Slimline or free walls.** Leave 1/16 inch margin on each side of nail plate. This makes a wide nail appear narrow.

5. **Half moon or lunula.** A half moon shape, the lunula, at the base of the nail is unpolished.

Polishing is very important. It is the last step to a perfect manicure and the last thing your client sees between visits. When your client looks at her nails polished perfectly, she will admire them, and you for doing a great job. (Figure 10–28).

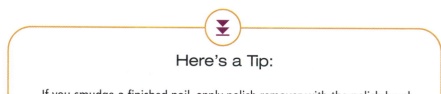

Here's a Tip:

If you smudge a finished nail, apply polish remover with the polish brush to the smudge before you put more polish on the area.

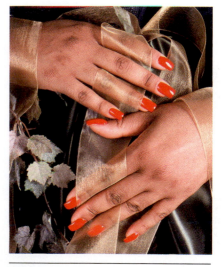

Figure 10-28 Finished manicure

Plain Manicure Post-service

Your plain manicure is complete. Refer to the post-service procedure previously explained on page 177.

◆ ◆ FRENCH AND AMERICAN MANICURES

French polish applications, as well as American polish applications, are both very popular and are often requested in the salon. These polish techniques create nails that appear clean and can have a natural appearance and are a good base for endless service designs that can be enhanced with the use of hand painted art, air-brushing, rhinestones, pearls, or stripping tape. The French, as well as the American, polish applications are sometimes referred to as a French manicure, but the procedures for both are the same as those described in the plain manicuring procedures. The only exception is the polish application. The French manicure usually has a

10

dramatic white on the free edge of the nail where the American manicure calls for a more subtle white. Perform the plain manicuring procedures up to the polish application.

1. **Apply base coat.** Apply a base coat to the nail. The base coat can be applied under the free edge as well. If the nail has pitting, striations, or ridges, use a ridge-filling base coat. It is self-leveling and will help the nail to appear smooth after the translucent polish is applied.

2. **Apply white polish.** Apply white polish to the free edge by starting at one side (usually left side of nail) and sweeping across toward the center of the free edge on a diagonal line. Repeat this on the right side of the nail. This will form a "V" shape. Some clients like this look. If not, fill the open top of the "V," so that you have an even line across the free edge. White may be applied under the free edge. Allow the white polish to dry (Figures 10–29, 10–30, and 10–31).

3. **Apply translucent polish.** Apply a sheer white, pink, natural, or peach color polish from the base to the free edge. Be careful not to get any on the cuticle. Most clients will prefer a pink shade, but choose the color according to skin tone and client preference.

4. **Apply top coat.** Apply a top coat over the entire nail plate and under the free edge if you chose to put it under the free edge previously (Figure 10–32).

For more information refer to Chapter 18, The Creative Touch.

◆ ◆ ◆ RECONDITIONING HOT OIL MANICURE

A reconditioning hot oil manicure is recommended for clients who have ridged and brittle nails or dry cuticles. It improves the hand condition and leaves the skin soft. It is suggested that a reconditioning hot oil manicure be performed once a week to add moisture to the skin and nails. Hot oil manicures are also beneficial to nail biters because it helps keep rough cuticles soft.

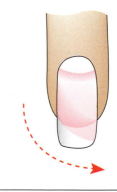

Figure 10-29 Apply white polish on free edge from the left side of the nail to the center.

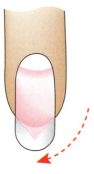

Figure 10-30 Apply white polish on free edge from the right side of the nail to the center.

10

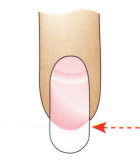

Figure 10-31 Fill in "V" with white polish.

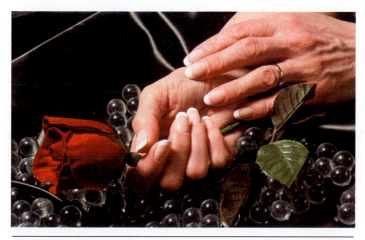

Figure 10-32 Finished French manicure

Supplies

In addition to your standard table set-up, you will need the following items.

1. **Hot oil heater.** This electric heater is used to heat the lotion in which you will soak your client's nails.

2. **Plastic cups to put in heater.** Most hot oil heaters are designed to hold a round or kidney-shaped disposable cup that is filled with lotion, cream, or oil. This cup comes in multiple packs and must be discarded after each manicure.

3. **Oil for the heater.** Most nail technicians use an oil or cream specially prepared for the hot oil heater. Olive oil or hand lotion can also be used. In this procedure, all of these items are referred to as lotion.

Reconditioning Hot Oil Manicure Pre-service

1. **Perform your Pre-service Sanitation Procedure.**

2. **Set up table.** Set up your standard manicuring table, hot oil heater with plastic cup, and lotion.

3. **Prepare heater.** Pour lotion into the disposable cup and place it in the heater.

4. **Preheat lotion.** Preheat lotion for 10-15 minutes before seating your client to begin your manicure.

5. **Greet client with a smile.**

6. **Wash hands.** Have the client remove jewelry and wash his or her hands while you are washing yours with a liquid soap.

7. **Do client consultation.**

8. **Begin manicure.** Begin working with the hand that is not the client's favored hand.

Reconditioning Warm Oil Manicure Process

During the procedure talk with your client about the products needed to maintain the manicure between salon visits.

1. **Remove old polish.**

2. **Shape nails.** Shape the nails on the hand that is not the client's favored hand.

3. **Apply warm oil with a cotton swab.** Then place fingertips in warm lotion while filing the other hand (Figure 10–33).

4. **Distribute lotion.** When you remove one hand from the lotion, place the other hand in the lotion. Spread lotion on the hand and arm to the elbow. This will give you enough lotion for the massage. If more lotion is required, use your spatula to dip more out of the heater and apply it to the hand or arm where needed.

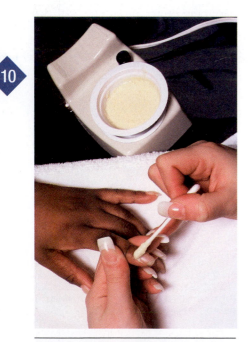

Figure 10-33 Apply warm lotion to fingertips

5. **Proceed with hand and arm massage.** Follow the procedure for hand and arm massage described on pages 192–194.

6. **Loosen cuticles.** Use orangewood stick covered with cotton at the tip to gently push back cuticles.

7. **Nip cuticles.** Use nippers to trim excess cuticle, if permitted in your state. Let client rest hand on a clean or disposable towel.

8. **Repeat on other hand.** Distribute lotion on the other hand. Proceed with steps 5–7.

9. **Wipe or have client wash hands.** If necessary, take a warm terry towel and wipe off excess lotion, or have client wash hands.

10. **Apply cold towel.** Close pores on arm and hand with a cold towel. Wrap towel around arm and hand and gently press.

11. **Remove all traces of oil from the nail plate.** Saturate cotton in alcohol or polish remover and wipe off oil from nails.

12. **Apply polish.**

13. **Complete manicure post-service.** Discard the plastic cup from the hot oil heater.

14. **Sanitize heater.** Use approved product to prepare the hot oil heater for the next client.

◆ ◆ ◆ PERFORMING A MAN'S MANICURE

Men are increasingly becoming more conscientious of the importance of having well-groomed nails and hands. Consequently, they are requesting the services offered by a professional nail technician more often. A man's manicure is executed using the same procedures as described under the plain manicure or reconditioning hot oil manicure. Follow each of the steps but omit the colored polish, replacing instead with either clear polish or buffed nails using a buffing cream.

Upon arrival, greet the client with a handshake and escort him to your station (Figure 10–34). Next, consult with the client to determine the type of service he is requesting, then complete the client information form. Evaluate the client's current nail condition to determine what products are needed (Figure 10–35).

Begin the service by removing old polish, if present from a previous manicure, and shaping the nails. The most common and requested shape for a male nail is round, but always ask if he has a preference. Next, soften the cuticles, wash and dry the nails and hands, and apply cuticle remover, following standard procedure. Most men will need a little more work done on their cuticles than women, so it may take more effort to loosen and trim cuticles.

If the client prefers, the manicure procedure can be shortened at this point by buffing the nails with a chamois buffer and buffing cream (Figure 10–36). After buffing, the client should wash hands to remove any traces of abrasive or cream.

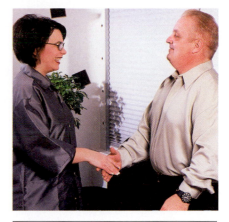

Figure 10-34 Greet client with a handshake.

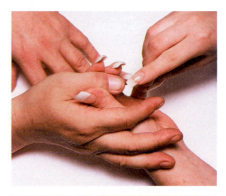

Figure 10-35 Evaluate client's nails.

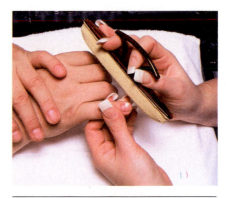

Figure 10-36 Buff nails with a chamois buffer, or a 3-way buffer.

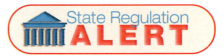

State Regulation ALERT

Buffing may not be allowed in your state. Check with your instructor or state board for regulations.

10

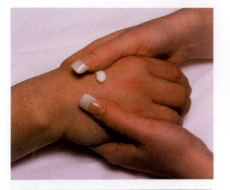

Figure 10–37 Apply hand lotion.

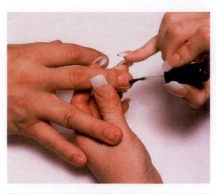

Figure 10–38 Polish with a matte or satin polish, if preferred.

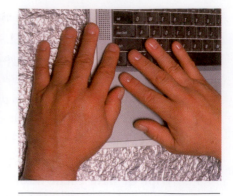

Figure 10–39 Finished man's manicure.

After cleansing and shaping nails, apply hand lotion and massage the hands and lower arms (Figure 10–37). A citrus- or spice-scented hand cream is recommended over a flowery scent for the male client.

If a polish application is requested, apply a base coat and a clear satin topcoat, followed with instant nail dry (Figure 10–38).

The man's manicure is complete (Figure 10–39).

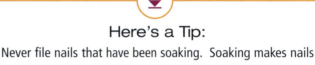

Here's a Tip:
Never file nails that have been soaking. Soaking makes nails soft and easy to break or split when filed.

B U S I N E S S **TIP**

The Male Nail

With today's emphasis on good grooming, more and more men are interested in taking care of their nails. Unfortunately, many are still not concerned about their nails. Alert the male public to your nail services by advertising in the business and sports pages of local publications. Since most men are new to nail care, don't forget to include a brief written description of what the services entail and a rundown of their benefits. You may also want to distribute flyers at local gyms, athletic stores and other places where men gather. Still another option is selling gift certificates to your female clients for their boyfriends and husbands. To make men feel more at home in your chair, have men's magazines on hand and be careful that your decor is unisex. Staying open later or opening earlier makes it easier for working men and women to schedule appointments.

◆◆ MANICURE USING AN ELECTRIC FILE

During a manicure, more advanced nail technicians may use a machine commonly referred to as an electric file. These files can be electric or battery-operated. The attachments, which are designed to work with the file, vary from manufacturer to manufacturer but most will have the following basic attachments (Figure 10–40).

- ❖ The **attachments for filing and shaping the nails** are similar to a traditional emery board. There are coarse and fine file attachments.
- ❖ The **buffer** simulates a chamois buffer, and is used to smooth corrugations and add shine to the nail.
- ❖ The **callous attachment** is designed to be used around the tip and side of the fingers to smooth any rough or callused growth.

Safety and Sanitation Requirements for Using an Electric File

- ❖ When using a file and attachments, extreme care must be taken to ensure that all safety and sanitation procedures are incorporated. Each attachment must be sanitized before use on each client, and all disposable attachments must be disposed of after use on each client.
- ❖ The file should never be used until you have received guidance from your instructor.
- ❖ Read all manufacturer's directions before using.
- ❖ Do not hold any attachments in one place on the nail area for extended times, as this will cause the client to experience a hot or burning sensation and can cause damage to the nail.
- ❖ All attachments must be checked regularly and replaced when necessary.

◆◆ PARAFFIN WAX TREATMENT

Paraffin wax treatments work by trapping heat and moisture in and opening up the pores of the skin. The heat from the warm paraffin increases blood circulation, softens and moisturizes the skin, and rejuvenates dry skin. The treatments were first used by doctors for therapeutic reasons and are beneficial for clients with arthritis. It is also considered to be a luxurious add-on service and can be safely performed on most clients.

Paraffin is a petroleum by-product that has excellent heat-sealing properties. Special units are utilized to melt solid wax into a liquid and then maintained at a temperature generally between 125 and 130 degrees Fahrenheit. When using this treatment always use the equipment that is designed specifically for the treatment. Never try to heat the wax in anything other than the proper equipment.

If proper procedures are followed, paraffin will not affect artificial nails, wraps, tips, gels, other artificial nail additions, or natural nails. There are several suggestions for the time preference to perform a paraffin treatment in conjunction with a manicure. Be guided by your instructor and your state regulations because some states require the service to be performed before the manicure.

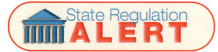

Some states do not permit the use of the electric file so be guided by your instructor and state regulations.

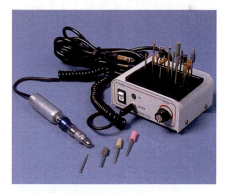

Figure 10–40 Electric file with bits

SAFETY CAUTION

Read and follow all operating instructions. Generally you should avoid giving paraffin treatments to anyone who has impaired circulation or skin irritations such as cuts, burns, rashes, warts, eczema, or swollen veins. The senior client may be more sensitive to heat because of medications or thinning skin. Patch test first to see if the temperatures can be tolerated.

PROCEDURE 10-4

Paraffin Wax Treatment (Performed Before a Manicure)

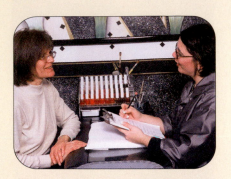

Figure 10-41 Client consultation

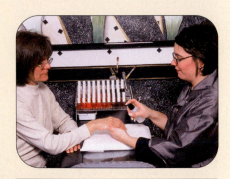

Figure 10-42 Spray hands with an antiseptic.

10

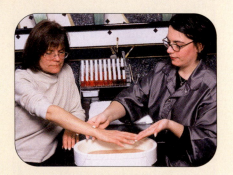

Figure 10-43 Position the hand for the dipping procedure.

1. Perform client consultation using health and record form paying particular attention to any listed health problems (Figure 10–41).

2. Wash your hands with liquid soap.

3. Have client remove his or her jewelry and place it in a safe and secure location.

4. Have client wash hands using a liquid soap and dry with a clean or disposable towel.

5. If applicable, have the client roll up long sleeves to avoid interference with the procedure and avoid damaging any clothing.

6. Check client's hands to insure that they are free from open wounds, diseases, or disorders. If it is safe to perform the procedures continue with the service.

7. Spray client's hands with an antiseptic (Figure 10–42).

8. Apply moisturizing lotion to client's hands and gently massage into the skin.

9. Test the temperature of the wax.

10. Position the hand for the dipping procedure (Figure 10–43). (The palm should be flat with the wrist slightly bent and the fingers slightly apart.)

Here's a Tip:

Several other procedures for applying paraffin wax include partially filling a plastic bag with the wax and inserting the client's hand, covering it with paraffin before placing the hand into the cloth mitt; or dipping cheesecloth into the paraffin wax and wrapping the client's hand before covering the hands with plastic and the cloth mitt.

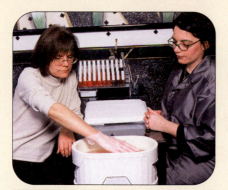

Figure 10-44 Aid the client in dipping one hand into the wax.

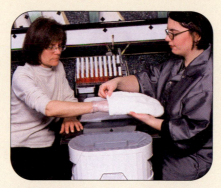

Figure 10-45 Wrap the hands in plastic wrap and cover with mitts.

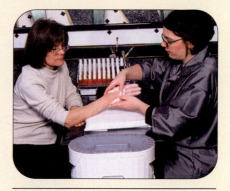

Figure 10-46 To remove the paraffin, start at the wrist, massage lightly to loosen wax, and peel paraffin from hand.

11. Aid the client in dipping one hand into the wax up to the wrist for about 3 seconds. Remove. Allow the wax to solidify before dipping again (Figure 10–44).

12. Repeat this process three to five times.

13. Wrap the hands in plastic wrap and cover with a cloth mitt (Figure 10–45).

14. Repeat this procedure on the other hand.

15. Allow the paraffin to remain on the hands for approximately 10 to 15 minutes.

16. To remove the paraffin, start at the wrist, massage the client's hands gently to loosen the wax, and peel the paraffin from the hands (Figure 10–46).

17. Properly dispose of the used paraffin.

18. Begin the manicuring procedure.

10

PROCEDURE 10-5

Paraffin Wax Treatment (Performed During a Manicure)

1. Perform all pre-sanitation and consultation required for manicuring services in Procedure 10–4, numbers 1–7.

2. Remove old polish and shape the nails to the desired shape. If any repairs are needed complete the procedures for necessary repairs before the treatment.

3. Apply moisturizer to client's hands and gently massage into skin.

4. Perform steps in Procedure 10–4, numbers 9–17.

5. Continue with the manicuring procedure.

Be guided by your instructor for the preferred time and state regulations.

◆ ◆ ◆ HAND AND ARM MASSAGE

A hand and arm massage is a service that can be offered with all types of manicures. They are included in all spa manicures, and can be performed on most clients.

A massage is one of the client's high priorities during the manicure, as most clients look forward to the soothing and relaxing effects. The massage manipulations should be executed with rhythmatic and smooth movements, never leaving the client's arm or hand untouched during the procedure.

During the manicure it is suggested that the massage be performed after the basic manicure procedure, just before the polish application. After performing a massage, it is essential that the nail plate be thoroughly cleansed to insure that it is free from any residue such as oil, cream, wax, or lotion. You can use alcohol or the selected nail polish remover to cleanse the nail.

Hand and arm massages are optional during a plain manicure but it will be to the advantage of the professional nail technician to incorporate this special, relaxing service to the client. This will show the client that you are giving them 100 percent of your time, knowledge, and service.

Hand Massage Techniques

1. **Relaxer movement.** This is a form of massage known as "joint movement." At the beginning of the hand massage the client has already received hand lotion or cream. Place client's elbow on a cushion covered with a clean towel. With one hand, brace client's arm. With your other hand, hold client's wrist and bend it back and forth slowly, about five to ten times, until you feel the client has relaxed (Figure 10–47).

2. **Joint movement on fingers.** Bring client's arm down, brace the arm with the left hand, and with your right hand start with the little finger, holding it at the base of the nail. Gently rotate fingers to form circles. Work towards the thumb, about 3–5 times on each finger (Figure 10–48).

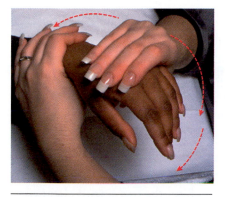
Figure 10–47 Relaxer movement

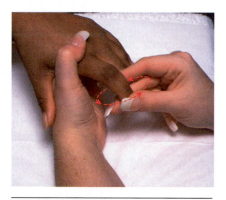
Figure 10–48 Joint movement on fingers

3. **Circular movement in palm.** This is **effleurage** (EF-loo-rahzh)—light stroking that relaxes and soothes. Place client's elbow on the cushion and, with your thumbs in the client's palm, rotate in a circular movement in opposite directions (Figure 10–49).

4. **Circular movement on wrist.** Hold client's hand with both of your hands, placing your thumbs on top of client's hand, your fingers below the hand. Move your thumbs in a circular movement in opposite directions from the client's wrist to the knuckle on back of the client's hand. Move up and down, 3–5 times. The last time you rotate up, wring the client's wrist by bracing your hands around the wrist and gently twisting in opposite directions. This is a form of friction massage movement that is a deep rubbing action and very stimulating (Figure 10–50).

5. **Circular movement on back of hand and fingers.** Now rotate down the back of the client's hand using your thumbs. Rotate down the little finger and the client's thumb and gently squeeze off at the tips of client's fingers. Go back and rotate down the ring finger and index finger, gently squeezing off. Now do the middle finger and squeeze off at tip. This restores blood flow to normal (Figure 10–51).

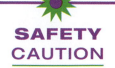

SAFETY CAUTION

DO NOT massage if client has high blood pressure, heart condition, or has had a stroke. Massage increases circulation and may be harmful to this client. Have client consult a physician first. Be very careful to avoid vigorous massage of joints if your client has arthritis. Talk with your client throughout the massage and adjust your touch to the client's needs.

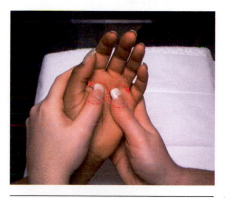
Figure 10–49 Circular movement – effleurage

10

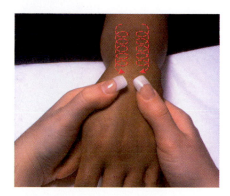
Figure 10–50 Circular movement on wrist

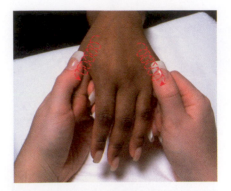

Figure 10-51 Circular movement on back of hand and fingers

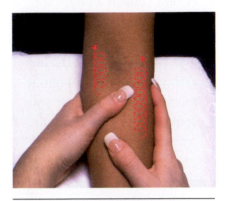

Figure 10-52 Effleurage on arms

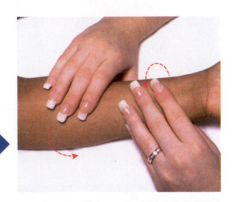

Figure 10-53 Wringing movement on arm – friction massage

Arm Massage Techniques

1. **Distribute cream or lotion.** Apply a small amount of cream to the client's arm and work it in. Work from the client's wrist toward the elbow, except on the last movement; work from the elbow to wrist, then squeeze off at fingertips, as you did at the end of hand massage. Apply more cream if necessary.

2. **Effleurage on arms.** Put client's arm down on the table, bracing the arm with your hands. Hold your client's hand palm up in your hand. Your fingers should be under the client's hand; your thumb side-by-side in your client's palm. Rotate your thumbs in opposite directions, starting at the client's wrist and working toward the elbow. When you reach the elbow, slide your hand down client's arm to the wrist and rotate back up to the elbow 3–5 times. Turn client's arm over and repeat 3–5 times on the top side of arm (Figure 10–52).

3. **Wringing movement on arm—friction massage movement.** A friction massage involves deep rubbing to the muscles. Bend client's elbow so the arm is horizontal in front of you, with the back of the hand facing up. Place your hands around the arm with your fingers facing the same direction as the arm, and gently twist in opposite directions as you would wring out a washcloth, from wrist to elbow. Do this up and down the forearm 3–5 times (Figure 10–53).

4. **Kneading movement on arm.** This technique is called the **petrissage** (**PE**-tre-sahza) **kneading movement**. It is very stimulating and increases blood flow. Place your thumb on the top side of client's arm so they are horizontal. Move them in opposite directions, from wrist to elbow and back down to wrist. This squeezing motion moves flesh over bone and stimulates the arm tissue. Do this 3–5 times. (Figure 10–54).

5. **Rotation of elbow—friction massage movement.** Brace client's arm with your left hand and, with cotton-tipped orangewood stick, apply cream to elbow. Cup elbow with your right hand and rotate your hand over the client's elbow. Do this 3–5 times. To finish the elbow massage, move your left arm to the top of the client's forearm. Gently slide both hands down the forearm from the elbow to the fingertips as if climbing down a rope. Repeat this 3–5 times (Figure 10–55).

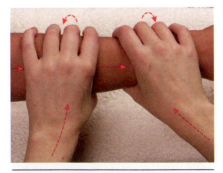

Figure 10-54 Kneading movement on arm

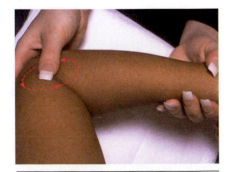

Figure 10-55 Rotation of elbow

◆ ◆ ◆ SPA MANICURE

Spa manicures are fast becoming a much-requested and desired salon service, but they are more advanced than basic manicures. Nail technicians who advance their education and knowledge necessary for implementing this service may find this area to be very lucrative. Spa manicures encompass not only extensive knowledge of nail care but skin care as well. They are known for their pampering, distinctive results, and skin-care based methods. All spa manicures should include a relaxing massage and some form of exfoliation for enhancing penetration of upscale products.

There are many types of spa manicures available, each recommended to the client after a thorough nail and skin analysis. Spa manicures have unique and distinctive names, which usually mirror the inventive ingredients and visual effects. For example, "The Rose Garden Rejuvenation Manicure" incorporates the use of hydrating rose oils and rose petals for ambiance. The "Alpha Hydroxy Acid Manicure" incorporates the use of an AHA- (alpha hydroxy acid) based products for exfoliation and skin rejuvenation.

Additional techniques that may be incorporated into a spa manicure consist of aromatic paraffin dips; aromatherapy; aromatic hand and arm massages with specifically recommended oils and lotions; reflexology; hand masks; and warm, moist towel applications. When performing any advanced procedures, which include any oils or cosmetics, always check with your client regarding their preference and any allergies.

During school it is imperative that you learn the basic procedures, as well as sanitation and safety requirements necessary for passing your state board examination. A license coupled with basic knowledge of professional manicuring procedures is the foundation needed to build advanced techniques.

Once you have completed, mastered, and become proficient in the basic manicuring procedures you can begin incorporating advanced techniques. These techniques may be learned from your instructor, through attending advanced nail care seminars, or from purchasing *Spa Manicuring for Salons and Spa* by Janet McCormick, published by Milady, an imprint of Delmar Learning.

10

bevel	To slope the free edge of the nail surface to smooth any rough edges.
chamois buffer	An implement that holds a disposable chamois, used to add shine to the nail and to smooth out corrugations or wavy ridges on nails.
effleurage	A light, continuous-stroking massage movement applied with fingers (digital) and palms (palmar) in a slow and rhythmic manner.
lacquer	A solution of nitrocellulose in a volatile solvent used on nails and hair to add shine.
mild abrasives	Substances such as tin oxide, talc, silica, and kaolin used for smoothing or sanding the nails and skin.
oval nail	A nail shape that is square with slightly rounded corners. This shape is attractive for most women's hands. The length of the nail can vary.
petrissage kneading movement	A kneading movement in massage performed by lifting, squeezing, and pressing the tissue.
pledgets	Small, fiber-free squares often used and by nail technicians to remove polish because the cotton fibers from the squares do not adhere to the nails, which can interfere with the polish application.
pointed nail	A nail shape suited to thin hands with narrow nail beds. The shape is tapered and somewhat longer; however, these nails are often weak and may break easily.
pumice powder	A hardened volcanic substance, white or gray in color, used for smoothing and polishing.
round nail	A nail shape that is slightly tapered and extends just a bit past the tip of the finger. This natural looking shape is common for male clients.
square nail	A nail shape that is completely straight across with no rounding at the edges. The length of the nail can vary.
squoval nail	A nail shape that extends slightly past the tip of the finger with the free edge rounded off.
styptic powder	An agent used to contract the skin to stop minor bleeding that may occur during a manicure.

10

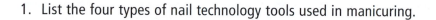

review questions

1. List the four types of nail technology tools used in manicuring.

2. Describe the procedures for sanitizing implements.

3. Briefly describe the procedures for handling blood in a salon.

4. List two types of polish removers and suggested use for each.

5. Why is having a material safety data sheet for all the products used in a salon important?

6. List the five basic nail shapes.

7. What should be considered when selecting the nail shape?

8. List and discuss the three-part procedure sequence required in manicuring.

9. Describe the correct procedures for polish application.

10. What is the purpose of a reconditioning hot oil manicure?

11. Discuss the basic differences between a female manicure and a male manicure.

12. List three safety precautions that should be taken when using the electric file.

13. What are the benefits of a paraffin wax treatment?

14. List the suggested procedures for performing a paraffin wax treatment.

15. Name five hand and arm massage techniques.

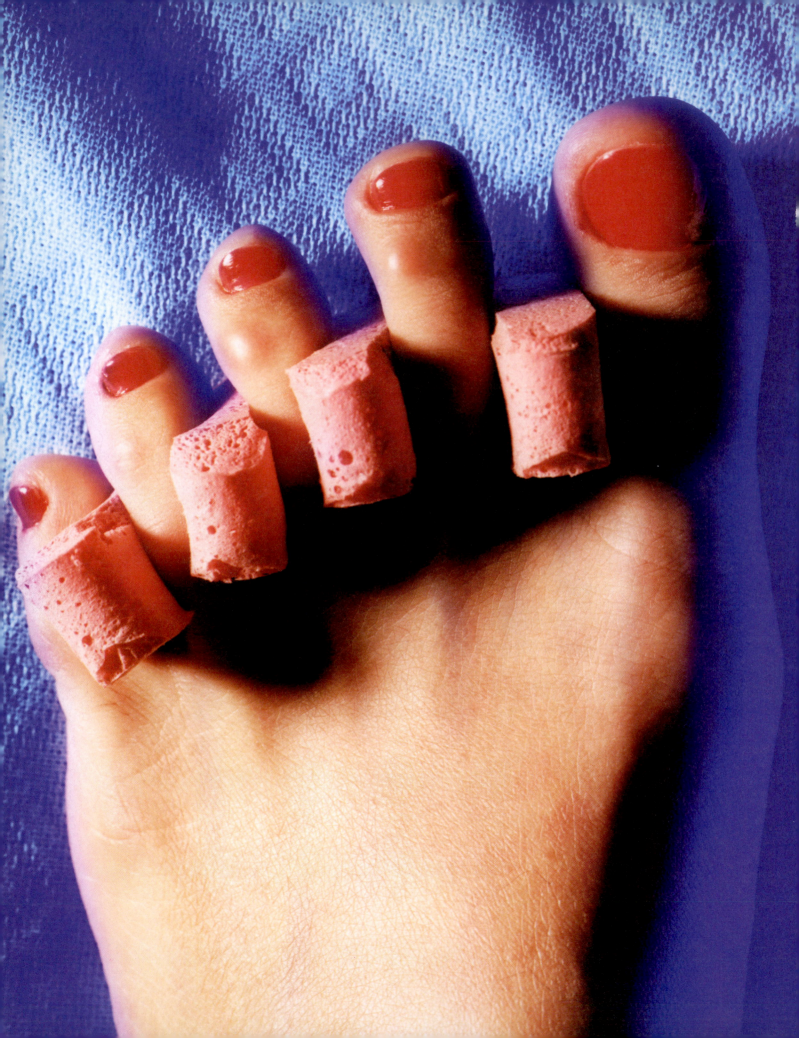

11

P E D I C U R I N G

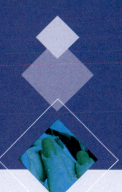

Author: Laura Mix

CHAPTER OUTLINE

Pedicure Supplies • Pedicures
Foot Massage • More About Pedicuring
Pedicure Instruments

PROCEDURES
11-1 Giving a Pedicure
11-2 The Full-service Pedicure

Learning Objectives

After you have completed this chapter, you should be able to:

1 Identify the equipment and materials needed for a pedicure and explain what they are used for.

2 List the steps in the pedicure pre-service procedure.

3 Demonstrate the proper procedures and precautions for a pedicure.

4 Describe the proper technique to use in filing toenails.

5 Describe the proper technique for trimming the nails.

6 Demonstrate your ability to perform foot massage properly.

Key Terms

Page number indicates where in the chapter the term is used.

curette
pg. 213

cuticle nippers
pg. 214

diamond nail file
pg. 214

effleurage
pg. 207

foot files (paddles)
pg. 214

friction movement
pg. 209

hand manipulation
pg. 207

massage
pg. 207

massage oils
pg. 211

nail rasp
pg. 213

pedicure
pg. 201

petrissage
pg. 207

scrubs
pg. 211

soaks
pg. 210

tapotement
pg. 207

toenail nippers
pg. 213

The information in this chapter will show you the pedicuring skills you need to care for clients' feet, toes, and toenails. A **pedicure** includes trimming, shaping, and polishing toenails as well as foot massage. Pedicures are a standard service performed by nail technicians. They are a basic part of good foot care and are particularly important for clients who are joggers, dancers, and cosmetologists. All these groups are particularly dependent on their feet for their livelihood or enjoyment. Once the client experiences the comfort and relaxation of a good pedicure they will return for more. If you really analyze it, pedicure services are for everyone. Not all clients will want or need a full pedicure service. Some only need a professional nail trimming. Do not limit yourself. Tailor your pedicure service to meet the needs of your entire clientele. Monthly pedicures should be promoted for healthy, happy feet, as they are in constant use and need routine maintenance. Proper foot care, through pedicuring, improves both personal appearance and basic foot comfort.

Here's a Tip:

When making an appointment for a pedicure, suggest that your client wear open-toe shoes or sandals so that polish will not smear. Also remind your client that hose will need to be removed before the pedicure can be performed.

◆ ◆ ◆ PEDICURE SUPPLIES

You will need the following supplies in addition to your standard manicure set-up to perform pedicures (Figures 11–1 and 11–2).

Pedicuring Station

A station includes a comfortable chair with armrests for the client, a footrest for the client, and a chair for the nail technician. Pedicure stations that combine all these items into one piece of furniture are available.

Pedicuring Stool and Footrest

A pedicuring stool is a low stool that will make it easier for you to work on your client's feet. Some pedicuring stools come with a footrest for the client, or a separate footrest can be used.

Pedicure Basin or Bath

The pedicure bath is filled with warm water and liquid soap to soak the client's feet. The bath must be large enough to completely immerse the client's feet.

Toe Separators

Foam rubber toe separators or cotton used to keep toes apart during the pedicure.

Foot File or Paddle

Used to remove dry skin or **callus** growths.

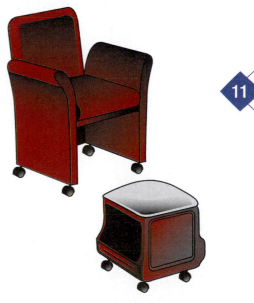

Figure 11–1 Pedicure station including client's chair, footrest and pedicuring stool

11

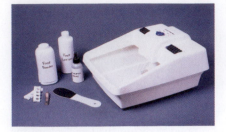

Figure 11-2 Supplies needed for pedicure

Toenail Clippers

Two types of toenail clippers are available; both are acceptable for a professional pedicure.

Antiseptic Foot Spray

This spray contains an **antifungal** (an-ti-FUN-gahl) agent as well as a mild antiseptic.

Liquid Soap

Liquid soap for pedicuring contains a soap or very mild detergent, an antifungal agent, and an antibacterial agent.

Foot Cream

Foot cream is used during foot massage. Hand lotion can also be used.

Foot Powder

Foot powder contains an antifungal agent for keeping feet dry after pedicure.

Pedicure Slippers

Disposable paper or foam slippers are needed for those clients who have not worn open-toe shoes.

◆ ◆ ◆ PEDICURES

As with other procedures, a pedicure involves three parts: the pre-service, the pedicure procedure, and the post-service. In the pre-service you will sanitize your implements, greet your client, and do a client consultation. Next you will do the steps involved in the actual procedure. Then, in the post-service, you will schedule another appointment for your client, sell the retail products you discussed during the service, sanitize your area, and disinfect all reusable implements.

Pedicure Pre-service

Your pedicure area should be close to a sink so it is convenient when you fill the pedicure baths with water.

1. Complete your pre-service sanitation procedure. (This procedure is described on pages 41–43.)

2. Your station should be set up to include a pedicuring stool, client's chair, and a footrest for your client.

3. Spread one terry cloth towel on the floor in front of client's chair to put feet on during the pedicure. Put another towel over the footrest to dry feet.

4. Set up your standard manicuring table at your pedicuring station. Add toe separators, foot file, toenail clippers, antiseptic antifungal foot spray, soap, foot cream, foot powder, and pedicure slippers to your table.

5. Fill basin with warm water. Add a measured amount of liquid soap to the bath (follow manufacturer's directions).

6. Greet your client with a smile.

7. Complete the client consultation. Use your client record/health form to record responses and observations. Check for nail disorders and decide if it is safe and appropriate to perform a service on your client. If infection or inflammation is present, refer your client to his or her physician. If athlete's foot is present, you must not perform a pedicure.

Pedicure Service

When using a manufacturer's product line, it is recommended that you follow those procedures. They have been tested and found to enhance the effectiveness of their product line. You should time the individual steps of the pedicure based on the time suggested by the manufacturer to complete the entire service economically and efficiently. Do not give the client the feeling of being rushed, but develop your procedures so there are no wasted motions. Have your instruments and products within easy reach (Figure 11–3). There should be no distractions for you or the client during the pedicure. You should, at all times during the pedicure, know what your client's expectations of the service are. Make the client feel that you have nothing more to do than to take care of their every wish. Talk to them if they want to talk, but if they want to drift off, give them the peace and tranquillity they are looking for.

Be gentle, but firm, when handling the foot. A gentle, light touch or hold will produce a tickling sensation, which is not relaxing. The client will become tense and pull away from the pedicurist during the service. Many people say that they cannot stand having their feet touched. A firm, but comfortable, grip on the foot will help to overcome this problem (Figure 11–4). In most instances, when working on the foot, it should be grasped between the thumb and fingers at the midtarsal area. This accomplishes two things. It locks the foot, making it rigid instead of being quite flexible and loose. It also allows the placing of the thumb or index finger at that point on the plantar aspect of the foot, where the two skin creases meet on the ball. This spot is usually located at the beginning of the longitudinal arch. Applying varying degrees of pressure to this point seems to have a calming effect on the client and overcomes any apprehension about someone touching his or her feet.

The actual performance of the pedicure can be divided into five basic steps: the soak, nail care, skin care, massage, and polishing of the nails (optional). Each of these steps is distinct from the other. Depending on client needs, some steps may not be necessary. For example, some clients may only need nail care. This should take approximately 15 minutes and other steps of the full pedicure may be eliminated. If you have a great massage technique, clients may want only the soak and a massage to relieve tension and stress after a day's work. Remember, be innovative and creative when it comes to your pedicure services.

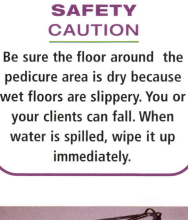

SAFETY CAUTION

Be sure the floor around the pedicure area is dry because wet floors are slippery. You or your clients can fall. When water is spilled, wipe it up immediately.

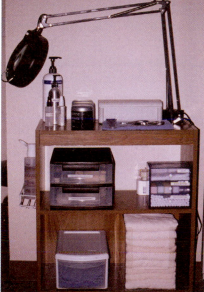

Figure 11-3 A portable pedicure supply cart containing all the instruments and supplies for a pedicure

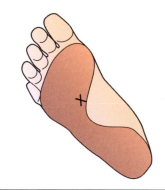

Figure 11-4 "X" marks the spot – Applying pressure to this area on a ticklish or apprehensive client will have a calming effect.

PROCEDURE 11-1

Performing a Pedicure

During the procedure, talk with your client about the products that are needed to maintain the service between salon visits. You might suggest polish, top coat, foot cream, and a foot file.

1. **Remove shoes and socks.** Ask your client to remove shoes, socks, and hose and roll pant legs to the knees.

2. **Spray feet.** Spray feet with foot spray or wipe them with antiseptic (Figure 11–5).

3. **Soak feet.** Put client's feet in soap bath for 5–10 minutes to wash and sanitize the feet before you begin the pedicure (Figure 11–6).

4. **Dry feet thoroughly.** Make sure you dry between the toes. Ask client to place both feet on the towel you have placed on the floor (Figure 11–7).

5. **Remove polish.** Remove polish from little toe on left foot working towards big toe. Repeat with the right foot (Figure 11–8).

6. **Clip nails.** Clip the toenails of the left foot so that they are even with the end of the toe (Figure 11–9). See more information on nail clippers on page 169.

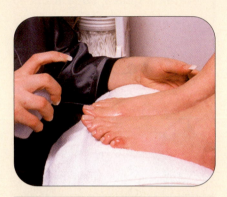

Figure 11-5 Spray feet with a foot spray.

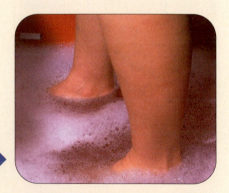

Figure 11-6 Soak feet for 5 to 10 minutes.

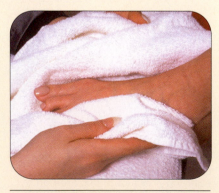

Figure 11-7 Dry feet thoroughly.

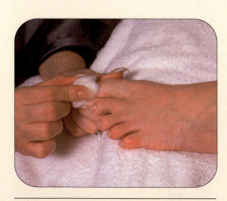

Figure 11-8 Remove old polish.

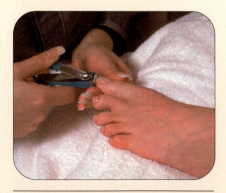

Figure 11-9 Clip toenails.

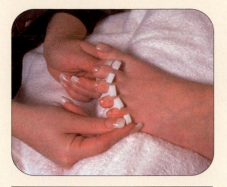

Figure 11–10 Insert toe separators.

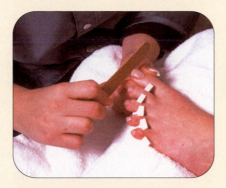

Figure 11–11 File nails.

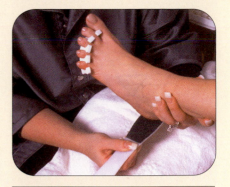

Figure 11–12 Use foot file.

7. **Insert toe separators.** Use both hands to carefully insert toe separators or cotton between the toes of the left foot (Figure 11–10). Repeat steps 6 and 7 on the right foot.

8. **File nails.** File the nails of the left foot with an emery board. File them straight across, rounding them slightly at the corners to conform to the shape of the toes. Smooth rough edges with the fine side of an emery board (Figure 11–11). Repeat this step on the other foot.

9. **Use foot file.** Use foot file on ball and heel of foot to remove dry skin and callus growths. Do not file too much because it can cause irritation and bleeding (Figure 11–12).

10. **Rinse foot.** Remove toe separators and place left foot in foot bath.

11. **Repeat steps 9 and 10 on right foot.**

12. **Brush nails.** While the left foot is in the foot bath, brush nails with nail brush. Remove the foot and dry thoroughly. Insert toe separators or cotton between toes (Figure 11–13).

13. **Apply cuticle solvent.** Use a new cotton-tipped orangewood stick to apply cuticle solvent to left foot. Begin with the little toe and work toward the big toe. You may apply solvent under free edge as well to soften excess skin beneath it (Figure 11–14).

14. **Push back cuticle.** On left foot, gently push cuticles with the new orangewood stick or metal pusher. If cuticle clipping is permitted in your state, clip only to remove a hangnail (Figure 11–15).

15. **Brush foot.** Remove toe separators. Ask your client to dip left foot into soap bath. With the left foot over the soap bath, brush with nail brush to remove bits of cuticle and solvent. Dry the foot thoroughly and place foot on towel.

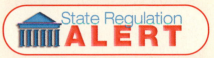

State Regulation ALERT

A credo knife is a holder that supports a razor blade. Some states do not allow the use of the credo knife to remove callus growths because it can easily cut the client's foot. Be guided by your instructor about the use of a credo knife in your state.

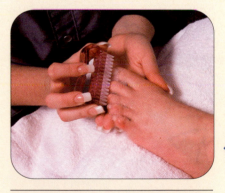

Figure 11–13 Brush nails.

11

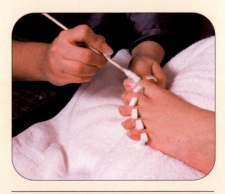

Figure 11–14 Apply cuticle solvent.

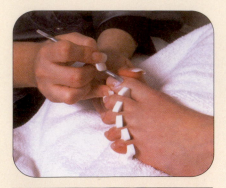

Figure 11-15 Push back cuticle.

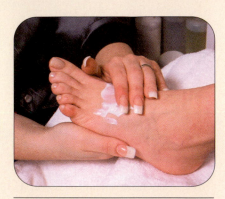

Figure 11-16 Apply lotion.

16. **Apply lotion.** Apply lotion to foot for massage. Use a firm touch to avoid tickling your client's feet (Figure 11–16).

17. **Massage foot.** Perform foot massage on the left foot. Then place foot on a clean towel on the floor. (See foot massage techniques on pages 208–209.)

18. **Proceed with steps 12–17 on the right foot.**

19. **Remove traces of lotion.** Remove traces of lotion from toenails of both feet with a small piece of cotton that has been saturated with polish remover.

20. **Apply polish.** Reinsert the toe separators. Apply base coat, two coats of color, and top coat to toenails. Spray with instant nail dry. Place feet on a towel to dry.

21. **Powder feet.** When polish is dry, powder feet before the client puts shoes on.

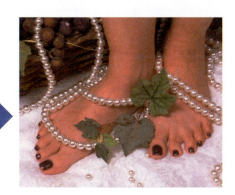

Figure 11-17 Finished pedicure

Pedicure Post-service

Your pedicure is not complete until you have performed the following (Figure 11–17).

1. **Make another appointment.** Schedule another pedicure appointment for your client.

2. **Advise client.** Advise client about proper foot care. Remind client that wearing tight shoes and very high heels can cause problems with the feet.

3. **Sell retail products.** Suggest that your client buy products you have discussed during the pedicure. Products such as polish, foot cream, and top coat help to maintain the pedicure.

4. **Clean pedicure area.** Drain or empty out basin and wipe it with a hospital-grade disinfectant to sanitize. Dry basin thoroughly. Wipe table and footrest with a hospital-grade disinfectant.

5. **Discard used materials.** Place all used materials in the plastic bag at the side of the table. If the bag is full, discard it in a closed pail.

6. **Sanitize table and implements.** Perform the complete pre-service sanitation procedure. In most states this procedure calls for 20 minutes of proper disinfection before implements can be used on the next client. Return your table to its basic set-up.

BUSINESS TIP

Pushing Pedicures During Cold Weather

It's relatively easy to sell pedicures during the summer. The weather is warm and clients want their bare or sandal-clad feet in tip-top shape. But in the winter, feet are bundled up in layers of socks and leather footgear. For many clients it's out of sight, out of mind. Pedicures should be promoted as a healthy service for the feet. They should also be promoted as a part of good grooming and a preventative health aid. Pedicures are not just a summer thing to do for the feet. Monthly pedicures should be promoted for healthy, happy feet. Feet that are confined uncomfortably in boots and often get wet from snow and sleet, can suffer from dryness, cracking, fatigue, and cramping. Remind clients that feet are in daily use and they need routine maintenance, for both men and women, even in winter.

◆ ◆ ◆ FOOT MASSAGE

Massage is defined in the medical dictionary as "a method of manipulation of the body by rubbing, pinching, kneading, tapping, etc." The art of massage has probably been around since the beginning of time. Touch is the first of our senses to develop and under normal circumstances the last to diminish. Most of us enjoy being touched and the art of massage takes touching to a higher level. Foot massage during a pedicure stimulates blood flow and is relaxing to the client.

There are three basic forms of **hand manipulation** utilized in therapeutic massage. These consist of

- ❖ light or hard stroking movements called **effleurage**.
- ❖ compression movements called **petrissage**, which includes kneading, squeezing, and friction.
- ❖ percussion or **tapotement**, where the sides of the hands are used to strike the skin and underlying tissues in rapid succession.

Effleurage relaxes muscles, and improves circulation to the small, surface blood vessels. It is also thought to increase blood flow toward the heart. Petrissage helps to increase movement by stretching muscles, tendons, and any scar tissue present from previous injuries. Tapotement is also a technique for improving circulation.

There are a number of massage styles and techniques. No matter what technique you use, perfect it so that it becomes second nature to you. Study and practice different methods to individualize the massage for different clients. During this part of the pedicure, be keenly aware of your client's needs and meet those requirements by giving a massage that fulfills them.

SAFETY CAUTION

DO NOT massage if client has high blood pressure, heart condition, or has had a stroke. Massage increases circulation and may be harmful to such a client. Have your client consult a physician before receiving a massage, then request a doctor's release.

The amount of pressure applied during the massage should be only as deep as is comfortable for you and your client. Ask the client whether they would like more or less pressure. Be aware of what areas or parts of the massage the client enjoys most and work those areas more. Work toward the heart to facilitate circulation. Keep your wrists straight in order to reduce stress and strain on yourself. Do not favor your dominant hand; always remembering to alternate the pressures from one to the other. Attention to the fine details will make your massage stand out from others.

Foot Massage Techniques

These techniques and illustrations provide directions for massage of the left foot.

1. **Relaxer movement to the joints of the foot.** Rest client's foot on footrest or stool. Grasp the leg just above the ankle with your left hand. This will brace the client's leg and foot. Use your right hand to hold left foot just beneath toes and rotate foot in a circular motion (Figure 11–18).
2. **Effleurage on top of foot.** Place both thumbs on top of foot at instep. Move your thumbs in circular movements in opposite directions down the center of the top of the foot. Continue this movement to the toes. Keep one hand in contact with foot or leg, slide one hand at a time back firmly to instep and rotate back down to toes. This is a relaxing movement. Repeat 3–5 times (Figure 11–19).
3. **Effleurage on heel (bottom of foot).** Use the same thumb movement that you did in the previous massage technique. Start at the base of the toes and move from the ball of the foot to the heel, rotating your thumbs in opposite directions. Slide hands back to the top of the foot. This is a relaxing movement. Repeat 3–5 times (Figure 11–20).

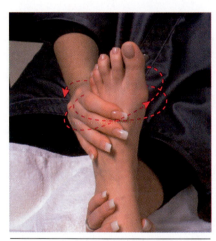

Figure 11-18 Relaxer movement to the joints of the foot

11

Figure 11-19 Effleurage on top of foot

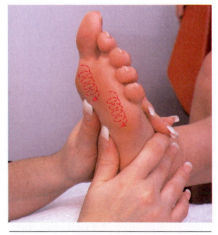

Figure 11-20 Effleurage on heel

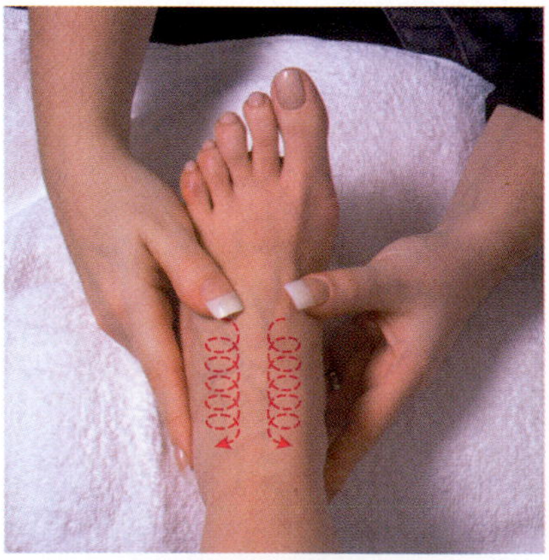

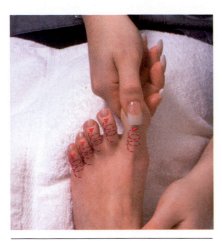

Figure 11–21 Effleurage on toe

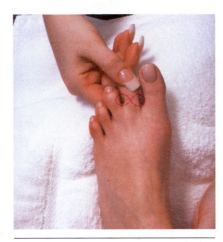

Figure 11–22 Joint movement for toes

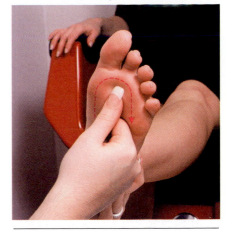

Figure 11–23 Thumb compression – "friction movement"

4. **Effleurage movement on toes.** Start with the little toe, using thumb on top and index finger on bottom of foot. Hold each toe and rotate with thumb. Start at base of toe and work toward the end of the toes. This is relaxing and soothing. Repeat 3–5 times (Figure 11–21).

5. **Joint movement for toes.** Start with the little toe and make a figure eight with each toe. Repeat 3–5 times (Figure 11–22).

6. **Thumb compression—friction movement.** Make a fist with your fingers, keeping your thumb out. Apply firm pressure with your thumb and move your fist up the heel toward the ball of the foot. Work from the left side of foot and back down the right side toward the heel. As you massage over the bottom of the foot, check for any nodules or bumps. If you find one, be very gentle because the area may be tender. This movement stimulates the blood flow and increases circulation (Figure 11–23).

7. **Metatarsal scissors (a petrissage massage movement, kneading).** Place your fingers on top of foot along the metatarsal bones with your thumb underneath the foot. Knead up and down along each bone by raising your thumb and lower fingers to apply pressure. This promotes flexibility and stimulates blood flow. Repeat 3–5 times (Figure 11–24).

8. **Fist twist compression (a friction movement, deep rubbing).** Place left hand on top of foot and make a fist with your right hand. Your left hand will apply pressure while your right hand twists around the bottom of the foot. This helps stimulate blood flow. Repeat 3–5 times up and around foot (Figure 11–25).

9. **Effleurage on instep.** Place fingers at ball of foot. Move fingers in circular movements in opposite directions. Massage to end of each toe, gently squeezing the tip of each toe (Figure 11–26).

10. **Percussion or tapotement movement.** Use fingertips to perform percussion or tapotement (tah-POT-mynt) movements to lightly tap over the entire foot to reduce blood circulation and complete massage.

SAFETY CAUTION

If the client has had any form of foot surgery, inquire as to whether or not massage is an acceptable procedure.

11

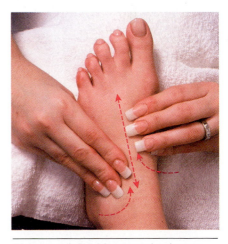

Figure 11–24 Metatarsal scissors

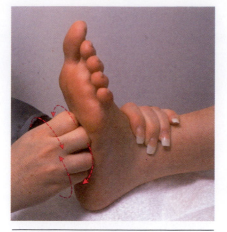

Figure 11-25 Fist twist compression

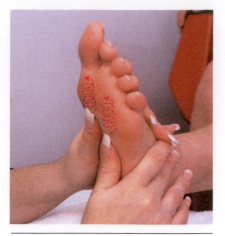

Figure 11-26 Effleurage on instep

◆ ◆ MORE ABOUT PEDICURING

The basic step-by-step pedicure procedure is a necessary learning tool to help you master a warranted and valuable service. There is, however, additional information needed to enable you to go beyond the basics. The products, implements, and equipment you will need to perform a pedicure are an important part of the service. The basic pedicure procedure is just the beginning. There is much more to come. When you become more proficient and begin to customize a pedicure, the following information will be indispensable in helping you accomplish that end.

Just as there are "systems" for nail enhancement products, so are there pedicure systems or lines available from many manufacturers of professional nail products. These manufacturers produce a complete line of products for the professional pedicure. It is recommended that you check out all of these lines. Compare them with each other and decide for yourself which is best for your clients. The educational support and commitment of the company is important in making this decision. Those companies that offer classes and training in the use of their line will be available when you have specific questions about individual client problems or their lines in general.

There are at least three basic product classes necessary for the pedicure service. Then, add-on products are available to enhance the pedicure service. The three basic product classes consist of

1. soaks.

2. scrubs.

3. massage preparations.

Soaks

Soaks are products used in the pedicure bath to soften the skin of the foot. A good soak should contain a gentle soap to sanitize the foot, moisturizers or hydrating agents, and a surface-active substance to allow for deeper penetration of the active ingredients. Dead sea salts are one of the ingredients often found in the better soaking agents. Because large amounts of therapeutic minerals, such as potassium, magnesium, calcium, and sodium, are found in soaks, they contribute to super hydration of the skin. They also contain antioxidants, to help counterbalance the surfactants, which can be harsh to the skin.

Natural antiseptics, such as tea tree oil, may be used as well as other antiseptic agents. If a soap is used it should be gentle on the skin. It should have more of a shampoo quality rather than that of a harsh cleaner. Other natural oils are used for their moisturizing and aromatherapy qualities. The soak really sets the stage for the rest of the pedicure. Be sure to purchase the one that meets all the requirements necessary to start the pedicure off on the right foot, so to speak.

Scrubs

Scrubs are used to help in the removal and smoothing of the dry, flaky skin and callus, which builds up on the foot. The scrub should be abrasive in order to do the job. However, if it is too abrasive, it will remove the living skin from the hands of the pedicurist who will be using it repetitively. A good scrub contains more softening agents, such as alpha hydroxy acids or oils, to further soften and penetrate the non-living areas of skin that need removal. The scrub will also contain an exfoliating agent, which acts as an abrasive. This helps to mechanically remove non-living tissue from the foot. Sea sand, ground apricot kernels, pumice, quartz crystals, and plastic beads are all exfoliating agents found in pedicure scrubs. Agents such as glycerin are also found in scrubs. These tend to bind with the flakes of tissue and assist in pulling them off the underlying living skin during the exfoliating process. Vitamins, essential aroma oils, and other moisturizers, which help to condition the skin, may also be found in various scrub preparations.

Massage Preparations

Massage oils are used to lubricate, moisturize, and invigorate the skin. They allow the hands of the pedicurist to glide soothingly over the skin during the massage part of the pedicure. They also help to promote a general feeling of relaxation and well-being in the client. A quality massage oil will not absorb into the skin too quickly. The molecular size of the oil determines the rate of absorption. Lanolin and mineral oil are examples of large-molecule oils. Most quality massage oils are a blend of therapeutic oils, which promote skin health. Jojoba oil and vitamin E oil are examples. Aromatherapy oils may also be incorporated for their relaxing and calming effects. Tea tree oil is often included for its antiseptic and antifungal qualities. The pedicurist, like some massage therapists, may want to formulate their own massage oil. Some massage therapy supply stores have base massage oils to which different essential or aromatherapy oils can be added. A number of massage oils can be formulated in this manner to match individual client needs. This will give a customized quality to the pedicure.

Massage lotions have smaller molecules, thus, are fast absorbing. These may be used at the end of the massage to further moisturize and invigorate the skin. Properly formulated, they help retard the growth of callus. Tea tree, vitamin E, jojoba, and other similar oils are also often found in massage lotions.

Add-on Products

These products are used to enhance and expedite the pedicure experience. Highly concentrated callus softeners are offered to help soften and remove the excess callus, which builds up around the heels and over pressure points. A 20 percent alpha hydroxy acid preparation is an example of this. It is applied directly to the callus and allowed to soak in to soften the excess callus buildup. This makes the callus easier to remove with the exfoliates and callus paddles.

Masks composed of mineral clays, sea extracts, hydrating alpha hydroxy acids, aromatherapy oils, and other therapeutic skin softeners, give the feet a special "mud facial" experience. These seem to be excellent products and the clients really enjoy them.

Hot paraffin baths for the feet are an excellent addition to the pedicure. The paraffin bath stimulates circulation and the deep heat helps to reduce inflammation and promote circulation to the affected joints. Aromatherapy oils can also be incorporated into the bath. Clients feel pampered and the hot paraffin wax service adds to the relaxation of the pedicure experience. **Do not** give this service to clients with impaired circulation, loss of feeling, or other diabetic-related problems. The hot wax may cause burns or skin breakdown in these situations.

Other items necessary for the best-ever pedicure could include

❖ pedicure slippers—Disposable paper or foam slippers are needed for those clients who have not worn open toe shoes.

❖ pedicure sandals—Sandals, with toe separators incorporated in their design, can be purchased by the client and brought in with them every time they have a pedicure.

◆ ◆ ◆ PEDICURE INSTRUMENTS

The use of quality, professional instruments and equipment by the nail professional is very important. A quality instrument will last the user many years and the proper tools make the job easy. This is particularly true when it comes to working on the foot. Improper, modified instruments used in the performance of foot services, by the nail technician, can easily cause injury to toenails and the soft tissues of the foot. The use of instruments and equipment made specifically for the purpose is, therefore, a major requirement in providing quality, professional foot services to your clients. Instruments and equipment made exclusively for pedicures will allow the nail technician to provide a safer service to clients. In addition, appropriate instruments and equipment will make foot services easier and quicker.

11

These services, thus, become a much more pleasant experience for the nail technician as well as the client and your client will view you as the professional you are. Additional instruments recommended for providing foot services include the following:

Toenail Nippers

These are not the modified enlarged fingernail clippers that are sold as toenail clippers. These are professional instruments made for cutting toenails. **Toenail nippers** come with either curved or straight jaws (Figures 11–27 and 11–28). The jaws of the nipper should come to a fairly fine point. Some come with a blunt point, which makes it very hard to trim out the small corners of a plicatured nail (one that is folded in along the margin). Yes, in certain circumstances a small corner of the nail should be trimmed out! Trimming the corner of a toenail, if done properly, which this nipper allows you to do, does not cause an ingrown toenail.

Curette

A **curette** is a small, spoon-shaped instrument that, if carefully used, allows for the removal of debris from the nail margins (Figures 11–29 and 11–30). With experience, the nail technician will find that it becomes an extension of the fingers in feeling for any rough edges or "hooks," which may have been left after the trimming process. Properly used, the curette is the ideal instrument for cleaning the debris from and feeling along the nail margins. In most clients, you will only have to use it along the margins of the great toenails. Only occasionally is it necessary to clean along the lesser toenail margins. Most curettes are quite sharp on their edges, while others are dull. A double-ended curette, which has a 1.5mm diameter on one end and a 2.5mm diameter on the other, is recommended. Some are made with a small hole making the curette easier to clean after it has been used. The curette, for the purpose of nail care, should not be used to cut out any tissue or debris adherent to the living tissues along the nail margin. The nail technician must, for safety purposes, use a curette that is not sharpened for the purpose of cutting tissue.

Nail Rasp

This metal file, or **nail rasp** as it is called in the medical field, is constructed so that it only cuts or files in one direction. The cutting part of the instrument is about 1/8th-inch wide and about 3/4-inch long (Figure 11–31). It is attached to a metal handle in a straight or angled manner. The angled file is recommended because it is easier to use along the nail groove.

This instrument smooths the edges of the nail in the nail groove. It should be placed in the nail groove against the free edge of the nail plate. The file is then gently pulled along the edge of the nail toward the end of the toe. This will smooth any rough edges of the nail plate, which may have been produced during the trimming or curetting procedures. This process

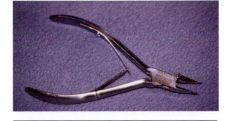
Figure 11-27 5-1/2-inch nail nippers with straight jaws

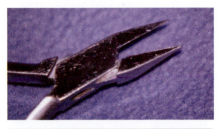
Figure 11-28 Close-up of jaws of nail nipper

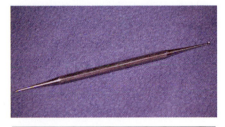
Figure 11-29 Double-ended curette

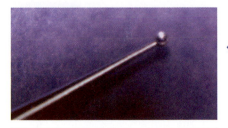
Figure 11-30 Close-up of curette

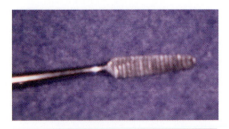
Figure 11-31 Close-up of nail rasp

11

may be repeated a number of times to make sure there are no rough edges remaining along the nail margin.

The nail rasp, like the curette, is mainly used along the nail margins of the great toenail. The lesser toenails do not usually require filing along their margins. By removing any sharp edges along the nail margin, the possibility of the nail cutting into the soft tissues is reduced. As you become proficient in the use of this file you will find it to be an invaluable and time-saving instrument. Properly used, it will add the professional finishing touch required in the care of toenails.

Diamond Nail File

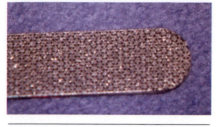

Figure 11-32 Close-up of diamond nail file

To file the free edge of the toenails and, in some cases, to thin them, a **diamond nail file** is an excellent instrument (Figure 11–32). It is metal with diamond dust impregnated into the metal. It comes in coarse, medium, and fine grits. For the toenails, the coarse grit seems to work best. It is constructed in such a manner that it does not fill up with nail debris during use. This file has the same shape as nail files used by the nail technician for fingernail filing. It is thin and flexible and can be used in the same manner as other nail files. *Major advantages of this file are that it is easily sanitized and can be kept in disinfectant solutions.* It, therefore, can be used safely on many clients. Because the file is metal and the cutting surface is made from diamond dust, it is not easily worn out, making the initial expense extremely cost effective.

Foot File or Paddle

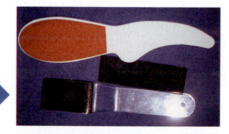

Figure 11-33 Two types of foot paddles and a replacement screen for one of them

Foot files or **paddles** are large sanding files made to remove dry, flaky skin and smooth callus from the foot. They come in many different grits and shapes (Figure 11–33). The main disadvantage is that most are not easily disinfected. You should pick a file that is advertised as being "sanitizable" and can be immersed in the disinfecting solution many times without falling apart.

A foot paddle that has a disposable, screen-like, abrasive sanding surface is available. This paddle is easily taken apart so the individual parts can be sanitized and disinfected, and a new abrasive surface can be applied when necessary.

Cuticle Nippers

This same instrument used for hand services, can be used for foot services. **Cuticle nippers** must be used carefully to avoid cutting the living skin. *Only on rare occasions* should it be used as its name implies—to cut cuticles. Sharp, close cutting of cuticles on toenails is not recommended for the same reasons discussed previously. This instrument can also be used to remove a small portion of the nail corner in the lesser toes (two through five). Having smaller jaws than the nail nippers described previously, it is easier to use, when necessary, on the smaller toenails.

Files

The electric file is an option when performing a nail service on thick, malformed toenails. Files come in four basic types: hand-held, cable-driven, belt-driven, and micromotor types. The secret of using any of these is to have a light touch and let the drill bit do the work for you. Improper use of the file by an untrained operator will cause injuries to the nail unit. With proper training and careful use, the file becomes an extension of the user's fingers, just as other instruments used to perform nail services.

Pedicure Equipment

When you enter the work force, your place of employment will undoubtedly provide the pedicure equipment needed to service your client. This section will discuss various large equipment necessary to provide a pedicure service. This can be as simple as a folding chair and a plastic dishpan to the elegant, fully plumbed pedicure unit. As with instruments, quality, well-manufactured, comfortable equipment will be cost effective and also will help to promote your foot care services. If you are uncomfortable and awkward in the provision of the service, this feeling will be transferred to your clients. When you are relaxed, your client can then relax and enjoy the pedicure. Let us discuss equipment that, in general, is not for home use.

Pedicure Carts

These units are basically a stool on wheels (Figure 11–34). The pedicurist straddles and sits on the cart. There are many different designs and manufacturers of these carts. Be sure the height of the cart is such that you will look down on the foot. This will tend to keep your back straighter and you will be more relaxed when giving the service. There is usually a built-in footrest for the client's feet. There are also drawers and shelves for storage of instruments and pedicure products. Some of these units even include a space for the footbath on the front of the cart. Most units are compact and take up little space.

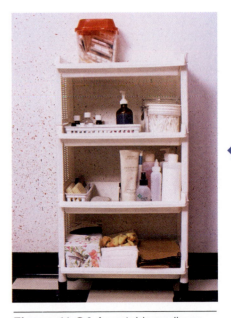

Figure 11–34 A portable pedicure cart has a place for the foot bath, storage area for supplies, and an adjustable foot rest.

Water Baths

There are small, portable water baths with vibrators and heaters built into them. They must be manually filled and emptied after each client service. If you use the portable type, be sure to have a comfortable chair or lounge in a private or semi-private area for the client to sit in while receiving the pedicure. Also, the chair should be on a platform to save your back during the service.

A step above the portable water bath is the custom-built pedicure unit, which has a removable foot bath built into the unit (Figures 11–35 and 11–36). These are constructed with both the client and the nail technician in mind. They add to the service and make it much easier for the nail technician to perform the pedicure. There are also pedicure units that have a pedestal design with a removable water bath.

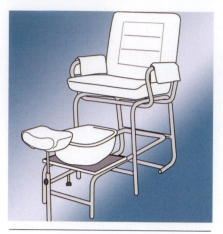

Figure 11–35 A semi-throne type pedicure station, well-built and affordable. It has an adjustable foot rest and a place for the water bath.

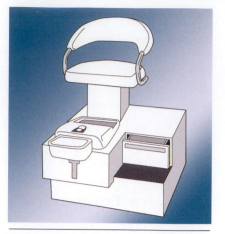

Figure 11–36 A pedicure center is well constructed with a removable foot bath, storage drawer, and adjustable foot rest.

There are portable foot basins available that have built-in whirlpools and can be filled from the sink (Figure 11–37). After the service, they are drained by pumping the water back into the sink drain. They have built-in foot rests and areas for storage of the pedicure materials. They add an extra touch to the service by the gentle massaging action of the whirlpool. These units can also have both a client's chair and the pedicurist's chair. These have been specifically designed to compliment the portable foot basin.

The ultimate pedicure foot bath is the fully plumbed pedicure basin chair (Figure 11–38). These units are not portable. The unit is attached to both hot and cold water as well as to a drain. If a floor drain is not available a pump option can be purchased to pump the water to an available drain. The units may also have a built-in massage feature as well as a warmer in the client chair, which adds to the relaxation of the pedicure. The units are easily sanitized and disinfected.

No matter which water bath unit you have, be sure the seat for yourself fits both you and the unit. If at all possible, look for a stool or chair that is adjustable for height and gives good support. Your back will love you for it.

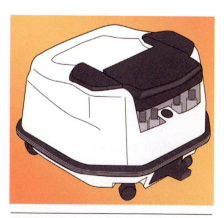

Figure 11–37 A fully self-contained portable foot basin

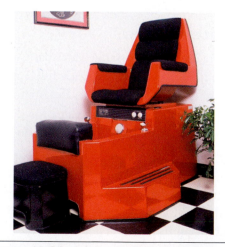

Figure 11–38 A fully-plumbed throne-type pedicure unit comes with many options including a massage unit built into the client chair.

PROCEDURE 11-2

The Full Service Pedicure

1. **The soak.** This service starts the procedure. It is important to soften and prepare the skin for what is to follow. It sets the stage, so to speak, for what is to come. The water should be about 104°F. If the client's circulation is compromised, it should not be over 100°F. Place the soaking product into the water according to manufacturer's recommendation. Allow the client to soak for approximately five minutes to sanitize the foot and begin the removal of dry skin and callus. You have time during this part of the service to make sure everything you will need for the rest of the pedicure is in place. You do not want to stop and hunt for something during the pedicure process.

2. **Nail care follows soaking.** Remove one foot from the bath and dry it with a towel. Remove any old nail polish from the toenails. At this point, if needed, apply callus and cuticle softeners to any areas of callus build up on the foot, as well as to the cuticles. This will give the product time to work while you care for the nails.

   Next, the curette is used, as an extension of the fingers, to gently push the soft tissue folds away from the lateral nail walls (Figure 11–39). This allows you to visually inspect the nail so that it can be trimmed without injuring the client. If there is extra build up of debris along the margin, blocking your view of the nail, it should be gently removed with the curette. To use this instrument, place the rounded side of the spoon toward the living skin. This allows the edge of the instrument to fall against the side or edge of the nail. A gentle scooping motion is then used along the nail plate to drag any loose debris or callus out of the nail groove. A gentle pressure against the nail plate and along the free edge of the nail margin is all that is necessary to accomplish the removal of the built-up debris. The pressure of this debris is quite uncomfortable if left in place. You may need to repeat this scooping motion a number of times to adequately remove enough of the loose debris. **Do not** use this instrument to dig into the soft tissues along the nail fold. These tissues are thin and may be easily injured. Any callus or other debris attached to the soft tissue, which is not easily removed in the manner described, should be removed by a podiatrist.

   The nails should now be carefully trimmed using the toenail nippers. The nippers are used like a pair of scissors (Figure 11–40). The nail is trimmed in a number of small cuts to avoid flattening it out and injuring the hyponychium during the process. Place the nipper over the free nail edge and slightly tilt

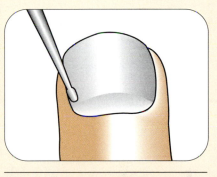

Figure 11-39 The curette is used as an extension of the fingers to gently push the soft tissue away from the nail margin.

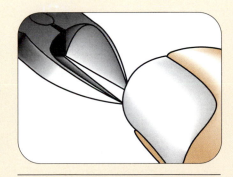

Figure 11-40 The nail nippers are used like a pair of scissors, making a series of small cuts across the nail.

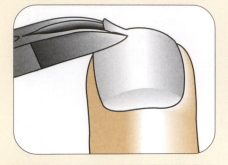

Figure 11-41 Trim the nail at a 45-degree angle. Notice the tilt of the nipper to reduce the possibility of injury to the underlying soft tissue.

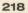

11

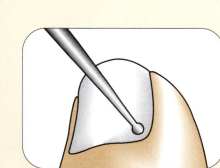

Figure 11-42 The curette is also used to remove the dead cuticle on the top of the nail plate.

the top of the nipper back toward the nail plate. This reduces the possibility of cutting the soft tissues of the hyponychium under the free edge (Figure 11-41). Give the nipper a slight squeeze before actually cutting the nail. The reaction of the client to this squeeze will tell you if you are cutting too deep. If you get a reaction, reposition the nipper on the nail and start the process over.

In most instances, you will trim the lesser toenails straight across, and later remove the small sharp corners with the file if they do not turn down into the soft tissue margins. The big toenail is usually the most challenging to trim. The nail margins, in most instances, turn down into the nail groove and, as a result, soft tissue debris, lint, soap, and other material build up occurs. Trim the great toenail just as described for the lesser toes but pay particular attention to the nail margins. Gently slip the point of the nipper under the sharp corner of the margin and trim it off at about a 45-degree angle. Remember not to trim it back too far. If you do, you will leave a "hook" of nail or a rough edge on the nail margin. If you can see the fine point of the nipper extending slightly beyond the edge of the nail before you cut it, you should not get into trouble. If you do leave a "hook" or rough edge it must be removed and smoothed to avoid an infection, which will most likely occur when the sharp point of nail penetrates the soft tissue. If the "hook" is not deep in the margin, gently remove it with the nipper. If it is difficult to remove with the nipper, move on to the next step and remove it with the small nail rasp or curette.

After the nails have been trimmed with the nipper, go back with the curette and gently remove any debris left along the nail margins. This is done, as previously described, by placing the cupped part of the curette against the lateral nail wall and edge of the nail. Gently draw the curette along the nail. This process may have to be repeated a number of times. In most instances this will remove an adequate amount of the non-living debris from the nail margins, thus, relieving the pressure and making the client comfortable. During this process also check the nail margins for rough areas and any "hooks" that may have been left behind after the trimming.

The curette is also used to remove dry cuticle from the top of the nail plate (Figure 11-42). The cuticle at the eponychium should not be pushed back on toenails. Any small break in the seal created by the true cuticle attachment to the nail plate at this level will allow fungal or bacterial infections to occur. To remove the cuticle from the top of the nail, the curette is drawn over the plate away from the eponychium in a sweeping "C" type motion from the nail fold toward the center of the nail plate. This motion is then repeated from the opposite side of the nail plate. You will need to repeat these motions a number of times to remove all of the cuticle debris from the top of the nail plate. Be careful not to injure the eponychium during this process.

The small nail rasp is then used to smooth the edges of the nail margins along the nail grooves (Figure 11–43). The rasp is made for this purpose. It is narrow and will only file the nail in one direction. It can be used to remove, smooth, and round off any sharp points present along these margins. Do not use it as a probe, but gently draw it along the edge of that portion of the nail that you have just trimmed. Small, short strokes with the file, from proximal to distal (back to front), will accomplish the task.

The diamond file should then be used to finally shape and smooth the rest of the nail. If the nail is thick, the file is also used to thin the nail plate. This file is used in the same manner as your regular nail files. Because of its construction, the diamond file is easily sanitizable and can be kept in the disinfectant solution. If you do not have a diamond file you can use the nail files that you use for fingernail services. However, remember that these files are not disinfectable and should be discarded after use. If some of the nails are quite thick you may choose to use the electric drills, discussed previously, to mechanically reduce the thickness. *You should only use the drill if you have had hands-on training in its use. This training must be provided by someone who is qualified and knowledgeable about the use of the drill for thinning the toenail.* The drill used by a qualified nail technician is a safe, timesaving tool, when it comes to thinning a thick toenail.

After completing the nail service on one foot place it back in the soak and repeat the process described above on the other foot. The entire nail trimming process should take approximately 15 minutes.

3. **Skin Care.** Care of the skin is the next step in the full service pedicure. The skin has been softened by the soaking solution. The thicker areas of dry skin and callus have been softened with the extra strength callus softeners during the nail trimming procedure. The exfoliative scrubbing product is now used to reduce and remove the unwanted skin. One foot is again removed from the bath and the scrub is liberally applied to the foot. Using a massaging motion, the pedicurist scrubs the dry skin off the foot. Use extra friction on the heels and other areas where more callus and dry skin builds up. During this process, the abrasive foot paddle is used to smooth and thin more of the thicker areas of callus. Remember that callus protects the underlying skin from irritation and is there for a purpose. Remove only enough to make the client comfortable. *Calluses should be softened and smoothed—not excessively removed.* You may need to educate your client about callus formation and the protective function it provides. Also discuss products for home use to help soften and condition calluses. The foot is then rinsed in the bath. Do not forget to clean between the toes. These areas are often missed.

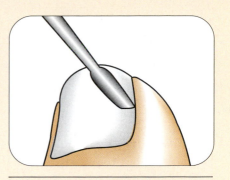

Figure 11–43 The small nail file or rasp is used to gently smooth the nail margin, removing any rough edges or hooks left behind after the trimming process.

11

SAFETY CAUTION

Hot wax services should not be provided to clients with poor circulation or to diabetic clients without a doctor's release.

If a mask product is to be used, this is the time to use it. After rinsing and cleaning the foot, apply the mask according to manufacturer's recommendations. Wrap the foot in a clean towel and place it on the foot rest. The scrubbing and callus smoothing process is then completed on the other foot. The entire process should take approximately 10 minutes. At this point approximately thirty-five minutes have been used for the pedicure. You may wish to allow the client to relax with the mask product (if used) for another five minutes. This will leave twenty minutes for the massage and polish.

The hot wax service may also be added at this point in the pedicure. It may be used in place of the mask or as a separate add-on part of the pedicure. The wax should be applied in accordance with manufacturer's instructions. By this time in the pedicure, the foot has been scrubbed and cleansed, and is as clean as it will ever be. Organisms, bacterial or fungal, will not live or survive in the hot wax. A plastic bag is placed over the foot and the foot is placed into a terry cloth boot or wrapped in a towel. The process is repeated on the other foot, and then the client should be allowed to relax in silence for five to ten minutes. This allows for the penetration of the heat and oils from the wax into the skin and underlying tissues. It can also be a nice prelude to the massage. Remember this is an add-on service which takes more time and requires special equipment and, therefore, warrants an extra charge.

4. **The massage** is a part of the professional pedicure where the nail technician can excel. This is what the client has been looking forward to. Often, a good massage will make the client come back for the next pedicure. The nail technician who perfects a good massage technique will build a good reputation with pedicure clients. Relaxation is the most important part of the massage. It will give the client a sense of well being and exhilaration. The massage also promotes increased circulation and muscle relaxation within the lower extremities. (See the massage section of this chapter.)

5. **Apply nail polish (optional).** After the massage, if the client desires, nail polish should be applied according to manufacturer's recommendations. Insert toe separators during this procedure. Remove traces of massage lotion from the toenails with polish remover. Apply base coat, two coats of color, and a topcoat (Figure 11–44). Place feet on a towel to dry.

6. **Post-pedicure procedures.** While you are doing this, recommend take-home products for the client to use between pedicures. Talk about proper foot care and why it is important for healthy feet. Ask what he or she liked or disliked about the pedicure and note it on the client health/record form after the client has gone. Also talk about the next appointment and rebook the client for the next pedicure.

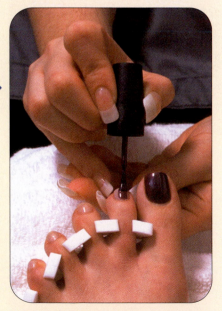

Figure 11–44 Apply nail polish after the massage.

Once the client is gone, sanitize (wash with soap and water) the equipment and instruments that were used for the pedicure and then place the instruments back into the disinfectant solution. If you are doing many pedicures, you may need two sets of instruments in order to allow for proper disinfection times. Spray disinfectant solution on the tub or water bath basin to disinfect all surfaces. You are now ready for your next pedicure client.

B U S I N E S S TIP

Service for the Elderly

The elderly also need care and maintenance for their feet on a year-round basis. There is a large segment of the elderly population who cannot reach their feet and need help in their foot care maintenance. It is estimated that 40 million Americans suffer from some form of arthritis. Many of them cannot reach their feet or cannot squeeze the nail nippers. They need proper foot care that a good pedicurist can provide. The nail technician who offers pedicure services for this segment of the population will be doing these individuals a great favor.

11

chapter glossary

curette	A small, spoon-shaped instrument used for cleaning debris from the edges of nail margins.
cuticle nippers	An instrument used for manicures and pedicures to trim dead and flaky skin from around the nail bed.
diamond nail file	A metal file with diamond dust, available in different grits, that is the same shape as other nail files. It can be easily sanitized and kept in disinfectant solutions.
effleurage	A light, continuous-stroking massage movement applied with fingers (digital) and palms (palmar) in a slow and rhythmic manner.
foot files (paddles)	Large sanding files made to remove dry, flaky skin and smooth callus from the foot.
friction movement	Firm pressure applied to the bottom of the foot using thumb compression to work from side to side and toward the heel.
hand manipulation	The process of skillfully treating, working, or operating with the hands.
massage	A method of manipulation of the body by rubbing, pinching, kneading, and tapping for therapeutic purposes.
massage oils	Blends of therapeutic oils used to lubricate, moisturize, and invigorate the skin during a massage or pedicure.
nail rasp	A metal file with an angled edge that can cut or file in only one direction.
pedicure	Standard service performed by nail technicians that includes care and massage of feet and trimming, shaping, and polishing toenails.
petrissage	A kneading movement in massage performed by lifting, squeezing, and pressing the tissue.
scrubs	Slightly abrasive products containing softening agents or oils to penetrate dry, flaky skin and callus that need to be removed during a pedicure.
soaks	Products containing gentle soaps, moisturizers, and deep penetrating, surface-active ingredients, used in the pedicure bath to soften the skin of the foot.
tapotement	A massage movement using a short, quick hacking, slapping, or tapping technique.
toenail nippers	Professional instruments with curved or straight jaws used for cutting toenails.

11

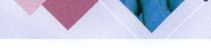
review questions

1. Name five pedicure supplies.

2. List the seven steps in the pedicure pre-service.

3. Briefly describe the pedicure procedure.

4. Describe the proper technique to use in filing toenails.

5. Describe the proper technique for trimming toenails.

6. List the six steps in the pedicure post-service.

7. Name six foot massage techniques.

8. What is a safety caution for pedicuring?

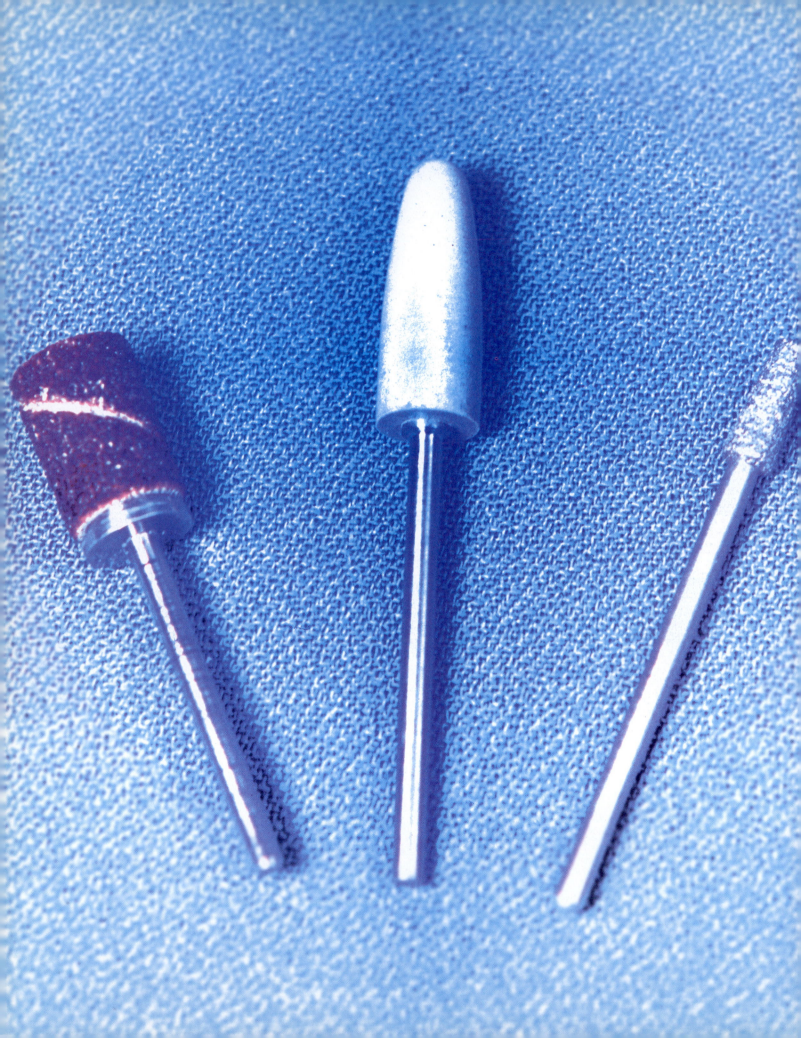

12

ELECTRIC FILING

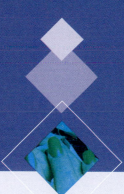

Author: Vicki Peters

CHAPTER OUTLINE

Are Electric Files Safe? • Types of Files
Choosing an Electric File • Bits
How to Use an Electric File • Troubleshooting
The Professional in You

Learning Objectives

After you have completed this chapter, you should be able to:

1. Determine if electric files are safe.

2. Identify which types of electric files have grown in popularity.

3. Define torque.

4. Define RPMs.

5. Explain "diamond" bit.

6. Determine the grits of a carbide bit.

7. Explain the application technique used to ensure safety.

Key Terms

Page number indicates where in the chapter the term is used.

bit
pg. 230

concentric
pg. 231

flutes
pg. 231

grit
pg. 231

revolutions per minute (RPMs)
pg. 228

rings of fire
pg. 227

torque
pg. 230

Electric files are professional machines made specifically for the nail industry, with educational support from the manufacturers who make them. Years ago, before the nail industry recognized the need for professional electric files, technicians used dental materials as nail enhancement products. Because they were difficult to use, technicians then resorted to craft tools purchased in hardware stores. Today, we have many electric file companies that provide much better equipment and education that allows us to use these machines safely. The Association of Electric File Manufacturers (AEFM), was formed in 1998 to establish the standards of electric filing. Today the AEFM educates nationally, and has created a non-product-related video on electric filing.

♦♦♦ ARE ELECTRIC FILES SAFE?

Yes, they are safe; however, in the hands of an unskilled technician, damage can be done. Learning how to use an electric file properly will stop the damage from happening. Education can be obtained from books and videos, as well as manufacturer education.

Do Electric Files Damage Nails?

They can damage nails if used incorrectly. When used properly, damage to the nails is not likely. The key is skill. Do not over file the artificial nails or use the electric file as a crutch to fix lumpy, acrylic applications.

Rings of fire and heat are the two most common ways to damage the nails. Rings of fire are created when using a barrel bit at the wrong angle near the cuticle, where the barrel's flat edge actually digs into the natural nail bed when refining the cuticle area. Heat is caused by too much friction. *Pressure causes friction and friction causes heat.* Too much pressure and leaving the bit on the nail too long will cause heat. Your goal should be to avoid client discomfort. Electric filing should not be painful and if you are doing something to cause discomfort to the client, you are doing something wrong.

♦♦♦ TYPES OF FILES

Belt-driven

This machine is one that dentists still use today. It is cumbersome and not found in the nail industry; you would have to purchase it from a dental supplier or directly from the manufacturer. It has belts on the arms that connect to the elbows of the arm and hand piece. If you have long hair, you must pull it back so it does not get caught in the belts when in use. The belts need to be replaced periodically.

Cable-driven

This is a hand-held micromotor that has a long cable with the hand piece at the end. The cable is not very flexible and is not a professional tool even though it is sold in some beauty supply stores. The file is a good one;

12

Practice Makes Perfect in Overcoming Your Fears

You will eventually need to practice on someone to understand pressure and how effective you are. In the meantime, glue a tip on a dowel or round clothespin and hold the dowel as you would a client's finger. Apply acrylic to the tip and practice. After you have gained some confidence, try practicing on a classmate or salon mate who can tell you about your pressure and guide you. The main thing is that you need to be comfortable holding the hand piece and must find a good working speed that is fast enough, but not too fast. You may want to start with a diamond bit that has a rounded tip so you can safely practice at the cuticle areas. The more you work with the file, the more comfortable you will become and this will build your confidence.

although, the **revolutions per minute (RPMs)** start too high. You must use it with a foot pedal to control the RPMs at a lower speed. There is no educational assistance for these machines and no nail industry support.

Micromotor

These machines are the most used files in the nail industry. They have small boxes with motors in them that sit on the manicuring table. There is a plug for the hand piece and some have plugs in the back for foot pedals, which are optional.

Hand-held Micromotor

This is a less expensive, but very effective, hand-held file in which the motor is in the hand piece with a cord that plugs into the wall. It runs through a direct-drive system and is portable, with a hand piece that can be cumbersome but is easy to use.

Portable

Inexpensive, battery-operated files are not worth the price you pay. They are cheap, do not run true, and can be difficult to control. An expensive portable, however, will give you the power, speed, and precision you need from an electric file.

◆◆◆ CHOOSING AN ELECTRIC FILE

When choosing an electric file make sure that the casing on the machine and its hand piece is sealed tight so that dust cannot get into the motor or the hand piece. An electric file can be a prominent addition to your inven-

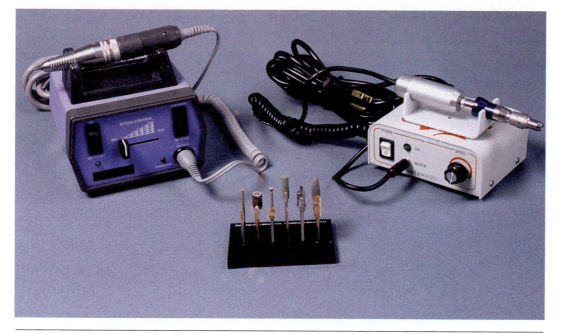

Figure 12-1 A selection of electric files with bits

tory of professional tools. When used properly, it can save you time and energy. The information provided in this chapter is geared toward helping you make an educated, well-informed decision on *how* to use, *when* to use, and *why* to use an electric file (Figure 12–1).

Power and Speed

Power and speed vary from file to file. Your needs and level of proficiency will determine which electric file is right for you.

❖ **RPMs.** Stands for **R**evolutions **P**er **M**inute. This is the number of times the bit rotates in a minute—how fast the electric file goes. For example, if the bit is rotating at 5,000 RPMs it is hitting the nail 5,000 times per minute.

❖ **Range of Speed.** This varies from file to file and, depending how smoothly the machine spins, will dictate how low the RPMs can spin. Most electric files start at 0–100 RPMs and can go as high as 35,000 RPMs. The average speed variations range from 1,000 to 30,000 RPMs. The average nail technician uses files between 5,000 and 15,000 RPMs, depending on skill level and what techniques are being used at the time. Most files have a speed dial; some are not numbered so you have to guess how fast you are going. Some electric files do not have a speed dial, which nail technicians need for speed adjustment.

❖ **Variable Speed.** Many electric files have a high- and low-speed setting like a hair dryer does. When purchasing an electric file, purchase one with a variable-speed dial, allowing you to adjust the speed to any RPM you desire.

❖ **Torque.** Torque is the amount of resistance in the electric file as the bit turns and is measured in pound-per-square-inch. Also called horsepower, when you bear down on the bit while it's in use, the torque will keep the bit spinning.

❖ **Direction of spin.** The electric file bit spins counterclockwise in the average file when in the forward position. However, if the nail technician is left-handed, it can be easier to learn to use the machine in reverse when first beginning. Most left-handed nail technicians use the file in forward. Some of the higher-end files offer reverse as an added feature. This is an advantage for a left-handed nail technician, when working on your own nails, or for reversing the direction of spin for underneath the nails.

❖ **Floor pedal.** Most electric files have a plug in the back for a foot pedal, which is sold as an option. Using a foot pedal allows you to adjust the speed as you work, saving time and making you more efficient.

Life Expectancy

How long should an electric file last? That depends on two things.

1. You get what you pay for, so if you purchase a good file it should last longer than an inexpensive one.

2. It depends on how much your file is used and how well you take care of it. If you keep your electric file in good working order, it should last many years.

Maintenance and Warranties

When purchasing an electric file be sure to ask about the warranties. Most manufacturers honor a one-year warranty and some will replace the file if necessary.

The average maintenance needed for an electric file will vary according to a number of factors, including the type and model you purchase and how often it is used. You should periodically replace the cords and have your file professionally cleaned once a year. The best time for maintenance is while you are on vacation, because most manufacturers can maintain and return the files within a week.

Cost

Cost will vary from file to file. The price for a low-end, hand-held micromotor can start at about $150, and the cost can go all the way to $600 for a high-end machine.

Bits

The term bit is used in the nail industry for what the dental industry called "burrs." The bits you choose are just as important as the file you buy (Figure 12–2). The best electric file will give you disappointing results when used with a poor quality bit. Spending the extra money on a well-

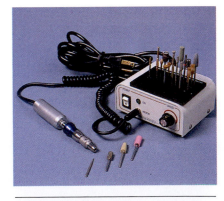

Figure 12-2 The bits are as important as the type of electric file you choose.

12

made bit will not only give you better results, but will last longer. Most bit styles are taken from the dental and jewelry industries, but several have been made specifically for nails, such as the backfill bits and a few others. Many come in carbides, as well as diamonds. Nail technicians choose which bit to use most often by preference and results. Other than some specific bits, such as the French backfill bit, there is no rule for what to use. The life expectancy depends on the quality and usage. A bit that is used all day, every day, will wear out faster than one that is used less often. Shapes vary extensively. There is the barrel, barrel with soft edges, cone, flat-tipped cone, football, bullet, and more. Some nail technicians use a cone at the cuticle, some use a flat-tipped cone, others use a football or a round-tipped barrel, all for the same technique. Again, personal preference is the key to making your choice.

The industry standard for shank size of bits is 3/32-inch. The 1/8th-inch shank is used for craft machines.

Changing the bits is very simple. A twist-lock chuck is available in most professional electric files. A simple twist of the hand piece opens the shank so you can easily remove and replace the bits.

Concentricity

Concentric is a word used for perfectly balanced bits. It means they are balanced so when they spin inside the drill motor chuck of the hand piece, they spin exactly centered. A bent bit, or one that is not concentric, will not spin correctly. The term "running true" means that the bit turns in the drill motor chuck perfectly, without being off center. If the bit is bent or the shank is damaged from being dropped, it will not run true; it will not rotate smoothly and will hit the nail unevenly on each revolution.

Finish

Each bit is cut with edges finished perfectly, so they are not sharp. However, you should feel the edges of the bit before use and if they are sharp, you can dull the edges using a smooth file while the bit is spinning at a slow speed.

Grits

Grit is measured the same way file grit is measured. Take a 1-inch square of file paper. It takes 100 grits to cover a 1-inch square, so the grits must be big, making it coarse. If the grit is 240, it takes 240 pieces of grit to cover, making each grit smaller and finer. The same applies to bits. However carbide bites are not measured this way. They are measured by the amount of **flutes** (cuts) in each bit. The larger and deeper the cuts, the coarser the bit. The more and less deep the cuts, the finer the bit. The cuts are in both directions (crosscut) and the right cuts are deeper than the left, so if you use the carbide bit in reverse it is not as effective.

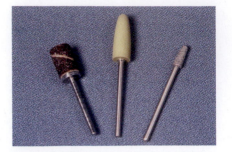

Figure 12-3 Sanding, natural, and diamond bits

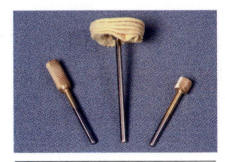

Figure 12-4 Carbide, buffing, and backfill bits

12

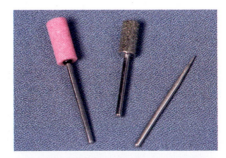

Figure 12-5 Abrasive stone, pedicure, and jewelry bits

◆ TYPES OF BITS USED ON THE NAIL

❖ **Natural nail bits.** These are synthetic rubberized bits that are used for smoothing and polishing jewelry. They come in a pointed-and-flat-tipped version. They can be disinfected when cleaned properly. On the natural fingernails and toenails, they can remove ptgyrium and smooth out ridges. They are also used for prepping the nails for a high shine (Figure 12–3).

❖ **Sanding bands.** These are round, black or brown, paper files that are slipped onto a mandrel and used on the nails. They are not sanitizable, so discard after each client. Because paper is a natural material, they can heat up faster than a metal bit. They come in extra-fine, fine, medium, and coarse grits. These are great for shortening an artificial nail (Figure 12–3).

❖ **Diamond bits.** These are bits made of metal that have diamond particles attached with adhesive. They work like a file with the grits on the surface. When purchasing a diamond bit, make sure the diamond particles are evenly distributed over the entire surface and they do not flake off when touching them. Diamond bits come in extra fine, fine, medium, and coarse grits, but are not quite as aggressive as a carbide bit (Figure 12–3).

❖ **Carbide bits.** Carbides are made of metal with flutes for cutting power. They can be very sharp, so it is important to make sure the edges are softened. Extra-fine, fine, medium, and coarse grits are available. The coarseness is measured by the amount of flutes (cuts) in each bit. The larger and deeper the cuts the coarser the bit. The less deep and the more cuts, the finer the bit. If the cuts are in both directions, it is called a crosscut bit. A one-cut bit usually has only right-sided cuts and is not as popular (Figure 12–4).

❖ **Backfill bits.** Originally, these smaller, shorter barrel bits were made to trench out the growth at the smile to replace the white tip powder. In theory they work well, but we all know that not replacing the entire white tip with white acrylic powder will make the free edge appear striped. Backfill bits come in many varieties today. Perhaps a combination of two will do the job. Experiment to find the one that best suits your technique (Figure 12–4).

❖ **Buffing bits.** These bits are usually made from natural materials, such as chamois, leather, goat's hair brushes, or cotton rag wheels. All are effective in applying buffing cream and bringing nails to a high-gloss shine. These bits cannot be disinfected, and should be disposed of between clients (Figure 12–4).

❖ **Abrasive stone bits.** These are white, pink, lavender, or blue ceramic stones usually in a barrel shape. They are made from natural materials, are not made concentric, are not disinfectable, and are not recommended for use on nails (Figure 12–5).

❖ **Pedicure bits.** These are usually diamond bits made in large barrel or cone shapes and are used on dry callus. Some traditional pedicure bits can be used to thin out thick toenails (Figure 12–5).

❖ **Jewelry bits.** A long, slender carbide has been made for drilling a hole into the free edge of an artificial nail to attach nail jewelry. It is the same shape as the hand tool, made into a bit for the electric file (Figure 12–5).

Sanitation and Disinfection of Bits

Disinfecting should be done the same as your implements. One should never use the same bit on two clients without disinfecting it. Start by removing the dust or acrylic with a wire brush or soaking it in acetone. Rinse with soap and water and submerge into the disinfection solution for the recommended time. Read the instructions on the label of your solution for proper disinfection.

Rinse and dry the bits and store in a clean dry container.

Here's a Tip:

You may want to purchase a plastic sink drain with holes in it. Place the bits inside the drain and then place it into your disinfection solutions. This way you don't have to dig around in the solution to find the bits!

Rusting

Two things can cause rusting of your bits.

1. inexpensive and cheaply made bits
2. leaving bits in disinfection solution too long

HOW TO USE THE ELECTRIC FILE

Using the fulcrum finger is a must for balancing and hand control. Start by balancing your hand on the table. Place the wrist of the hand that holds the client's hand on the table. Do not work suspended above the table. Take the hand piece and hold it as you would a pencil. Balance the pinky finger of your right hand on the tip of the left pinky you extend out. This may seem awkward at first, but, in the long run, will give you better stability as you work. By balancing your hands this way, it takes the negative pressure off the tip of the bit and gives you better control as you work.

Application Techniques

❖ **The right angle.** When using an electric file it is important to always keep the bit, no matter what shape you prefer, flat to the nail and not at an angle.

❖ **Rings of fire.** Rings of fire are the ridges created when using a bit at the wrong angle near the cuticle area. Each ring of fire usually represents the electric filing done at each fill.

❖ **Heat.** Pressure causes friction, friction causes heat. The bits do not cause the heat, the nail technician does. Try working one direction, from right to left, picking the bit up off the nail from the left to right, allowing the nail to cool. Going back and forth, when inexperienced, can cause the nail to heat up. If the nail gets hot, stop working and slow down. Realize that it is the heat reaching the natural nail that causes discomfort to the client.

❖ **Correct speed.** This varies from nail technician to technician. As long as you are working safely, the speed you choose is fine. If the bit grabs and wraps around the finger or squeals, this is an indication you are working too fast. If the file bogs down when working slowly, try raising your RPMs.

❖ **Natural nail prepping.** A synthetic, natural nail bit is the only bit recommended for prepping the natural nail and removing the shine for an artificial service. Never use sanding bands or metal bits on the natural nail.

❖ **Artificial nail maintenance.** A bullet or cone is recommended for prepping the nails for a fill. Use it flat to the nail and remove any lifted product without damaging the natural nail.

❖ **Cuticle work.** Use a cone or a flat-tipped cone with the bit flat to the nails for cuticles. Work the finger and bit together, starting from the right side nail groove, to the top of the cuticle, to the left side of the nail groove. Move the finger to meet the bit as you work.

❖ **Lifted product.** If your client has lifting, you can take the sharp edge of a barrel bit, or the French backfill bit, and cut a trench into the lifting right below the spot where the lifting ends. Cut about 75 percent into the lifting, then bend the lifted piece back and break it off, without pulling up any of the unlifted product. Bevel the rest of the lifting flush with the natural nail.

❖ **Cracks.** Use a slender barrel or bullet bit and place sideways into the crack. Slowly bevel a wide trench with the body of the bit, exposing the crack. Then repair the crack.

Shaping Under the Nail and C-curves

With a pointed or flat-tipped cone, turn the nails over and gently refine the undersides. You can file in the forward motion to do one side of all the undersides, then place the file in the reverse mode to do the other side.

For the c-curves, look down the barrel of the nail. Place a barrel bit up under the nail to refine the c-curves and the undersides of the free edges.

Backfills

Backfills can be done a number of ways, with a number of bits. For example after you have prepped the nails for a fill, thin out the tip's edges with a barrel bit to make cutting in the smile line easier. You can also thin out the entire free edge of the nail and, instead of cutting in the smile lines, replace the area with the white tip powder and smile lines as you would a new nail.

When cutting in the smile line you can also use a pencil to draw a line as a guide. Take three cuts, one from the right groove wall, across the center, then the third from the center cut to the left groove wall. So the first cut would be from 3 o'clock to 5 o'clock, the center from 5 o'clock to 7 o'clock, and the third from 7 o'clock to 9 o'clock.

12

Next, turn the nail so you can see the profile and, with a barrel bit, remove 75 percent of the remaining acrylic. When removing the acrylic make sure you are consistent so the white tip powder you replace will have the same density from nail to nail. Also, place the white tip powder against the new smile line wall you cut with your bit and do not overlap. Gently wipe any excess white product at the smile line. Do all ten nails with the white powder and let all dry before applying the pink or clear. This way, you will preserve your new smile lines.

Finishing

Graduating your grits is the key to finishing your nails without file marks. If you start with a coarse bit, graduate to a medium, and then to a fine, making sure you have total coverage with each bit and do not leave any deeper scratches behind. Removing the dust between the use of each bit will help with smoothing the nails as well. Using enough pressure, that is safe and not damaging, for good coverage will aid in your work. Lighten the pressure as you lighten the grits. Using an electric file is definitely an asset to any nail technician; however, there is one technique that you cannot do with an electric file. That is, to shape the perimeter of the nails. You must use a hand file to complete this process.

You may use a fine bit or a buffer bit to go over those edges after filing the shape. The important aspect of finishing the nails is to ask yourself if all the edges are absolutely perfect and if nothing has been left unfiled, even the underside edges of the extensions.

Buffing Oils

The use of buffing oils can enhance your finish work and provide slippage, which can keep the nails a bit cooler as you work. Do not use a mineral-based oil. Use a pure and thin oil that is specifically made for this procedure. Thicker oils are scented and can clog the hand piece. You will have to send it back to the manufacturer for maintenance and cleaning more often.

❖ **High shine buffing.** After you have graduated your grits properly and have a smooth finish, you can high shine the nails with a buffing bit made from cotton rag wheels, chamois or leather. Be careful not to apply too much pressure because these materials are natural and heat up quickly. If you do not get a high shine go back to the second bit you used and start over, making sure you are covering the entire nail and using the correct bits to graduate your grit. Otherwise you will be high shining scratched nails. Again be careful not to apply too much pressure.

❖ **Buffing creams.** The use of buffing creams enhances your high shine power. Most creams come with pumice and can be used with any buffer bit. Apply the buffing cream with a goat's hair brush and slowly work in the cream before using a buffer bit. The goat's hair brush brings up most of the shine before you even use a buffer bit.

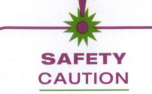

◆◆◆ TROUBLESHOOTING

Heat

If your electric filing is causing too much heat and discomfort to your client, you must slow down the RPMs and use less pressure. Try working from the left side of the nail to the right and then picking the bit up off the nails as you return to the right side of the nail. Going back and forth, without taking the bit off the nail, may cause heat. Remember, pressure causes friction, friction causes heat. Find the combination of speed and pressure that works best for you and your client. Sometimes going too slowly causes heat and sometimes going too fast does, so it is important to find your perfect speed.

Left-handed Technicians

Unless you start from the very beginning using the reverse mode of your electric file, you will find it difficult to get used to it in reverse. Most left-handed nail technicians work in the forward mode. They hold the hand piece in their left hand and work in the forward mode. Either way is correct.

▼ Here's a Tip: Carbide Grabbing

If your bit grabs and wraps around your client's finger, you are working too fast or applying too much pressure. Slow down and use less pressure. This happens more frequently with the silver bits that do not have a finish on them and are very sharp. Use 75 percent less pressure with these bits at a slower RPM.

Carpal Tunnel

For many nail technicians who experience carpal tunnel syndrome using an electric file can help, only because of the change in hand position. Although, some technicians find holding the hand piece can be more straining on the hands.

Speed

Using an electric file does not mean you can go faster. Some nail technicians are faster with a hand file than an electric file because they are not as adept with an electric file. So, the speed comes with practice, as does safety.

◆◆◆ THE PROFESSIONAL IN YOU

A true professional nail technician will understand safety when using an electric file. Educating your clients and never hurting them will increase their confidence in you. An electric file is a safe tool in the hands of a skilled user. Remember, practice safety, good sanitation, and proper use of the electric file and you will find that using an electric file can enhance your work.

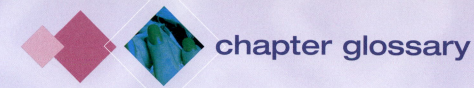

chapter glossary

bit	The replaceable part of the electric file, usually carbide or diamond, that does the actual filing of the nail. It comes in different shapes and sizes for various nail styles and techniques. Sample shapes include barrel, cone, flat-tipped cone, football, and bullet.
concentric	Perfectly balanced and centered bits that spin inside the drill motor chuck to make sure the file rotates smoothly and hits the nail evenly.
flutes	Long, slender cuts or grooves found in carbide file bits.
grit	The amount of abrasive material used on files and bits. The smaller the number, the larger amount of grits used; for example, it the grit is 240, it takes 240 pieces of grit to cover a 1" square; therefore, the grit is finer than a grit of 100.
revolutions per minute (RPMs)	The number of times a bit rotates in one minute. In nail technology, how fast an electric drill goes.
rings of fire	Ridges in the nail caused by using a barrel bit at the wrong angle near the cuticle, where the barrel's flat edge actually digs into the natural nail bed.
torque	Also known as horsepower; the amount of resistance (measured in pounds-per-square-inch) in a file as the bit turns.

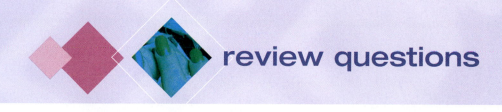

review questions

1. Are electric files safe?

2. What types of electric file have grown in popularity?

3. What is torque?

4. What are RPMs?

5. What is a diamond bit?

6. What grits does a carbide bit come in?

7. What application techniques ensure safety?

8. How do you disinfect bits?

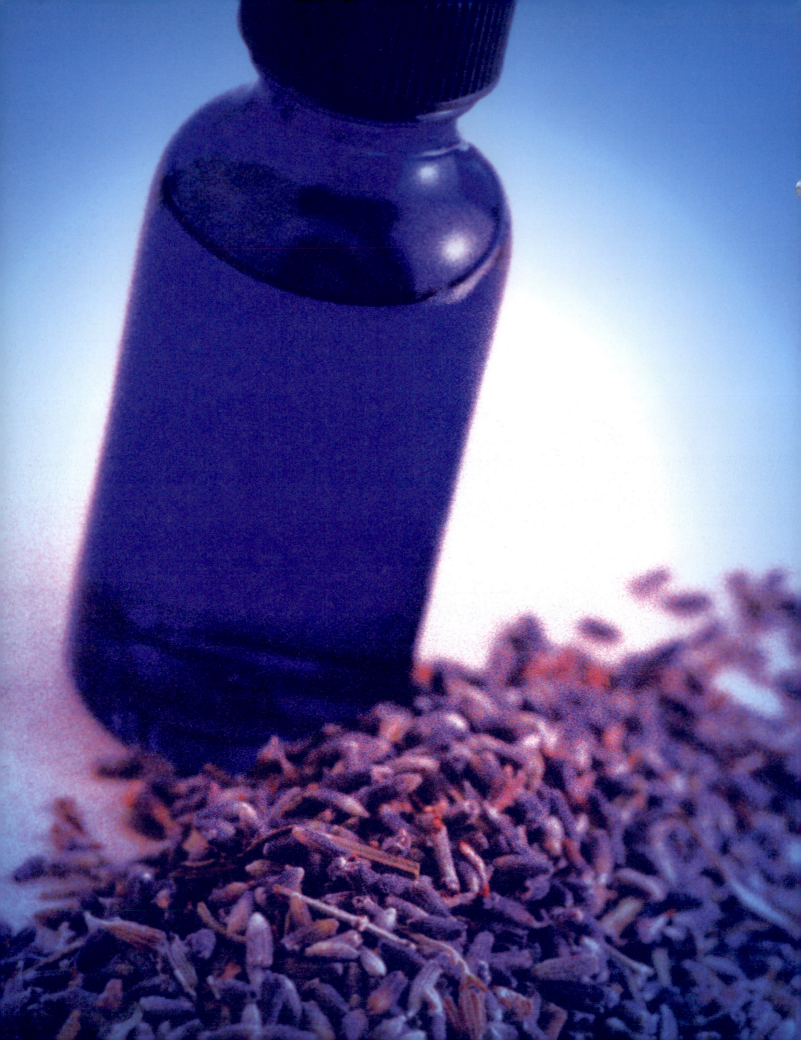

13

AROMATHERAPY

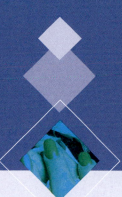

Author: Jewell Cunningham

CHAPTER OUTLINE

What Is Aromatherapy? • Essential Oils • Carrier Oils
The Hands and Manicures • The Feet and Pedicures
Choosing an Aroma

Learning Objectives

After you have completed this chapter, you should be able to:

1 **Define and understand aromatherapy.**

2 **Explain where essential oils come from.**

3 **Name the essential oils most commonly used in the beauty industry.**

4 **Identify carrier oils and understand their use.**

5 **Understand how aromatherapy can be incorporated into a service.**

Key Terms

Page number indicates where in the chapter the term is used.

aromatherapy
pg. 241

carrier oil
pg. 244

essential oils
pg. 242

As you embark on this journey into the world of aromatherapy, you may be inspired to add aromatic liquids, known as essential oils, and the practice of aromatherapy into your salon services. By adding essential oils, you will have taken a new direction in providing a calm, sweet-smelling environment to work in, as well as for your clients to enjoy. Aromatherapy is for everybody, young, old, male, and female. Everyone can benefit from its incredible healing properties.

In this chapter you will learn what aromatherapy is, where it came from, and what the first documented uses of aromatherapy were. The chapter covers essential oils, including the top ten oils, what they do, and what they are derived from, as well as other oils used in the beauty industry. You will find information about carrier oils including what they are, their properties, and why they are used. Most importantly, you will learn how easy it is to incorporate aromatherapy and essential oils into your services for increased income. Easy ideas for new services you can add to your current salon menu, some recipes to try, and suggestions on pricing of these services are discussed. Aromatherapy continues to be one of the fastest growing services being added to the salon menu today.

◆ ◆ ◆ WHAT IS AROMATHERAPY?

The literal translation is just what it says, *Aroma Therapy*, therapy through aromas. The term **aromatherapy** was coined by the French chemist René-Maurice Gattefossé in 1928. He was fascinated by the therapeutic possibilities of oils after a burn on his hand was healed rapidly while working with lavender oil. He also noticed that the scarring was not as prominent as was thought to be. This led him to do research on the benefits of such oils.

The word "aromatherapy" conjures up images of people alleviating their depression, ailments, illnesses, and/or insecurities with wonderful scents. Aromatherapy is more than that; by adding aromatherapy to your life, your overall health, beauty, and psyche can be enhanced. Aromatherapy can improve your sleep, giving you more energy. It can help eliminate skin conditions, giving you relief, as well as improve your general mood and the mood of those around you (Figure 13-1).

"The rose distills a healing balm, the beating pulse of pain to calm."
Thomas Moore

The most wonderful thing about aromatherapy is that it is so easy to use and be a part of. Most people love to receive fragrant oils to use in their bath or rub on their body. Many of us love the aroma of an orange or a rose. As children, we were drawn to the wonderful smells around us. Some of our most distinctive memories are associated with those smells. Think, for just a moment, of . . . chocolate chip cookies baking . . . freshly baked bread . . . a full-blown red rose . . . the squeeze of a lemon. Few things can move us so deeply or have such a profound impact on our psyche, as the memories evoked by specific smells.

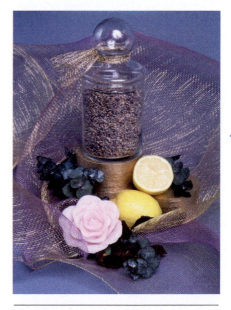

Figure 13-1 Aromatherapy comes in various forms, including candles and essential oils.

13

"Look in the perfumes of flowers and of nature for peace of mind and joy of life"
Wang-Wei

Smell is our most direct means of communication with nature. We smell with every breath we take, constantly monitoring the world around us. Exactly how aromatherapy works is still unclear. Some researchers speculate that odors influence feelings because the nasal passage opens directly into the part of the brain that controls emotion and memory. Others believe that fragrance compounds interact with receptor sites in the central nervous system. What we do know is that the mere smell of a fragrance can influence us physically and emotionally, which is why aromatherapy is practiced in many forms.

There are vast uses for aromatherapy, ranging from medicinal to preventive health to beauty to massage. The use of essential oils for beauty and skin care go back as far as Ancient Egyptians 5,000 years ago. Aromatic herbs and oils were carefully incorporated into cosmetic ointments and other beauty preparations, even embalming. Many countries, such as China and India, have practiced aromatherapy for many years. Remember the three wise men? The gifts they were bearing were frankencense and myrrh (Figure 13–2). One of the first perfume formulas, dating back to 1,800 B.C. in Babylon, was a combination of cedar, myrrh, cypress, labdanum, and storax. Some newer formulations you might be more familiar with are a blend of sandalwood, amber, bergamot, musk and civet, or a blend of frankencense, patchouli, vetivert, clove, and musk. There continue to be more and more essential oils being used in the world around us—more than we ever thought. Remember the song verse: parsley, sage, rosemary, and thyme?

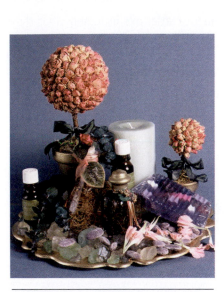

Figure 13-2 Essential oils are extracted from botanical sources, such as fruit, flowers, and herbs.

◆◆ ◆ ESSENTIAL OILS

The practice of aromatherapy involves the use of essential oils. What exactly are essential oils? **Essential oils** are the oils that are extracted, by various forms of distillation, from botanical sources in various parts of the plant, including seeds, bark, roots, leaves, wood, and resin. Each part produces a different aroma. Some examples are the Scotch pine which, yields a different aroma from the needles than from the resin and wood. The time of day the plant was harvested will also change the aroma. A rose petal that is harvested early in the morning will have more dew on its petals than one harvested in the evening. The dew content will alter the aroma.

Each batch of essential oils can also differ due to weather conditions. Even the countries that produce the same plants will have different aromas. Lavender that comes from France is different from Bulgarian lavender. Some essential oils you can actually feel without distillation or any processes. Take the lemon for instance. When you hold it in your hand and gently press the skin, you feel the oil it produces. That oil is the aroma of lemon. The same types of oils are released when you touch a lime or orange.

"Aromatherapy—The art of combining life-giving forces of plants into oils and transferring their benefits to humans."
Jewell Cunningham

Not all plants contain essential oils that are easy to detect. The aromatic content in rose petals is so small that it takes over one ton of rose petals to produce one pound of essential rose oil. It is the wide range of aromatic materials obtained from natural sources and the art of extraction that has developed over the course of time to give us the essential oils we currently use.

The use of essential oils is limitless. You can use them in manicures, pedicures, massage, reflexology, and facials. They can be used to soften cuticles or as an additive to hand creams as a hand conditioner. Use them in light rings or diffusers to help clear the mind, for a quick lift, or to change the mood of a room.

Following is a partial list of oils used today in the cosmetic and beauty industry.

Bergamot	Bitter Almond	Black Pepper	Bulgarian Rose
Camphor	Cedar	Cedarwood	Chamomile
Citrus	Clary Sage	Clove	Cypress
Eucalyptus	French Lavender	Gardenia	Geranium
Grapefruit	Jasmine	Lavender	Lemon
Lemon Verbena	Lemongrass	Lime	Marjoram
Neroli	Orange	Peppermint	Petigrain
Rose	Rosemary	Sandalwood	Spearmint
Tangerine	Tea Rose	Tea Tree	Vanilla
Vetivert	White Birch	Ylang Ylang	

Ten Basic Essential Oils

Lavender   Herbaceous (having the characteristics of an herb), overall first-aid oil, antiviral and antibacterial, boosts immunity, antidepressant, anti-inflammatory, relaxant, balance, and antispasmodic

Chamomile   Fruity, anti-inflammatory, digestive, relaxant, PMS, soothes frayed nerves, migraine, stamina, and antidepressant

Marjoram   Herbaceous, antispasmodic, anti-inflammatory, headaches, comfort, menstrual cramps, and antiseptic

Rosemary   Camphoraceous (from the wood or bark of the camphor tree), stimulating to circulation, relieves pain, a decongestant

Tea Tree   Camphoraceous, antifungal, and antibacterial

Cypress   Coniferous (mostly from evergreen trees with cones, such as pine) astringent, stimulating to circulation, and antiseptic

Peppermint   Minty, digestive, clears sinuses, antiseptic, energy, decongestant, and stimulant

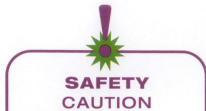

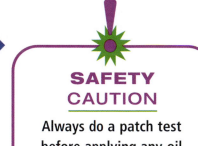

Eucalyptus	Camphoraceous, decongestant, antiviral, antibacterial, and stimulant
Bergamot	Citrus aroma, antidepressant, antiviral, antibacterial, water retention, and anti-inflammatory
Geranium	Floral, balancing to mind and body, tranquility, antifungal, and anti-inflammatory

We must emphasize that each essential oil has benefits, as well as cautions, that need to be taken into consideration before you decide to incorporate their use in your services. This is a general overview of a highly complex subject. The nail industry can employ the use of aromatherapy and enjoy its benefits. As such, we urge you to continue your education by reading books like *Milady's Guide to Aromatherapy* by Shelley Hess, taking classes, and seeking information on the Internet.

◆ ◆ CARRIER OILS

Depending on the type of service for which you use essential oils, you will need a carrier oil. A carrier oil is a base oil with an essential oil added. This creates an oil that is not so concentrated and easier to use. Direct contact with essential oils can sometimes cause skin irritations. For any massage, always use a carrier oil, as it adds slippage and makes the massage much easier to perform. The only times it is not necessary to use a carrier oil is when the essential oil is being added to water, lotion, or any substance that will reduce the concentration or if you use pure essentials in a diffuser to add an aroma to the air.

There are three oils that are the exception to the rule. They are lavender, for use on cuts, burns and abrasions, ylang ylang, and sandalwood, both used as perfume when applied directly to the skin.

Following is a partial list of carrier oils used today in the cosmetic and beauty industry.

Sweet Almond Oil	This is an excellent lubricant and is softening. It is a medium- to light-weight multipurpose massage or skin oil.
Apricot Oil	Especially for prematurely aged, dry skin, a light-weight massage oil
Avocado Oil	Recommended for dull and dehydrated skin, highly nutritious, a medium- to heavy-weight oil
Grapeseed Oil	A very popular massage oil with a fine texture and low odor, a light-weight massage oil.
Jojoba Oil	The only oil that resembles the same structure as our skin's own sebum, giving it excellent moisturizing and emulsifying properties; one of the most versatile carrier oils with the longest shelf life; a light- to medium-weight oil.

13

Ways To Use and Apply Essential Oils and Practice Aromatherapy

There are many salon services and methods in which essential oils can be used including:

manicures	pedicures	hand massage	foot massage
spa manicures	spa pedicures	care of natural nails	cuticle repair
stress relief	hand care	reflexology	diffusers
nail strengthener	candles	full body massage	salt rubs

◆ ◆ ◆ THE HANDS AND MANICURES

Our hands are one of the most precious parts of our bodies. They wipe away tears, hug and hold, discipline, touch, heal, and caress. They wash dishes, change diapers, plant flowers, and build buildings. They hold hands in comfort, hold our children, and wear the symbol of a marriage. Our hands are one of the first places we begin to show our age. The back of the hand becomes loose and wrinkled. What can we do to aid our hands? Get a manicure. Encourage everyone you know to get a manicure. They are great for children, as well as men and the elderly, and everyone in between.

Our nails are a sure sign of the care we take of our hands. Some are bitten beyond repair (or so it is thought), others are the signs of working nails with dirt and grease. All of these hands need loving care.

The manicure is one of the most underrated services available. There is a definite art in performing a proper and relaxing manicure. In the last few years with the evolvement of spa services, we have learned to perfect the manicure. Adding essential oils to the manicure is a natural progression. The exact translation of the word manicure is "hand heal." A manicurist is a hand healer. Essential oils are healers; therefore, they go hand in hand. The best lotions have essential oils added to them for healing but if your lotion does not have an essential oil as an ingredient, you may add a few drops of your favorite oil. Some of the best oils to incorporate into your manicures (and pedicures) are:

Lemongrass	Orange	Lemon
Lavender	Jasmine	Lime
Chamomile	Rose	Peppermint
Spearmint	Bergamot	Vetiver
Carrot	Eucalyptus	Rosemary
Grapefruit	Cypress	

These oils can be used alone or in any combination. Remember, there are many oils to choose from. Make sure the essential oil you are using will aid in the remedy, for example, for stress relief, use Lavender and Chamomile. For invigoration, use Peppermint or Lemongrass and so on.

BUSINESS TIP

IN THE SALON

As a nail technician, there are ways to incorporate a massage into every one of your services. One idea is to offer the *TLC 60-second Stress Relief Massage*. This massage is performed at the beginning of the service. Have the client sit in the chair and close their eyes. Stand behind the chair and use a calming essential oil, such as lavender (a very small amount used with a lotion or carrier oil), on your middle fingers and massage their temples. This 60 seconds is only about the client. Not about their day, or their nails, or anything else except making them feel better. A little TLC goes a long way, and this will be the best 60 seconds they have spent all day. The client will be calmer, easier to work on, and they will also feel better.

Always do your best to make the hand massage as relaxing as possible. *Try not to talk to the client during this time of the service.* This will allow the client to enjoy the massage part of the manicure even more.

Recipes for Manicures

Try some unique recipes for manicures as well as pedicures. Not only do these kinds of services set you apart, they will increase your income. Just add a dollar or two to the cost of your custom services. The following recipes are some ideas that your client might enjoy.

Nail Strengthening Treatment

> 20 drops Lemon
>
> 15 drops Carrot Oil
>
> 13 drops Grapeseed Oil
>
> 13 drops Rosemary
>
> 13 drops Avocado Oil
>
> 2 oz. Jojoba Oil

Blend all oils together and keep in a light-sensitive bottle (dark in color) with a dropper. Use it on your client after you have polished the nails by adding one drop around the cuticle and allowing it to just absorb into the matrix. This strengthener can be used on clients practicing natural nail care as well as clients with nail enhancements.

Cuticle Softener

> 15 drops Carrot Oil
>
> 12 drops Peppermint
>
> 12 drops Eucalyptus
>
> 2 oz. Jojoba Oil

Mix all ingredients together and store in a light-sensitive bottle. Use one drop on each nail and massage well into the cuticle.

Age Deterrent

> 15 drops Lemon
>
> 10 drops Lime
>
> 5 drops Rosemary
>
> 5 drops Lavender
>
> 1 drop Spearmint
>
> 1 oz. Grapeseed Oil

Blend all ingredients together and put in a light-sensitive bottle. This hand treatment will help with spots on the back of the hand, which is a tell-tale sign of aging. Use 2–3 drops of this mixture on the back of the hand. Try to keep the oil only on the skin and not on the nails. The Lemon and Lime are natural pigment lighteners. The Rosemary and Lavender are calming. The Grapeseed Oil is quick in penetration and hydration and the Spearmint is invigorating, bringing blood to the surface, which promotes healing. Gently massage the back of the hand for 3–4 minutes and within 4–5 treatments you should see some of the discoloration begin to fade.

Decadent Manicure

> 1/4 C. heavy cream
>
> 10 drops of a pure or blended essential oil of your choice
>
> 1 bowl of fragrant salts for aroma only (same aromas as soak)
>
> A few candles (if permitted)
>
> Some spa music in the background
>
> 1 client

Light the candles and/or prepare the aromatics in the room. Next add the heavy cream, essential oils, and the hands of the client to the manicure bowl and let soak for 5–10 minutes. Have the client smell the essential oil that is in the cream. You can use all Lavender for stress or Peppermint for revitalization. This will aid the olfactory system in beginning to assimilate the aroma. This could be the time to do the TLC massage on the client's temples. Proceed with normal manicure. Make sure to wipe off the nails before applying polish.

As a variation to this manicure, try using Vanilla, just because it smells wonderful and makes people feel cozy. This makes a great new service for the winter months.

"Why not take care of this body, which is the receptacle of our soul, so that it may remain as healthy, strong, and perfect as possible . . ."
Paracelsus

THE FEET AND PEDICURES

Some people feel that feet are one of the most sensuous parts of the body. Yet, they are often the most neglected area of the body. Just think about what we put our feet through and the weight they carry. We abuse our feet like no other part of our body. Some people think feet are ugly, and if you think how neglected they are, it's no wonder. If we think our feet are too large, we cram them into a size shoe that is one size smaller, just in case someone asks us, "What size shoe do you wear?" It is only when they finally hurt us that we begin to notice them. A wise person once said, "If you take care of your feet, the rest of your body will take care of itself."

There are actually more than 50,000 nerve endings in our feet, which is why a foot massage can make the entire body feel relaxed. A massage during the pedicure is the client's favorite part. A great pedicurist is like an accomplished musician. They can make music from the type of massage they do on the client. When a massage is done with the utmost of care and quality products, the clients will feel as though they are walking on air when they leave the salon. And that is worth a lot of business to you.

Recipes for Pedicures

Dry and Cracked Heels

> 10 drops Rose
>
> 5 drops Chamomile
>
> 5 drops Geranium
>
> 5 drops Pettigraine

Combine ingredients and pour into a light-sensitive bottle. Add 8–10 drops to the pedicure water before adding anything else. Let the client soak for 10 minutes. Proceed with pedicure, including adding any other products you use. Near the end of the pedicure, before the massage, add 3–4 drops on each heel and massage as normal. Take your time and really massage the oils into the heels until they are completely penetrated. A few treatments like this will have the heels soft and supple in no time.

Swollen Feet

> 15 drops Lavender
>
> 15 drops Chamomile
>
> 15 drops Rosemary
>
> 15 drops Fennel
>
> 4 oz. Jojoba Oil

Combine ingredients and pour into a light-sensitive bottle. Use about 25–30 drops as a massage oil. The massage is very important with this treatment. You are urging the blood to the feet to increase the circulation. Allow the feet to rest for five minutes and then, if possible, have the client elevate his or her feet for 10–15 minutes above the heart. Your clients will feel like a million bucks when they leave the salon and they will be yours for life.

Decadent Pedicure

> 1–2 C. heavy cream
>
> 25 drops of a pure or blended essential oil of your choice
>
> Or 3 fragrant salt crystals in the pedicure bath

1 bowl of fragrant salts for aroma only (same aroma as the soak) or
   a candle, if permitted

Spa music in the background

1 client

Add heavy cream, essential oils, and the client's feet to the pedicure bath
and let soak for 5–10 minutes. This could be another time to use the TLC
massage on the client's temples. Proceed with normal pedicure. Make sure
to wipe off the toes before applying polish. You can use Lavender for stress
or Peppermint for revitalization, or try Vanilla just because. This makes a
great new service for the winter months. Make sure to always have your spa
music playing. It helps set the mood of the technician, as well as the client.

◆ ◆ ◆ CHOOSING AN AROMA

In addition to the recipes included in this chapter, you might need the
client's help in deciding which aromas to use in your service. When
choosing oils for the service, talk to the customers and see how they are
feeling. Also, consider the time of the year. Use lighter oils for spring and
summer and heavier oils for fall and winter. Let the client experience the
essential oils you have to offer. Gently pass the uncovered oil under her
nose so she is aware of the aroma. Do not allow the client to see the names
of the oils or she will choose them by name instead of aroma. This can
cancel their benefit. Suggest that she close her eyes, relax, and take a
"cleansing breath" between choices. She will enjoy having participated in
the aroma selection and you can be assured of her enjoyment and pleasure
when you use the one she chose.

Recommended Oils for Pedicures

Peppermint	Tea Tree	Lavender	Lemon Rose
Jasmine	Calendula	Geranium	Sandalwood

Oils for Calming

Lavender	Rosemary	Sandalwood	Ylang Ylang
Vetiver			

Oils for Ambiance

Vanilla	Pine	Bayberry	Cherry
Cinnamon	Jasmine	Rose	Lemon
Orange	Lavender		

Oils For Energy

Eucalyptus	Peppermint	Spearmint	Lemon
Orange	Geranium	Jasmine	Fennel

13

Other Useful Blends

Invigorating	Spearmint - Peppermint - Lemon - Rosemary
Stress Relief	Lavender - Chamomile - Vetivert
Clear Minds	Rosemary - Cypress
Romance	Ylang Ylang - Sandalwood - Jasmine
Foot Odor	Sage - Baking Powder
Bactericide	Cinnamon - Clove - Lemon - Eucalyptus Lavender - Pine - Grapefruit - Lime
Cuts & Scrapes	Tea Tree - Lavender - Eucalyptus
Barber's Rash	Lemongrass - Peppermint - Geranium
Nail Infections	Tea Tree
Oily Skin	Bergamot - Geranium - Clary Sage - Petigrain Cedarwood

Here's a Tip:

For a unique service idea, try this recipe on one of your clients.

Aromatic Whipped Cream

1/2 pint whipping cream

1–2 drops of a pure or blended essential oil of your choice

Whip cream to desired consistency, add essential oil, and mix well.

This is just a really decadent idea. Add this mixture to your pedicure and watch the reaction of the clients. Be creative. WOW!

SAFETY CAUTION

There are some oils to be used with caution: allspice, aniseed, sweet basil, borneol, caraway, cinnamon, and ginger just to name a few. These oils can cause irritation to the skin. Do not use peppermint on pregnant women. Always be careful when using oils on clients. Don't try to come up with a medical "diagnosis" or "prescription."

By using essential oils you give clarity to the mind, healing and care to the hands and inspiration to the feet. The body, as a whole, has received many benefits as well, and the soul has been fed essential oils—"the nourishment of the gods."

Essential oils are like medicine, so use them with care. Make sure you know and understand what you are using. When using essential oils for beauty services, purchase them from beauty industry suppliers and follow all manufacturer's instructions. Those oils were manufactured specifically for the services you are performing. The oils in the health food stores may be good, but remember, they are not designed specifically for use in the salon. Always make sure the oils you are purchasing are the quality you are looking for.

Aromatherapy has an addictive quality—once hooked you will find it hard to let go. There is *always more* to learn and discover.

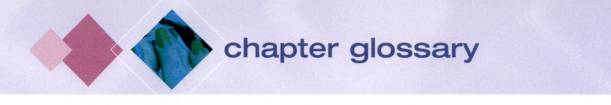

chapter glossary

aromatherapy	The use of aromatic fragrances to induce relaxation; therapy through aroma.
carrier oil	A base oil used in aromatherapy that is added to an essential oil to dilute the concentration of the essential oil. The carrier oil adds slippage and makes the massage easier to perform.
essential oils	Oils used in aromatherapy that are extracted, by various forms of distillations, from various parts of plants, including seeds, bark, roots, leaves, wooks, and resin.

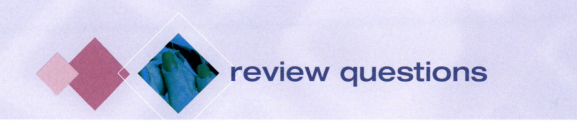

review questions

1. What is aromatherapy?

2. How are essential oils used?

3. List five basic essential oils and give their uses.

4. Why is a carrier oil sometimes necessary?

5. Why is aromatherapy a helpful tool in our industry?

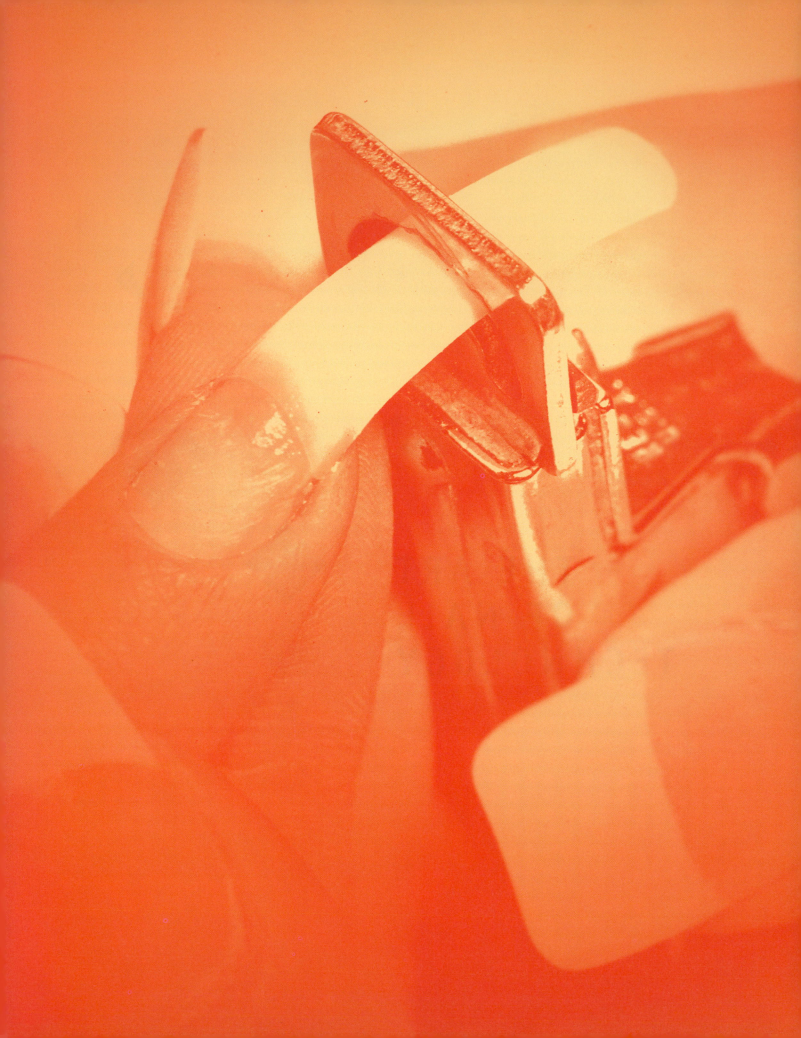

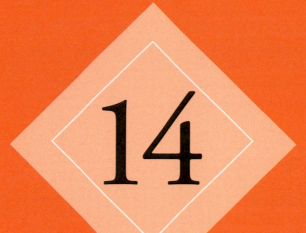

14

NAIL TIPS

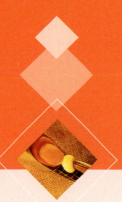

Author: Vicki Peters

CHAPTER OUTLINE

Supplies for Nail Tips • Nail Tip Application
Alternative Tip Applications
Maintenance and Removal of Tips

PROCEDURES

14-1 Nail Tip Application
14-2 Tip Removal

Learning Objectives

After you have completed this chapter, you should be able to:

1 Identify the supplies needed for nail tips and explain what they are used for.

2 Identify the two types of nail tips.

3 Demonstrate the proper procedure and precautions to use in applying nail tips.

4 Describe the proper maintenance of tips.

5 Demonstrate the proper removal of tips.

Key Terms

Page number indicates where in the chapter the term is used.

acrylic
pg. 263

abrasive
pg. 257

buffer block
pg. 257

nail adhesive
pg. 257

nail tip
pg. 257

tip cutter
pg. 262

tip well cutting
pg. 262

A **nail tip** is an artificial nail made of plastic, nylon, or acetate. Tips are adhered to the natural nail to add extra length. Usually tips are combined with another artificial service, such as a fabric wrap or sculptured nail, since a tip worn with no overlay is very weak. If a client chooses to wear a tip with no overlay, the tip is considered a temporary service.

◆ ◆ ◆ SUPPLIES FOR NAIL TIPS

In addition to the materials on your basic manicuring table, you will need the following supplies for nail tip application (Figure 14–1).

Abrasive

A rough surface that is used to shape or smooth the nail and remove the shine is an **abrasive**. It usually looks like a large emery board or disk, but it can be any shape or color.

Buffer Block

Lightweight rectangular block that is abrasive and used to buff nails is a **buffer block**.

Nail Adhesive

Glue or bonding agent used to secure the nail tip to the natural nail is a **nail adhesive**. It usually comes in a tube with a pointed applicator tip, a one-drop applicator, or as a brush on. Even the smallest amount of glue in the eyes can be very dangerous and can blind a person. A nail technician should always wear safety goggles when using and handling nail adhesives. Goggles should be offered to the client, as well.

Nail Tips

All tips have a well that serves as the point of contact with the nail plate. The position stop is the point where the nail plate meets the tip before it is glued to the nail. Tips are designed with either a partial or full well (Figure 14–2) The tip should never cover more than one-half of the natural nail plate. Tips come in large boxes that have an assortment of sizes. Some nail technicians prefer to have tips from several different manufacturers, since they vary slightly in size, shape, and color. With a wide assortment, it is easier to fit each client with precisely the right size and shape tip.

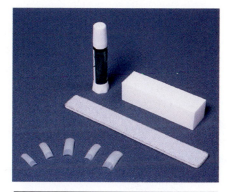

Figure 14-1 Supplies needed for tip application

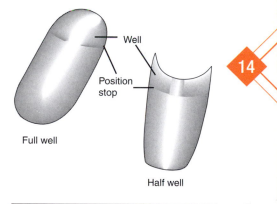

Figure 14-2 Tip with full well and tip with half well

14

◆ ◆ NAIL TIP APPLICATION

Nail Tip Application Pre-service

1. **Complete pre-service sanitation procedure.** (This procedure is described on pages 41-43.)

2. **Set up your standard manicuring table.** Add abrasives, buffer blocks, nail adhesive, and nail tips to your table.

3. **Greet client and ask her to wash hands with antibacterial soap.** Thoroughly dry hands with a clean or disposable towel.

4. **Do client consultation, using client record/health form to record responses and observations.** Check for nail disorders and decide if it is safe and appropriate to perform a service on this client. If the client should not receive service, explain your reasons and refer her to a doctor.

PROCEDURE 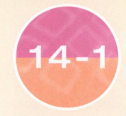 14-1

Nail Tip Application

During the procedure, discuss products such as polish, top coat, and lotion that will help your client maintain the service between salon visits.

1. **Remove old polish.** Begin with your client's left hand, little finger and work toward the thumb. Then repeat on the right hand.

2. **Push back cuticle.** Use a new cotton-tipped orangewood stick or sanitizable pusher to gently push back cuticle.

3. **Buff nail to remove shine.** Buff lightly over the nail plate with medium/fine abrasive to remove the shine and natural oil. Do not use a coarse abrasive and be careful not to apply extreme pressure. Remove the dust (Figure 14–3).

4. **Size tips.** Select the proper size tips. Make sure the tips you choose completely cover the nail plate from sidewall to sidewall but never cover more than half the length of the nail (Figure 14–4). Trim tips to the right size if the well covers too much of the nail. Nail tips should be pre-beveled along the edge closest to the cuticle to thin out the plastic. Tips that are pre-beveled require less filing on the natural nail after application. This cuts down the potential for damage to the natural nail. Put all sized tips on towel in order of finger size.

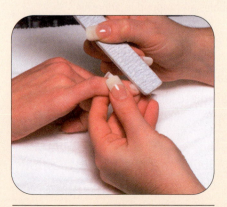

Figure 14-3 Remove shine from nails.

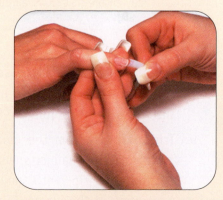

Figure 14-4 Size tips.

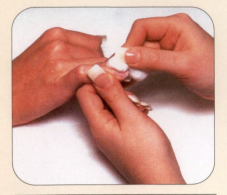

Figure 14-5 Apply nail antiseptic.

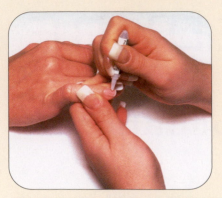

Figure 14-6 Apply adhesive.

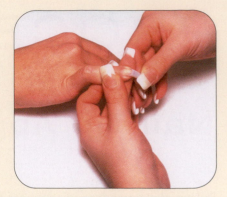

Figure 14-7 Slide on tips.

> ## ! SANITATION CAUTION
>
> **If you accidently touch the nails after you apply antiseptic, you must clean them again and reapply antiseptic.**

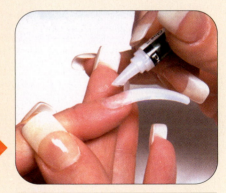

Figure 14-8 Apply adhesive bead to seam.

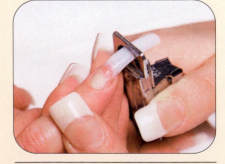

Figure 14-9 Trim nail tip.

5. **Apply nail antiseptic dehydrator.** Use a cotton-tipped orangewood stick or spray to apply nail antiseptic to nails. Begin with the little finger on the left hand. The antiseptic will remove more of the remaining natural oil and dehydrate the nail for better adhesion (Figure 14–5).

6. **Apply adhesive.** Place enough adhesive on nail plate to cover area where tip will be placed, or apply glue to well of tip. Do not let adhesive run onto the skin. Apply adhesive from the middle of the nail plate to free edge (Figure 14–6).

7. **Slide on tips.** Remember the stop, rock, and hold procedure. *Stop*—find stop against free edge at 45-degree angle. *Rock*—rock tip on slowly. *Hold*—hold in place 5 to 10 seconds until dry (Figure 14–7).

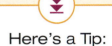

Here's a Tip:

An alternate method of applying adhesive is to apply to the well of the tip. This may ensure that fewer air bubbles are trapped in adhesive.

8. **Apply adhesive bead to seam.** Apply a bead of adhesive to seam between the natural nail plate and the tip to strengthen the stress point (Figure 14–8).

9. **Trim nail tip.** Trim the nail tip to desired length using a tip cutter or large nail clippers. Cut from one side to the other. Cutting the tip with nail clippers straight across causes weakening of the plastic (Figure 14–9).

14

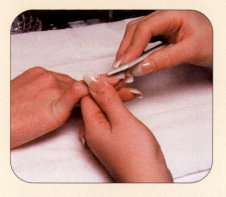

Figure 14–10 Blend tip into natural nail.

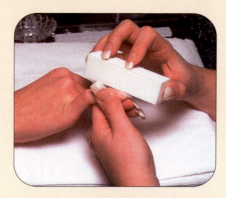

Figure 14–11 Buff tip.

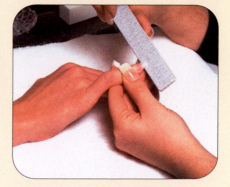

Figure 14–12 Shape tip.

10. **Blend tip into natural nail.** Sand the shine off the tip with a semi-coarse abrasive. Make sure you keep the file flat on the nail at all times. Never hold file at an angle because filing at an angle can make a groove in the nail plate (Figure 14–10).

11. **Buff tip for perfect blend.** Use the buffer block to gently buff down the area between the natural nail plate and the tip extension. The tip should blend with the natural nail so that there is no visible line or cloudiness between the two (Figure 14–11).

12. **Shape nail.** Use abrasive to shape the new, longer nail (Figure 14–12).

13. **Proceed with desired service.** Your tip application is now complete. Although your client's tips blend perfectly with natural nails, tips are very seldom worn without an additional nail service such as wraps, acrylic nails, or gel nails. You are ready to proceed with the service that your client has chosen (Figure 14–13).

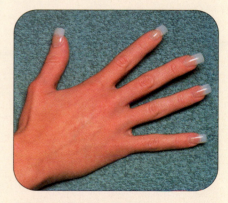

Figure 14–13 Finished tip application.

Nail Tip Post-service

If your client is only wearing tips as a temporary service, add a drop of cuticle oil to each nail and buff.

1. **Make another appointment.** Schedule another appointment with your client to remove tips and condition nails and cuticles.

2. **Sell retail products.** Suggest that your client buy products necessary to maintain her nails throughout the week. Polish, lotion, top coat, etc. are valuable maintenance tools for her to have.

3. **Clean up around your table.** Take the time to restore the basic set-up of your table. Cap glue and clean applicator tips in acetone.

4. **Discard used materials.** Place all used materials in the plastic bag at the side of the table. If the bag is full or contains used materials from artificial nail services, discard it in a closed pail.

5. **Disinfect table and sanitize implements.** Perform the complete pre-service sanitation procedure. Implements need to be sanitized 20 minutes before they can be used on the next client.

◆ ◆ ◆ ALTERNATIVE TIP APPLICATIONS

Tip Well Cutting Application

Tip well cutting is a new, alternative method of achieving the perfect smile lines with white tips or with traditional tips with no tip blending. Size out the tips for the nails, keeping in mind you're removing the well and where you cut should fit from side wall to sidewall.

With your **tip cutter**, not a nail clipper, place the tip into the cutter at a slant so your cut is not flat. It will be rounded like a smile line. Place the blade of the tip cutter above the well, removing the well completely. Cut quickly and evenly. Once you have cut the well off the tip, finish any uneven edges with a file. Put a small amount of acetone on your little finger and wipe the edge of the smile line for a perfect finish to the edge. Do this on all ten tips.

One by one, turn each tip over and brush a thin layer of glue on the edge of the underside from smile line edge to smile line edge. Place the tip right on the edge of the free edge and attach the tip to the nail. Do all ten tips; then cut and shape the nails. Apply the overlay as you normally would.

If you are applying a resin or gel overlay, build up the arch with a thicker resin or building gel first to cover the smile line thickness of the tip. Then overlay the entire nail for support. If you apply acrylic, keep in mind that you must build up the arches of the nail because it needs the extra strength. In this procedure, do not blend the tip down flush to the nail plate because that may ruin the smile line.

In theory, this procedure sounds like it would not support the nail, but remember that glue breaks down in water; gel and acrylics do not Placing the tip on the very edge of the nail and overlaying it, gives you strength. There is more product on the nail plate, not the tip. Blending a tip well takes more time so the tip well cutting is giving you a clear smile line with barely any effort.

Here's a Tip:

Before you apply the tips, spray one hand at a time with glue activator. You will have an immediate bond and won't have to waste time holding the tip in place as the glue dries.

BUSINESS TIP

Profit with Temporary Tips

Consider selling tips as a temporary service. Tips have long been favored by individuals who desire length but can't seem to grow their nails, or by those who want longer nails without the wait. However, tips have a third following—women who want temporary length for a special occasion, such as a wedding or the prom. These people might work in jobs where long nails are a hindrance or they may find that longer lengths don't fit their lifestyle, but they still want the look for a day or two. For them, create a two-appointment service. During the first visit you apply and paint the tips. Schedule the second appointment to remove the extensions, then condition and manicure the client's own, natural nails.

Tip Application with Acrylic

For added strength, you can apply tips with **acrylic**. Prep the nail plate as you normally would, prime, and let dry. One nail at a time, take a dry ball of clear acrylic. Place the ball on the very tip of the nail and spread from sidewall to sidewall. You can also apply the acrylic to the back of the tip. Let the acrylic set a bit, then take your tip and place it into the acrylic and hold in place until the acrylic is dry and secure. This definitely takes more time, but for the client who tends to pop off her tips easily or has "ski jump" nails, it is the perfect solution.

If you place the well of the tip tightly against the free edge, the excess acrylic will be pushed out onto the nail plate. Remove the excess, before it entirely sets up, with a new orangewood stick or a disinfected implement. If you leave the excess acrylic and it makes a ledge, it may make the nail appear too thick.

◆ ◆ MAINTENANCE AND REMOVAL OF TIPS

Maintenance

Clients wearing tips will need weekly or biweekly manicures for regluing and rebuffing. Reglue at the seam between the natural nail and the temporary tip. Most tips need non-acetone polish remover because acetone remover dissolves the tips.

PROCEDURE 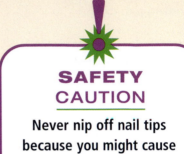 14-2

Tip Removal

Tips that have been glued to the nail plate can cause damage if removed improperly. Use a glue remover or acetone to remove tips.

1. **Complete nail tip application pre-service.** You will only need to add a buffer block to your manicuring table.

2. **Soak nails.** Place enough remover in a small glass bowl to cover nails. Soak nails for a few minutes.

3. **Slide off tip.** Use a new orangewood stick to slide off the softened tip. Be careful not to pry the tip off because you can damage the nail bed and mantle.

4. **Buff nail.** Gently buff the natural nail with a fine block buffer to remove any glue residue.

5. **Condition cuticle and surrounding skin.** Condition the cuticle and surrounding skin with cuticle oil and massage cream.

6. **Proceed to desired service.**

SAFETY CAUTION

Never nip off nail tips because you might cause permanent damage to the nail bed.

chapter glossary

abrasive	A rough surface used to shape or smooth the nail and remove the shine.
acrylic	A substance that is mixed with liquid and applied to an artificial nail tip to strengthen the natural nail and the tip.
buffer block	A lightweight, rectangular block that is abrasive and used to buff nails.
nail adhesive	A glue or bonding agent used to secure a nail tip to the natural nail.
nail tip	An artificial nail made of plastic, nylon, or acetate that is adhered to the natural nail to add length.
tip cutter	An implement similar to a nail clipper used exclusively to trim artificial tips.
tip well cutting	An alternative method of achieving the perfect smile lines using white tips or traditional tips with no tip blending.

review questions

1. List the four supplies, in addition to your basic manicuring table, that you need for nail tip application.

2. Name the two types of nail tips.

3. What portion of the natural nail plate should be covered by a nail tip?

4. What type of tip application is considered a temporary service? Why?

5. Briefly describe the procedure for a nail tip application.

6. Describe the proper maintenance of nail tips.

7. Describe the procedure for the removal of tips.

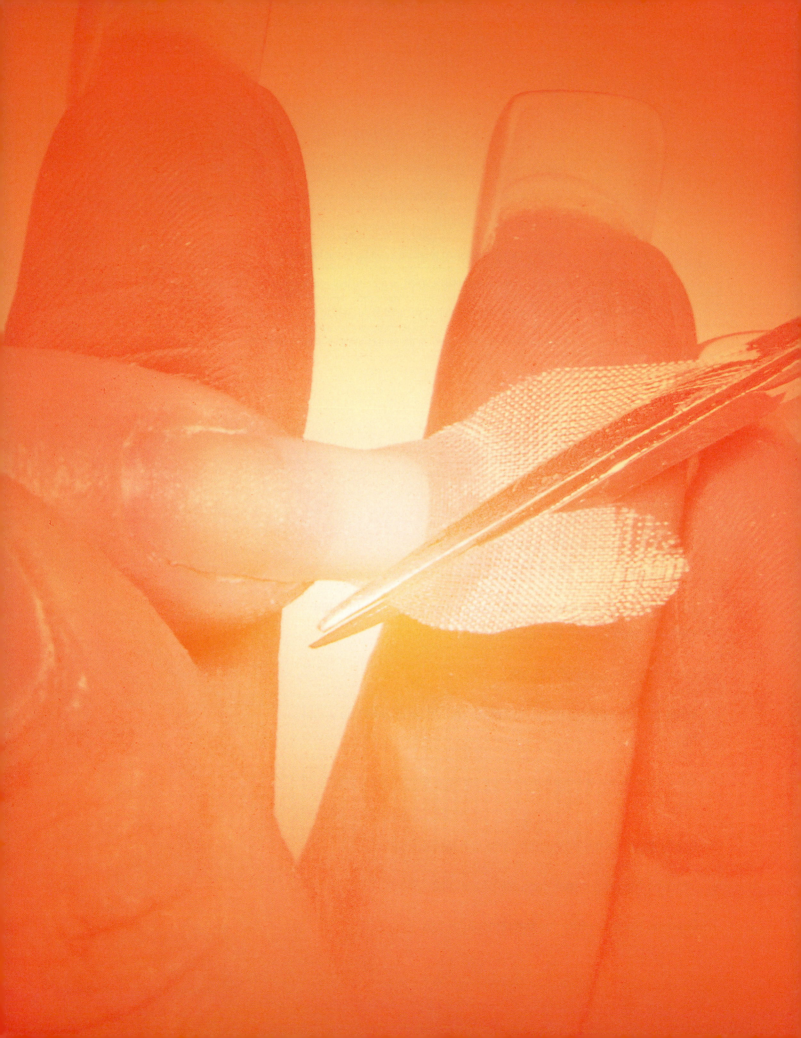

15

NAIL WRAPS

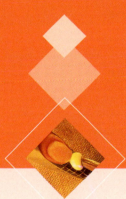

Author: Terri Lund

CHAPTER OUTLINE

Fabric Wraps • Fabric Wrap Maintenance, Removal, and Repairs
Paper Wraps • Liquid Nail Wrap

PROCEDURES

15-1 Nail Wrap

15-2 Two-Week Fabric Wrap Maintenance

15-3 Four-Week Fabric Wrap Maintenance

15-4 Paper Wrap Application

Learning Objectives

After you have completed this chapter, you should be able to:

1 List four kinds of nail wraps and what they are used for.

2 Explain benefits of using silk, linen, fiberglass, and paper wraps.

3 Demonstrate the proper procedures and precautions to use in fabric wrap application.

4 Describe the maintenance of fabric wrap. Include a description of the two-week and four-week follow-up.

5 Explain how fabric wrap is used for crack repair.

6 Demonstrate the proper procedure and precautions for fabric wrap removal.

7 List the supplies used in paper wrap.

8 Demonstrate proper procedures for paper wrap application.

9 Define liquid nail wrap and describe its purpose.

Key Terms

Page number indicates where in the chapter the term is used.

fabric wraps
pg. 269

fiberglass
pg. 269

linen
pg. 269

liquid nail wrap
pg. 280

nail wraps
pg. 269

paper wraps
pg. 269

repair patch
pg. 277

silk
pg. 269

stress strip
pg. 277

Nail wraps are nail-size pieces of cloth or paper that are bonded to the top of the nail plate with nail adhesive. They are used to repair or strengthen natural nails or nail tips. Wraps can be cut from a swatch of cloth, rolls of fabric, or a piece of paper to fit a client's nail size and shape, or they can be purchased pre-cut. Pre-cut overlays have an adhesive back.

Fabric wraps are made from silk, linen, or fiberglass. **Silk** is a thin natural material with a tight weave that becomes transparent when adhesive is applied. A silk wrap is lightweight and smooth when applied to the nail. **Linen** is a closely woven, heavy material. It is much thicker than silk or fiberglass. Because it is opaque, even after adhesive is applied, a colored polish must be used to cover it completely. Linen is a strong wrap. **Fiberglass** is a very thin synthetic mesh with a loose weave. The loose weave makes it easy for adhesive to penetrate. It is especially strong and durable.

Paper wraps are made of very thin paper and dissolve in both acetone and non-acetone remover. For this reason, paper wraps are temporary and must be reapplied when polish is removed. Paper wraps are glued both on top of the nail and under the free edge.

◆ ◆ ◆ FABRIC WRAPS

Supplies

In addition to the materials on your basic manicuring table, you will need the following items (Figure 15–1).

Fabric

Small swatches of linen, silk, or fiberglass material can be cut to fit a client's nail size and shape. You may also find pre-cut wraps with an adhesive backing.

Nail Adhesive

Glue or a bonding agent is used to secure the nail tip or fabric to the natural nail. It usually comes in a tube with a pointed applicator tip called an **extender tip** or in brush-on form. When working with adhesives, be sure to protect your eyes with goggles; offer them to your client, as well.

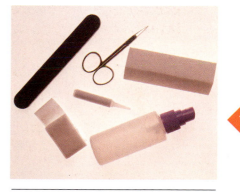

Figure 15–1 Materials necessary for fabric wrap application

Small Scissors

Small and sharp for cutting fabric.

Nail Block Buffer

Abrasive

Adhesive Dryer

Drop-on, brush-on, or spray that dries nail adhesive quickly.

Small Piece of Plastic

Nail Wrap Pre-service

Use the following preparation for all nail wrap procedures.

1. Do the pre-service sanitation procedure. (This procedure is described on pages 41–43.)

2. Set up a standard manicuring table. Add fabric, nail adhesive, small scissors, nail block buffer, abrasive, adhesive dryer, and a small piece of plastic to your table.

3. Greet your client and ask her to wash her hands in liquid soap. Dry hands and nails thoroughly with a clean or disposable towel.

4. Do client consultation, using client health/record form to record the responses and your observations. Check for nail disorders. Decide if client's nails and hands are healthy enough for you to perform a service. If the client has a nail or skin disorder and should not receive a service, explain the reasons and refer the client to a doctor. If you proceed with the service, discuss your client's needs and wants.

PROCEDURE 15-1

Nail Wrap Application

During the procedure discuss with your client the products needed to maintain the service between salon visits.

1. **Remove old polish.** Begin with the client's left hand, little finger. Saturate cotton with polish remover. If client is wearing artificial nails, use non-acetone remover to avoid damaging them. Hold saturated cotton on nail while you count to ten in your mind. Wipe the old polish off the nail with a stroking motion towards the free edge. If all polish is not removed, repeat this step until traces of polish are gone. It may be necessary to put cotton around the tip of a new orangewood stick and use it to clean polish away from cuticle area. Repeat this procedure on each finger of both hands.

2. **Clean nails.** Dip nails in a fingerbowl filled with warm water and liquid soap. Then use a nail brush to clean nails over the fingerbowl. Rinse nails briefly in clear water or have client wash in sink. DO NOT soak client's nails in water before you apply a nail wrap. Natural nails are porous and retain water.

3. **Push back cuticle.** Use the same cotton-tipped orangewood stick, with new cotton applied to the tip, to gently push back cuticle. Use a light touch because the cuticle has not been soaked.

4. **Etch nail to remove shine.** Etch lightly over nail plate with fine abrasive to remove the natural oil. Do not use a coarse file and be careful not to apply extreme pressure. Nail wraps can be done over natural nails or over a set of tips. If you are using tips, shape the free edges of the nails to fit the shape of the tip wells.

5. **Apply nail antiseptic.** Spray or wipe antiseptic onto the nails. The antiseptic will remove the remaining natural oil and dehydrate the nail for better adhesion.

6. **Apply adhesive.** Apply adhesive to the entire surface of all ten nails. This prepares them to receive wraps. Let adhesive dry. Use activator if needed to speed up process.

7. **Apply tips if desired.** Blend out the tip well with a file or tip blender.

> **! SANITATION CAUTION**
>
> Remember: do not use the same orangewood stick on more than one client. They are not sanitizable.

15

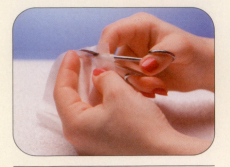

Figure 15-2 Cut fabric.

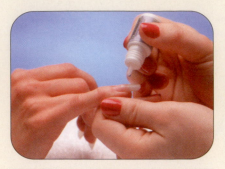

Figure 15-3 Apply fabric adhesive if using non-adhesive backed fabric.

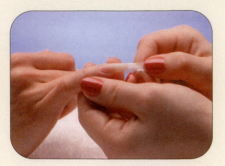

Figure 15-4 Apply fabric.

8. **Cut fabric.** Cut fabric to the approximate width and shape of the nail plate or tip. Be careful to keep the dust and oils from your fingers from contaminating the adhesive-backed fabric. This could prevent the fabric from adhering to the nail (Figure 15–2).

9. **Apply adhesive.** If you are using a non-adhesive backed fabric, you will need to apply a drop of adhesive to the center of the nail. Remember to keep adhesive off the cuticle. It could cause the wrap to lift or separate from the nail plate (Figure 15–3).

10. **Apply fabric.** Gently fit fabric over the nail, 1/16-inch away from the cuticle. Press to smooth, using a small piece of thick plastic (Figure 15–4).

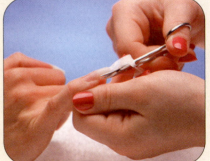

Figure 15-5 Trim fabric.

15

Here's a Tip:

Using a 6″ x 4″ piece of plastic sheet to press fabric onto nail will prevent the transfer of dust and oil from you to your client. It is necessary to constantly change to a fresh area on the plastic for each finger.

11. **Trim fabric.** Use small scissors to trim fabric 1/16-inch away from sidewalls and free edge. Trimming fabric slightly smaller than nail plate prevents fabric from lifting and separating from the nail plate (Figure 15–5).

12. **Apply fabric adhesive.** Draw a thin coat of adhesive down the center of the nail using the extender tip to apply. Do not touch the cuticle. The adhesive will penetrate the fabric and stick to the nail surface (Figure 15–6). Use the plastic again to make sure there are no bubbles or areas of fabric that missed the adhesive.

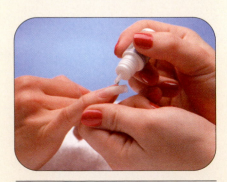

Figure 15-6 Apply adhesive.

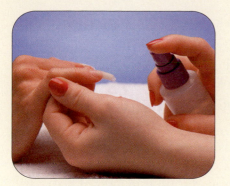
Figure 15-7 Apply adhesive dryer.

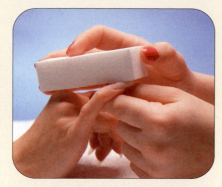
Figure 15-8 Buff tip.

13. **Apply adhesive dryer.** Spray, brush, or drop on adhesive dryer. Keep adhesive dryer off skin to prevent overexposure to the product (Figure 15–7).

14. **Apply second coat of adhesive.** Apply and spread adhesive with extender tip. Seal free edge with adhesive by running the extender tip on the edge of the nail tip to prevent any lifting.

15. **Apply second coat of adhesive dryer.**

16. **Shape and refine nails.** Use medium/fine abrasive to shape and refine nails.

17. **Buff nails.** Apply cuticle oil and buff to a high shine with block buffer. Use the block buffer to smooth out rough areas in fabric. Do not buff too much or too hard because you can wear through the wrap and weaken it (Figure 15–8).

18. **Remove traces of oil.** Send your client to thoroughly wash at the sink with a nail brush and soap, to remove not only oil, but any dust or nail chemicals.

19. **Apply polish** (Figure 15–9).

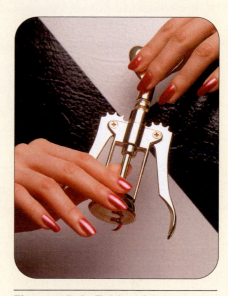
Figure 15-9 Finished fabric wraps

Nail Wrap Post-service

Follow this post-service for all your nail wrap services.

1. **Make another appointment.** Schedule another appointment with your client to maintain the nail wrap she has just received or for another service.

2. **Sell retail products.** Suggest that your client buy products necessary to maintain her nails throughout the week. Polish, cuticle cream, lotion, top coat, etc. are valuable maintenance tools for her to have.

3. **Clean up around your table.** Take the time to restore the basic set-up of your table. Cap adhesive and adhesive dryer to prevent

evaporation. Apply oil to the neck of adhesive bottle to keep the cap from sticking.

4. **Clean extender tips.** To clean clogged extender tips, place them in a covered glass jar with acetone. Poke a clean toothpick through hole.

5. **Store fabric.** Store fabric in a sealable plastic bag to protect from dust and soil.

6. **Discard used materials.** Place all used and nonsanitizable materials in the plastic bag at the side of the table. If the bag is full or contains used materials from artificial nail services, discard it in a closed pail.

7. **Sanitize table and implements.** Perform the complete pre-service sanitation procedure. Implements need to be sanitized 20 minutes before they can be used on the next client.

B U S I N E S S TIP

Host Nail Fashion Nights

Whoever coined the phrase "seeing is believing" must have known that a person is more likely to purchase something she is familiar with. To acquaint customers firsthand with the latest manicure looks, try hosting a nail fashion night. For a $10.00–$15.00 admission fee, you showcase the latest nail looks by giving each attendee a manicure—using the season's most popular fashion colors and hottest new products, of course. To top off the evening, offer each client a nail care fashion kit comprised of trial-sized products and a gift certificate for 15 percent off the next nail care purchase or service. Spending an entire night focused on the products creates a buzz about them and shows clients how to use them. The sample size gets them hooked and the gift certificate gives them an incentive to return to you.

FABRIC WRAP MAINTENANCE, REMOVAL, AND REPAIRS

Fabric wraps need regular maintenance to keep them looking fresh. In this section you will learn how to maintain fabric wraps after two weeks and after four weeks. You will also learn how to remove fabric wraps and how to use fabric wraps for crack repair.

Fabric Wrap Maintenance

Fabric wraps are maintained with glue "fills" after two weeks and with glue and fabric "fills" after four weeks.

PROCEDURE

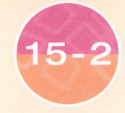

15-2

Two-Week Fabric Wrap Maintenance

After two weeks use the following procedure to maintain fabric wraps. You will need to add nail adhesive, a block buffer, and adhesive dryer to your standard table set-up.

1. **Complete nail wrap pre-service.**

2. **Remove old polish.** Use a non-acetone polish remover to avoid damaging wraps.

3. **Clean nails.**

4. **Push back cuticle.**

5. **File nail to remove shine.** Make sure the line between the new growth and the existing wrap is smooth. There should be no sign of the bottom of the wrap near the cuticle.

6. **Apply nail antiseptic.**

7. **Apply adhesive to new nail growth area.** Brush on or apply a small drop of adhesive to new nail growth. Spread with the extender tip, taking care not to touch skin.

8. **Apply adhesive dryer.**

9. **Apply adhesive to entire nail.** Apply a second coat of adhesive to entire nail to strengthen and reseal the wrap.

10. **Apply adhesive dryer.**

11. **Shape and refine nail.** Use medium/fine abrasive over surface of nail to remove any peaks and imperfections.

12. **Buff nails.** Apply cuticle oil and buff to a high shine with the block buffer.

13. **Apply hand lotion and massage hand and arm.**

14. **Remove traces of oil.** Use a small piece of cotton to remove traces of oil from the nail so polish will adhere.

15. **Apply polish.**

16. **Complete nail wrap post-service.**

PROCEDURE 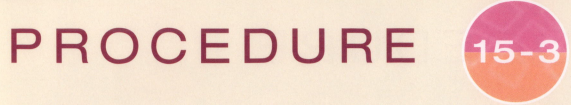 15-3

Four-Week Fabric Wrap Maintenance

After four weeks use the following maintenance procedure to apply fabric and adhesive to new growth. You will need nail adhesive, a block buffer, fabric, small scissors, and adhesive dryer in addition to your standard table set-up.

1. **Complete nail wrap pre-service.**
2. **Remove old polish.** Use a non-acetone polish remover to avoid damaging wraps.
3. **Clean nails.** Use a nail brush and liquid soap to gently clean nails or have the client wash hands at the sink using the same procedure.
4. **Push back cuticle.**
5. **Buff nail to remove shine.** Lightly buff over nail plates to remove natural oil and any small pieces of fabric that may have lifted. Buff the end of the wrap until smooth, without scratching the natural nail plate. Totally refine the nail until there is no line of demarcation between new growth and fabric wrap.
6. **Apply nail antiseptic.**
7. **Cut fabric.** Cut a piece of fabric large enough to cover the new growth area and slightly overlap the old wrap.
8. **Apply adhesive to regrowth area.** Apply a small drop of adhesive to the fill area. Spread throughout the new growth area with the extender tip or fill in the area with brush-on adhesive. Be careful to avoid touching cuticle or skin (Figure 15–10).
9. **Apply fabric.** Gently fit fabric over new growth area and smooth (Figure 15–11).
10. **Apply adhesive.** Apply another drop of adhesive, again avoiding the cuticle.
11. **Apply adhesive dryer.** Spray, brush, or drop it on the adhesive to dry adhesive more quickly.
12. **Apply adhesive.** Apply a second coat of adhesive to regrowth area.

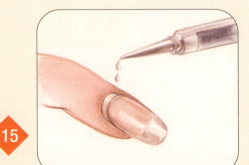

Figure 15-10 Apply adhesive to regrowth area.

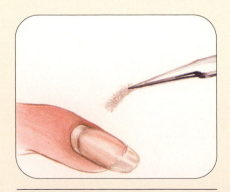

Figure 15-11 Apply fabric.

15

13. **Apply second coat of adhesive dryer.**

14. **Apply adhesive to entire nail.** Apply a thin coat of adhesive to entire nail to strengthen and seal wrap.

15. **Apply adhesive dryer.**

16. **Shape and refine nail.** Use medium/fine abrasive over surface of nail to remove any peaks and imperfections. Carefully stay away from cuticle so you do not cut and damage skin.

17. **Buff nails.** Apply cuticle oil and buff to a high shine with block buffer.

18. **Apply hand lotion and massage hand and arm.**

19. **Remove traces of oil.** Use a small piece of cotton and acetone to remove traces of oil from nail so polish will adhere.

20. **Apply polish.**

21. **Complete nail wrap post-service.**

Repairs with Fabric Wraps

Small pieces of fabric can be used to strengthen a weak point in the nail or repair a break in the nail. A **stress strip** is a strip of fabric cut to 1/8 inch. The strip is applied to the weak point of the nail, using the four-week maintenance procedure. A **repair patch** is a piece of fabric that is cut so it completely covers the crack or break in the nail. Use the four-week fabric wrap maintenance procedure to apply your repair patch.

Fabric Wrap Removal

Be careful not to damage the nail plate when removing fabric wraps.

1. **Complete nail wrap pre-service.**

2. **Soak nails.** Put enough acetone in a small glass bowl to cover the nails. Immerse client's nails in the bowl and soak for a few minutes. The acetone should be approximately one inch above the nails.

3. **Slide off softened wraps.** Use an orangewood stick or metal pusher to slide softened wraps away from nail.

4. **Buff nails.** Gently buff natural nails with a fine block buffer to remove the glue residue.

5. **Condition cuticles.** Condition cuticles and surrounding skin with cuticle oil and lotion.

15

◆ ◆ ◆ PAPER WRAPS

Paper wraps are applied as a temporary method of strengthening the nail. Mending tissue, a thin paper, is applied over the nail plate to add strength to a nail just as a fabric does. Paper wraps are temporary because they are applied with mending liquid, which dissolves in polish remover. Therefore, the wrap is removed each time the polish is removed. Paper wraps provide added strength for a short period of time. These wraps are not recommended for extra long nails because they do not provide the strength that long nails require.

Supplies

Mending Tissue

A lightweight thin tissue paper.

Mending Liquid

A heavy liquid adhesive that dissolves in polish remover. It is applied with a brush.

Ridge Filler

◆ ◆ LIQUID NAIL WRAP

Liquid nail wrap is a polish made of tiny fibers designed to strengthen and preserve the natural nail as it grows. It is brushed on the nail in several directions to create a network that, once hardened, protects the nail. It is similar to nail hardener, but thicker because it contains more fiber.

PROCEDURE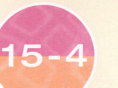

Paper Wrap Application

1. **Complete nail wrap pre-service.** Add mending liquid, mending tissue, and ridge filler to your table.

2. **Remove old polish.**

3. **Clean nails.** Use nail brush and liquid soap to gently scrub nails or have client wash hands at the sink following the same procedure.

4. **Push back cuticle.**

5. **Buff nails to remove shine.** Use medium/fine abrasive to gently remove shine from nails.

6. **Apply nail antiseptic.** Use a piece of cotton or spray to apply nail antiseptic to all nails.

7. **Tear mending tissue.** Tear tissue to fit the shape of the nail, making sure it is feathered at the edges. The tissue should be long enough to tuck under the free edge (Figure 15–12).

8. **Apply mending liquid to tissue.** Saturate each piece of tissue with mending liquid.

9. **Apply tissue.** Place wrap over the nail using two fingers (Figure 15–13).

10. **Smooth the wrap.** Use a steel pusher or orangewood stick to push tissue toward the free edge and sidewalls. Dip pusher into polish remover repeatedly and pat tissue until it is smooth.

15

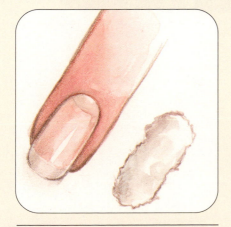

Figure 15-12 Tear mending tissue.

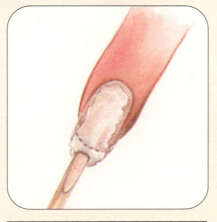

Figure 15-13 Apply tissue.

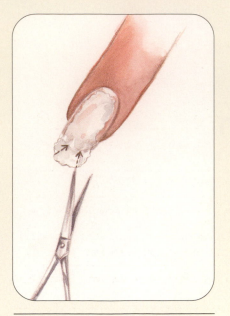

Figure 15-14 Cut slits into tissue.

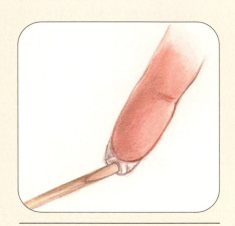

Figure 15-15 Smooth wrap under free edge.

15

11. **Trim excess tissue.** Trim tissue 1/16 inch from the sidewalls. Leave enough tissue at the end to wrap under free edge (Figure 15–14).

12. **Apply mending liquid under free edge.** Turn the finger over and apply mending liquid under free edge.

13. **Smooth wrap.** Use a pusher to smooth wrap under free edge. (Figure 15–15).

14. **Refine nail.** Gently smooth top of the wrap with the fine side of an emery board. This removes any minute particles that may cause bubbling.

15. **Apply mending liquid.** Apply two or three coats of mending liquid to the top and underside of the free edge of the nail.

16. **Apply ridge filler.** Apply a thin coat of ridge filler to top of nails to smooth surface. Allow filler to dry completely before applying polish.

17. **Apply polish.**

18. **Complete nail wrap post-service** (Figure 15–16).

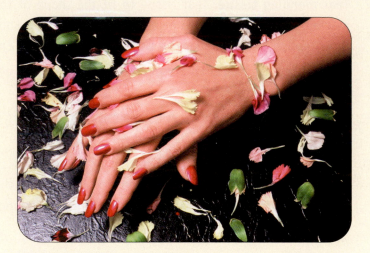

Figure 15-16 Finished paper wrap

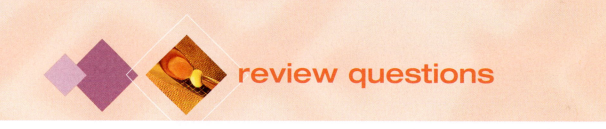

chapter glossary

fabric wraps	Nail wraps made of silk, linen, or fiberglass.
fiberglass	A very thin synthetic mesh with a loose weave used for nail wraps because it is especially strong and durable.
linen	A closely woven, heavy material used for nail wraps because it stays opaque, even after the adhesive has been applied.
liquid nail wrap	A thick polish made of tiny fibers designed to strengthen and preserve the natural nail as it grows.
nail wraps	Nail-size pieces of cloth or paper that are bonded to the top of the nail plate with nail adhesive; often used to repair or strengthen natural nails or nail tips.
paper wraps	Temporary nail wraps made of very thin paper that dissolves in acetone and non-acetone remover.
repair patch	A piece of fabric cut to completely cover a crack or break in the nail during a four-week fabric wrap maintenance procedure.
silk	A thin, natural material with a tight weave, that is sometimes used for nail wraps; becomes transparent when adhesive is applied.
stress strip	A strip of fabric, 1/8" long, applied during a four-week fabric wrap maintence, to repair or strengthen a weak point in a nail.

review questions

15

1. List four kinds of nail wraps.

2. Explain the benefits of using silk, linen, fiberglass, and paper wraps.

3. Describe the procedure for fabric wrap application.

4. Explain how a fabric wrap is used as a crack repair.

5. Describe how to remove fabric wraps and what to avoid.

6. Describe the purpose of paper wraps and explain why they are not recommended for very long nails.

7. List the materials used for paper wraps.

8. Define liquid nail wrap and describe its purpose.

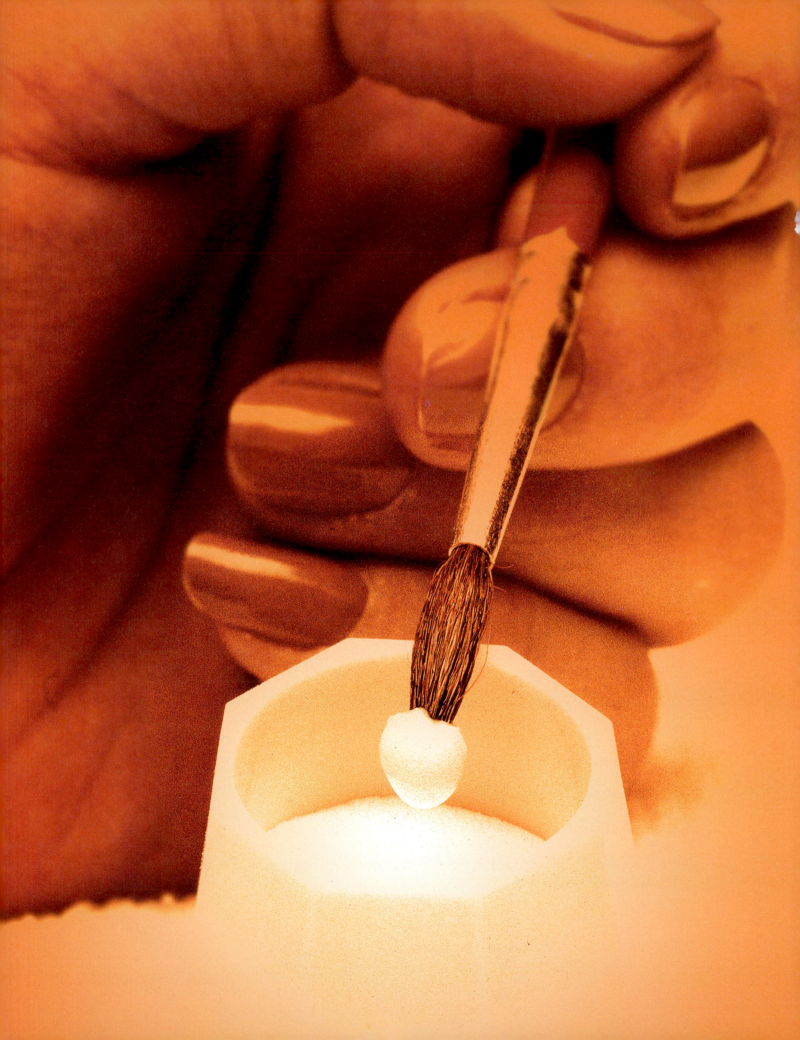

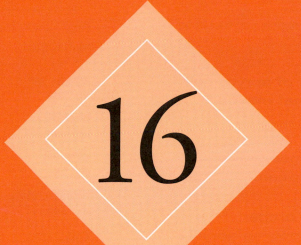

16

ACRYLIC NAILS

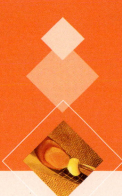

Author: Lin Halpern

CHAPTER OUTLINE

Acrylic Nails Over Forms • Acrylic Backfill • Acrylic Nail Maintenance and Removal Odorless Acrylics • Light-Cured Acrylics • Colored Acrylics • Dipping Methods

---

PROCEDURES

16-1 Acrylic Nails Using Forms • 16-2 Acrylic Nails Over Tips or Natural Nails

16-3 Acrylic Backfill Using an Electric File

16-4 Acrylic Backfill Without Using an Electric File

16-5 Acrylic Nail Application Over Bitten Nails • 16-6 Acrylic Nail Refills

16-7 Acrylic Nail Crack Repair • 16-8 Acrylic Removal

Learning Objectives

After you have completed this chapter, you should be able to:

1 Explain the origin of acrylic nail chemistry and what makes it work.

2 List the supplies needed for acrylic nail application.

3 Demonstrate the proper procedures for applying acrylics, using forms, over tips, on natural nails, and on bitten nails.

4 Practice safety precautions involving the use of primer.

5 Describe the proper procedure for maintaining healthy acrylic nails.

6 Demonstrate the proper procedure and precautions for acrylic nail application over bitten nails.

7 Perform regular maintenance procedures and repairs.

8 Implement the proper procedure for removal of acrylic nails.

9 Explain how the application of odorless and light-cured acrylics differs from the application of traditional acrylics.

10 Describe how the dipping method of using acrylics differs from all other methods.

Key Terms

Page number indicates where in the chapter the term is used.

acrylic nails
pg. 285

backfill
pg. 296

catalyst
pg. 285

cyanoacrylate
pg. 307

fills
pg. 301

odorless acrylics
pg. 306

photo initiators
pg.306

polymer
pg. 285

polymerization
pg. 285

reaction
pg. 285

rebalancing
pg. 301

Acrylic nails (a-KRYL-yk), often referred to as sculptured nails or enhancements, are created by combining acrylic liquid and acrylic powder. They can be applied directly onto the natural nail or can be sculpted on a form using a brush. The brush hairs are immersed into the acrylic liquid (monomer - MON-oh-mehr). The natural hair bristles absorb and hold the monomer like a reservoir. The tip of the brush is then touched to the surface of the acrylic powder (polymer - POL-i-mehr), and a wet ball of product collects on the tip of the brush. The product ball is then placed onto the nail surface and molded into shape with the use of the brush. Acrylic chemistry is manufactured from Ethylmethacrylate Monomer liquid.

For acrylic nails, Ethylmethacrylate Monomer liquid plus added ingredients are mixed together and then put into a reactor similar to a pressure cooker. When the reactor completes its process, it is called a **reaction**. A transformation occurs during the reaction, changing the liquid monomer into a powdery substance called **polymer**. Reacted polymer comes from this process shaped like tiny round beads, which are not all the same size. To sort the polymer and take out the large chunks, it is poured through a mesh screen. The polymer beads are then packaged for use.

The liquid starts out as Ethylmethacrylate Monomer liquid too. Special additives are blended into the liquid to insure color stabilization, strength, and flexibility, and to prevent the liquid from becoming hardened on its own. The polymers are then blended together with pigments to change clear to pink, white, or natural. The latest colored polymers are for artistry and full nail color like reds, blues, greens, and purples.

The polymer and monomer are exactly the same chemistry except one remains in liquid form and one is in powder form. The two like chemistries, now separate from each other, need a helper to make them whole again. The helper is called a **catalyst** (KAT-a-list). The catalyst is added to the polymer during one of the blending processes and coats each of the polymer beads. When the liquid from the brush picks up the powder from the jar, another reaction begins. The catalyst "explodes" when it makes contact with the monomer, causing heat. The heat starts a chain reaction like a set of dominos set up on edge; as you tap the first domino it hits the next, and so on, and so on. The heat caused by the explosion of the catalyst sets off a chain of movements. Heat transfers from one polymer bead to another and continues until the last polymer bead receives heat. This process is called **polymerization** (POL-i-mehr-eh-za-shun).

16

◆ ◆ ◆ ACRYLIC NAILS OVER FORMS

Today's acrylic powders come in many colors, including variations of basic pink, white, clear, and natural. Artistic acrylic colors are also available for nail extensions to create patterns and florals within the overlay acrylic nail structure. Acrylics can be done by either using one-color powder over the entire nail surface or using pink powders on the nail bed and white powder on the free edge area to replicate the French manicure look. The finished surface can then be polished with nail enamel or given a high-gloss shine for a more natural look.

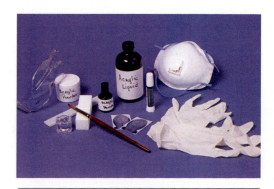

Figure 16–1 Materials needed for application of acrylic nails

Supplies for Acrylic Nails

In addition to the supplies in your basic manicuring set-up, you will need the following items (Figure 16–1).

Acrylic Liquid

Combined with the acrylic powder to form the sculptured nail. Also referred to as a monomer.

Acrylic Powder

Powder in white, clear, natural, pink, and many other colors is available. The color(s) you choose will depend on the acrylic nail method you are using. Also referred to as polymer.

Sanitizer

Your entire work area needs to be sanitized before beginning acrylic service.

Antiseptic

Spray your hands and your client's hands before beginning, or both of you should wash with a liquid soap. Dry hands thoroughly with a clean or disposable towel.

Dehydrater

Apply liberally to natural nail plate only, to cleanse and remove surface moisture on the nail plate prior to acrylic application.

Primer

Acid primer (methacrylate acid) is widely used to enhance the adhesion of the acrylic to the natural nail. This product should be used with caution. Using a tiny applicator brush, insert the brush tip into the primer. Touch the brush tip to the edge of the bottle's neck to release the excess primer back into the bottle. Using a light dotting action, dab the brush tip to the prepared natural nail only. The acid leaves a residue molecule behind. The open-ended molecule connects with the acrylic molecules to form a better bond to each other. *Be sure to read the label for manufacturer's suggested use and cautions.*

Non-acid Primer

The chemistry of a non-acid primer contains adhesive additives. It is *not* glue. These formulas vary from manufacturer to manufacturer. They work similarly to double-sided sticky tape, attaching one product to another. They are non-invasive to the natural nail and non-corrosive to the skin, but they may not be as effective as acid primer.

Abrasives

Select a coarse (100) grit for natural nail preparation and initial shaping. Choose a medium (180 to 240) grit for smoothing and a fine block buffer of 350 or more grit for final buffing. A three-way shiner file is used when no polish is worn. This shiner file brings the acrylic surface to a high-gloss shine. (Nail files come in coarse, medium, and fine grits.)

Nail Forms

These are placed at the fingers' ends to extend acrylic past fingertip. They are made of paper/mylar coated, adhesive-backed, or pre-shaped plastic or aluminum. Remember to sanitize the plastic and aluminum forms and dispose of the adhesive-backed ones for each client.

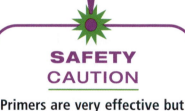

SAFETY CAUTION

Primers are very effective but can cause serious, sometimes irreversible, damage to the skin and eyes. Never use primer without plastic gloves and safety glasses.

16

Nail Tips

These are preformed nail extensions (available in a variety of shapes and colors like natural, white, and clear).

Nail Glue

There are many types of glue for securing nail tips to the natural nails. Choose a small size (4–6 gms maximum) because glue has a shelf life of up to six months depending on usage. Be sure to close cap securely, set upright, and store at room temperature between 60–85°F.

Dappen Dish

The monomer is poured into the dappen dish. During use, the monomer can become contaminated as the brush redips into the liquid, so *never* pour your unused portion of monomer back into the original container. Refill your dappen dish as needed while you work. Wipe clean with acetone before storing in a dust-free location. Dappen dishes can also be used as small containers for your powders.

Brush

For use with acrylics, the best brush is made of sable hair. Synthetic and less expensive brushes do not pick up enough liquid or release the acrylic properly. Choose the brush shape and size with which you feel the most comfortable.

Safety Glasses

Optional (Use plastic eyeglasses for protection.)

Safety Mask

Optional. This is worn over nose and mouth to prevent inhalation of dust (available in disposable soft paper or preformed cup-style).

Plastic Gloves

Acrylic Nail Pre-service

1. **Complete the pre-service sanitation procedure on pages 41–43.**
2. **Set up your standard manicuring table.** Add the acrylic materials to your table. Always have enough supplies to prevent running out while performing the service.
3. **Greet client and ask her to wash hands with soap.** Be sure to dry hands thoroughly with a clean disposable towel.
4. **Do client consultation, using client health/record form to record responses and observations.** Check for nail disorders and decide if it is safe and appropriate to perform a service on this client. If the client should not receive a service, explain your reasons and refer her to a doctor. Record any skin or nail disorders, allergies, and medications being taken. Make a note if the client is a nail biter or does heavy work in her daily routine. Write a brief notation alerting you of abusive activity to the new acrylic. Write down specific information about the service you will perform (e.g., acrylic overlay with polish, acrylic pink and white with gloss coat, the color polish the client chooses).

PROCEDURE 16-1

Acrylic Nails Using Forms

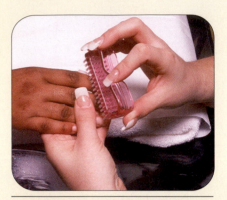

Figure 16-2 Clean nails.

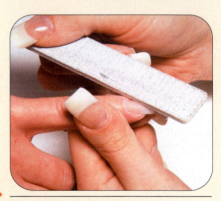

Figure 16-3 Buff nails to remove shine.

1. **Clean nails and remove polish.** Begin with your client's left hand, little finger, and work toward the thumb. Then repeat on the right hand (Figure 16–2).
2. **Push back cuticle.** Use a cotton-tipped orangewood stick to gently push back cuticle.
3. **Remove shine from natural nail surface.** Buff lightly over nail plate with medium/fine abrasive to remove the natural oil. Brush off filings (Figure 16–3).
4. **Apply nail antiseptic.** Apply nail antiseptic to nails with cotton-tipped orangewood stick, cotton, or spray. Begin with the little finger on the left hand and work toward the thumb (Figure 16–4).
5. **Position nail form.** Position nail form on nail. If you are using disposable forms, peel a nail form from its paper backing and, using the thumb and index finger of each of your hands, bend the form into an arch to fit the client's natural nail shape. Slide the form onto your client's finger and press adhesive backing to sides of the finger. Check to see that the form is snug under the free edge and level with the natural nail.

   If you are using reusable forms, slide the form onto the client's finger, making sure the free edge is over the form and that it fits snugly. Be careful not to cut into the part of the skin under the free edge. Tighten the form around the finger by squeezing lightly (Figure 16–5).
6. **Apply primer.** Put on plastic gloves and a pair of safety glasses and offer a pair of safety glasses to your client (Figure 16–6). Most primer bottles have self-contained brushes. These brushes

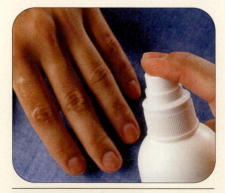

Figure 16-4 Apply nail antiseptic.

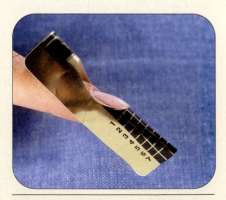

Figure 16-5 Position nail form.

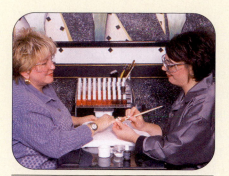

Figure 16–6 Always wear safety glasses when applying primer.

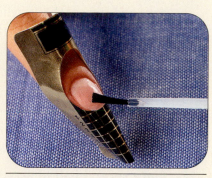

Figure 16–7 Carefully dot on primer. Allow to spread.

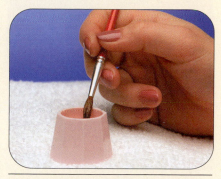

Figure 16–8 Dip brush into acrylic liquid.

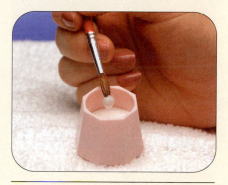

Figure 16–9 Form ball of acrylic.

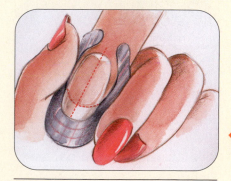

Figure 16–10 The center line and free edge of the nail

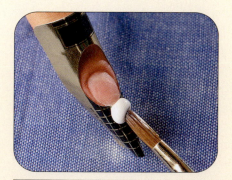

Figure 16–11 Place ball of acrylic on nail form.

hold too much primer and can cause primer burn. Use a separate primer brush to apply a dot of primer to the natural nail surface. The primer prepares the nail surface for bonding with the acrylic material. Primer will spread evenly without moving the brush over the entire nail surface. Avoid overusing primer. Overly primed nails can become too slick and cause acrylic to lift. Do not use hair dryers or wave hands in the air. Allow primer to dry naturally to a chalky white appearance (Figure 16–7).

7. **Prepare acrylic liquid and powder.** Pour acrylic liquid and acrylic powder into separate small containers. If you are using the two-color method, you will need three small containers—one for the white tip powder, one for the clear, natural, or pink powder, and one for the acrylic liquid. (Throughout this chapter, pink and white acrylic powders are used for the two-color method. Your client may select the one-color method or may pick clear or natural powder instead of pink.)

8. **Dip brush into acrylic liquid.** Dip brush fully into the liquid and wipe on the edge of the container to remove the excess (Figure 16–8).

9. **Form acrylic ball.** Dip the tip of the same brush into the acrylic powder and rotate slightly. You will pick up a ball of acrylic product of medium-dry consistency that is large enough for shaping the entire free edge extension. If you are using the two-color acrylic method, use the white powder at this point (Figure 16–9).

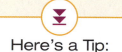

Here's a Tip:

Do not touch primed area of the nail with wet brush until you apply acrylic on the area. The acrylic will lift if the area has been touched with the wet brush.

10. **Place ball of acrylic.** Place acrylic ball on the nail form at the point where the free edge joins the nail form (Figures 16–10 and 16–11).

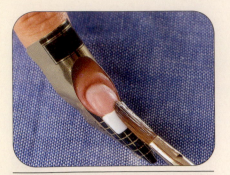

Figure 16-12 Press acrylic ball flat, keeping brush flat to nail.

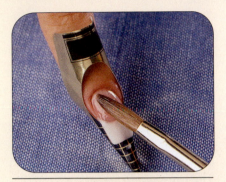

Figure 16-13a Shape white acrylic into a "smile."

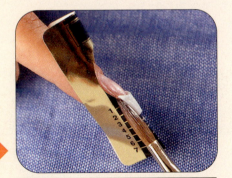

Figure 16-13b Check sidewalls.

11. **Shape free edge.** Use the middle portion of your sable brush to dab and press the acrylic to shape an extension. Do not "paint" the acrylic onto the nail. Dabbing and pressing the acrylic is more accurate than "painting" and produces a more natural-looking nail. Keep sidewall lines parallel and shape acrylic continuously along free edge line. If you are using the two-color acrylic method, make sure you follow the natural free edge line with the white powder to produce the French manicure look (Figures 16–12 and 16–13).

12. **Place second ball of acrylic.** Pick up a second ball of acrylic of medium consistency and place it on natural nail next to the free edge line in center of nail (Figure 16–14).

13. **Shape second ball of acrylic.** Dab and press product to sidewalls, making sure the product is very thin around all edges. If you are using a two-color acrylic product, use the pink powder in this step (Fig 16–15).

14. **Apply acrylic beads.** Pick up small, wet beads of pink acrylic powder on your brush and place at cuticle area. Use the moisture in the brush to smooth these beads over entire nail plate. Glide brush over nail to smooth out imperfections. Acrylic application near cuticle, sidewall, and free edge should be extremely thin for a natural-looking nail (Figure 16–16).

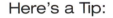

Here's a Tip:
Acrylic applied too thickly near cuticle can cause the acrylic nail to lift.

15. **Apply acrylic to remaining nails.** Repeat steps 5–14 on remaining nails.

16. **Remove forms.** When nails are thoroughly dry, loosen forms and slide them off. Nails are dry when they make a clicking sound when lightly tapped.

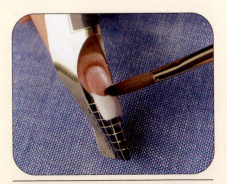

Figure 16-13c Wipe clean above smile line.

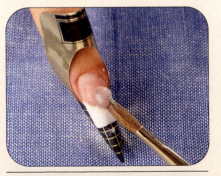

Figure 16-14 Place ball above smile line onto natural nail.

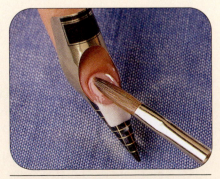

Figure 16-15 Shape second ball of acrylic.

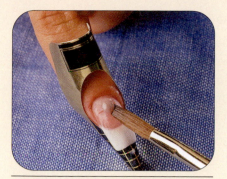

Figure 16–16 Apply smaller acrylic bead below cuticle area.

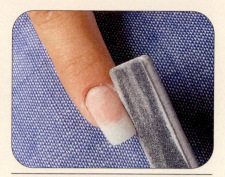

Figure 16–17a File sidewalls evenly toward free edge.

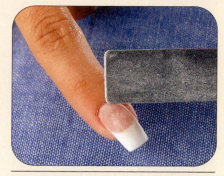

Figure 16–17b Smooth and thin out cuticle area.

17. **Shape nails.** Use coarse/medium abrasive to shape free edge and to remove imperfections. Glide abrasive over each nail with long sweeping strokes to further shape and perfect nail surface. Make nails thinner toward cuticles, free edge, and sidewalls (Figure 16–17).

18. **Buff nails.** Buff nails with block buffer until entire surface is smooth (Figure 16–17d).

19. **Apply cuticle oil.** Use a cotton-tipped orangewood stick to apply cuticle oil to cuticles, surrounding skin, and nails (Figure 16–18).

20. **Apply hand cream and massage hand and arm.**

21. **Clean nails.** Ask client to wash with soap and use a nail brush to clean nails. Rinse with water. Dry thoroughly with a clean, disposable towel. If your client selected the two-color method, her acrylic nails are finished except for a brush-on sealer or a buffed shine.

22. **Apply polish.** If your client selected one-color acrylic nails, apply the polish she has chosen (Figure 16–19).

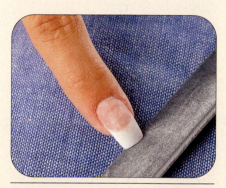

Figure 16–17c Shape and contour free edge thickness.

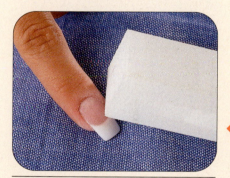

Figure 16–17d Buff entire surface with a white block buffer.

16

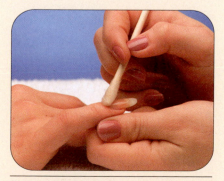

Figure 16–18 Apply cuticle oil.

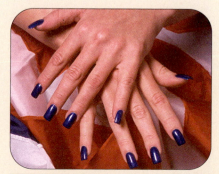

Figure 16–19 Finished acrylic nails

Acrylic Nail Post-service

1. **Make another appointment.** Schedule another appointment with your client for maintaining her acrylic nails. A fill-in will be necessary in two or three weeks, depending on how quickly the nails grow. Encourage your client to return for a plain manicure between acrylic maintenance appointments if her acrylic nails are polished.

2. **Sell retail products.** Suggest that your client buy products necessary to maintain her acrylic nails between appointments. Polish, lotion, and top coat may be helpful.

3. **Clean up around your table.** Take the time to restore the basic set-up of your table. Be sure that all your acrylic product bottles are closed tightly. Dispose of any item that cannot be disinfected or sanitized.

4. **Clean brush.** Clean brush in acetone or in manufacturer's cleaner. Never pull out bristles of brush because you will loosen the remaining bristles. Clip one stray hair if necessary but never trim bristles because you will ruin the accuracy of the brush. Do not allow brush to sit in acetone, as it will start to dissolve the glue that holds the bristles in the ferrule.

5. **Store acrylic products.** Store acrylic powders in covered containers. Store all primers and acrylic liquids in a cool, dark area. Do not store products near heat.

6. **Discard used materials.** Never save used primer or liquid that has been removed from original bottle. Use on one client only. In order to dispose of leftover liquid or primer, pour it into a very absorbent paper towel or cloth and then place the towel or cloth in a plastic bag. Never pour the liquid directly into the plastic bag! Place all used materials in the plastic bag at the side of the table. After all used materials have been placed in the bag, seal it, and discard it in a closed pail. It is important to remove items soiled with acrylic product from your manicuring station after each client. Dispose of these items according to your local rules and regulations.

7. **Sanitize table and disinfect implements.** Perform the complete pre-service sanitation procedure. Implements must be disinfected for 20 minutes before they can be used on another client. Reusable forms must be sanitized for at least 20 minutes in an approved disinfectant since they will be used again.

16

PROCEDURE 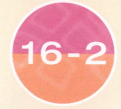 16-2

Acrylic Nails Over Tips or Natural Nails

1. **Complete acrylic nail pre-service on page 287.**

2. **Remove polish.** Begin with your client's left hand, little finger, and work toward the thumb. Then repeat on the right hand.

3. **Clean nails.** Ask the client to dip nails in a fingerbowl filled with liquid soap. Then use a nail brush to clean the nails over a fingerbowl. Rinse nails briefly in clear water and dry thoroughly with a clean, disposable towel.

4. **Push back cuticle.** Use a cotton-tipped orangewood stick or metal pusher to gently push back cuticle.

5. **Buff nail to remove shine.** Buff lightly over nail plate with medium/fine abrasive to remove the natural oil. Brush off filings with a sanitized brush.

6. **Apply nail antiseptic.** Apply nail antiseptic to nails with cotton-tipped orangewood stick, cotton, or spray. Begin with the little finger on the left hand and work toward the thumb.

7. **Apply tips.** Apply tips if your client desires them, using the technique described in Chapter 14.

8. **Apply Primer.** Put on plastic gloves and a pair of safety glasses, and offer a pair of safety glasses to your client. Most primer bottles have self-contained brushes. These brushes hold too much primer and can cause primer burn. Use a separate primer brush to apply a dot of primer to the natural nail surface. Primer will spread evenly without moving the brush over the entire nail surface. Avoid overusing primer. Overly primed nails can become too slick and cause acrylic to lift. Do not use hair dryers or wave hands in the air. Allow primer to dry naturally to a chalky white appearance.

9. **Prepare acrylic liquid and powder.** Pour acrylic liquid and acrylic powder into separate small containers. If you are using the two-color system, you will need three small containers—one for the white tip powder, one for the pink powder, and one for the acrylic liquid.

16

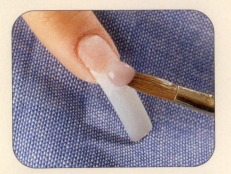

Figure 16–20a Place ball of acrylic on free edge.

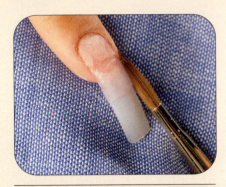

Figure 16–20b Pat and press one ball over stress and free edge area.

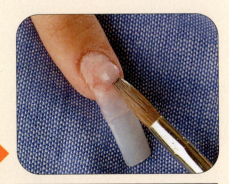

16

Figure 16–21a Place second ball of acrylic on nail bed.

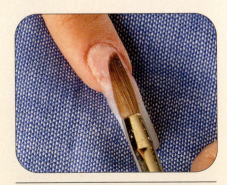

Figure 16–21b Press out second ball over nail bed area.

10. **Dip brush into liquid.** Dip brush fully into the liquid and wipe on the edge of the container to remove the excess.

11. **Form acrylic ball.** Dip the tip of the brush into white acrylic powder if you are using the two-color acrylic method, or dip the tip of the brush into clear or natural acrylic for a one-color overlay. Make a small circular pattern, then lift the brush from the powder. The ball should be medium, moist, and firm. For a smaller nail free edge, use less liquid on the brush to pick up a small product ball. For a larger nail free edge, use more liquid to pick up a larger product ball. Adjust as needed.

12. **Place ball of acrylic on free edge.** Place acrylic ball on the free edge of tip or natural nail (Figure 16–20a).

13. **Shape free edge.** Use the middle portion of your sable brush to dab and press the acrylic to shape the free edge. Keep sidewall lines parallel. Do not "paint" acrylic onto nail. If you are using the two-color acrylic method, make sure you follow the natural free edge line with the white powder to produce a French manicure look (Figure 16–20b).

14. **Place second ball of acrylic.** Pick up a second ball of acrylic of medium consistency and place it on the nail bed next to the free edge line in center of nail (Figure 16–21a).

15. **Shape second ball of acrylic.** Dab and press product to sidewalls and cuticle, making sure the product is very thin around all edges. If you are using a two-color acrylic product, use the pink powder in this step (Figure 16–21b).

16. **Apply acrylic beads.** First, cut tip to proper length (Figure 16–22a) Pick up small, wet beads of acrylic powder on your brush and place at cuticle area. Use the moisture in the brush to smooth these beads over entire nail. Glide brush over nail to smooth out imperfections. Keep acrylic application near cuticle, sidewall, and free edge extremely thin for the most natural-looking nail. For the two-color method use pink powder to form acrylic beads (Figure 16–22b-d).

17. **Shape and refine nail.** Use coarse abrasive to shape free edge and to remove imperfections. Then refine with medium/fine abrasive (Figure 16–23).

18. **Buff nails.** Buff nail with block buffer until entire surface is smooth (Figure 16–24).

19. **Apply cuticle oil.** Rub cuticle oil into cuticles surrounding skin and nail surface.

20. **Apply hand cream and massage hand and arm.**

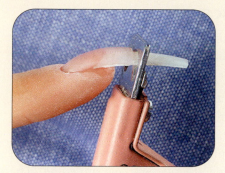

Figure 16-22a Cut tip to proper length.

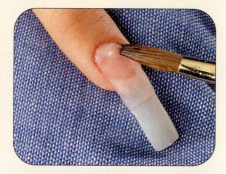

Figure 16-22b Apply small wet ball at cuticle area.

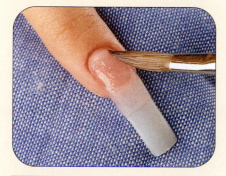

Figure 16-22c Press ball out at cuticle area.

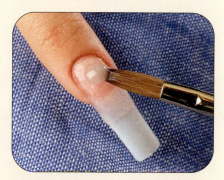

Figure 16-22d Apply stress ball (usually clear ball) over entire nail surface.

21. **Clean nails.** Ask client to dip nails in fingerbowl filled with liquid soap. Then use nail brush to clean nails over fingerbowl. Rinse with water. Dry thoroughly with a clean, disposable towel. If your client selected the two-color method, her acrylic nails are finished except for a brush-on sealer or a buffed shine.

22. **Apply polish.** Polish one-color acrylic nails (Figure 16–25).

23. **Complete acrylic post-service procedure.**

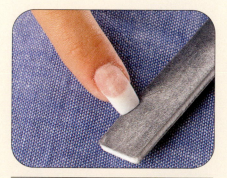

Figure 16-23 Shape and contour free edge.

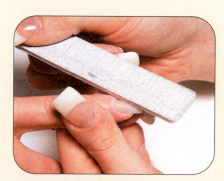

Figure 16-24 Buff nails.

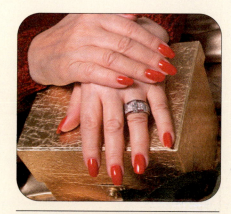

Figure 16-25 Finished acrylic.

◆ ◆ ◆ ACRYLIC BACKFILL

The term **backfill** applies to the repositioning of the white free edge. The backfill should be combined with a refill appointment. Allow extra time to complete both services.

Four to six weeks after your client receives a new pink and white French manicure acrylic application, the free edge area moves too far forward (away from the cuticle), creating a see-through space. This space now reveals the natural nail under the pink acrylic covering. The backfill procedure removes the grown out area and replaces a new smile line. The appointment rotation for an acrylic pink and white French manicure service is

❖ first revisit—refill

❖ second revisit—backfill

❖ third revisit—refill

❖ and so on

Supplies

In addition to your basic acrylic application kit, you will need the following:

Gauze Wiping Pads (or Similar Wiping Pads)

Pencil

Electric File

**Barrel Carbide Bit (or Any Other Bit
You Feel Comfortable Using)**

PROCEDURE

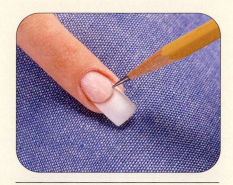

16-3

Acrylic Backfill (Using an Electric File)

1. **File entire nail surface to remove shine.** Remove clear polish, if needed, with acetone.

2. **Push back cuticle.**

3. **Prepare new nail growth area for refill.**

4. **Dust entire nail surface.**

5. **Using a pencil, draw a new smile line approximately 1/16-inch in front of the previous smile line** (Figure 16–26).

6. **Use a cylinder carbide bit on a medium speed.** Hold the bit at a 45-degree angle. With moderate pressure, score out a groove along the penciled smile line (Figure 16–27).

7. **Reposition the file parallel to the nail surface.** Grind out the area to be backfilled using the score line as your guide. Remove enough of the previously applied white acrylic to allow for application of fresh, new, white acrylic (Figure 16–28).

8. **Dust off nail filings.** Wipe with acetone to remove pencil marks (Figure 16–29).

9. **Wet backfill area with monomer.** (The wet surface will grab the product ball off the brush and pull it up to the smile line.) Pick up a white product ball and place it below the smile line onto the new backfill area. Holding your brush flat, push and guide the product toward the sidewall areas. Pat to even out the level of the white with the pink nail bed area (Figure 16–30).

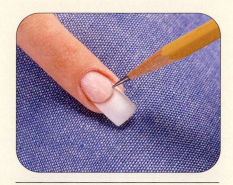

Figure 16-26 After removing shine with a file, draw a smile line with pencil.

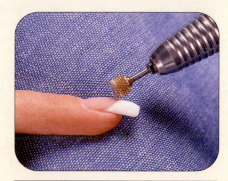

Figure 16-27 Hold bit at a 45-degree angle on medium speed. Trench out smile line.

16

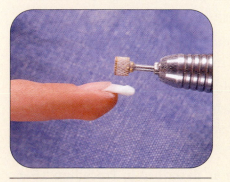

Figure 16-28 Reposition bit and remove area below smile line.

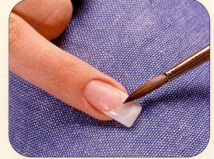

Figure 16-29 Dust. Remove pencil line using acetone swab. Moisten area with monomer.

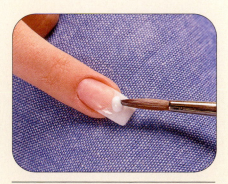

Figure 16-30 Pick up white ball and place below smile. Pat into place, covering entire free edge.

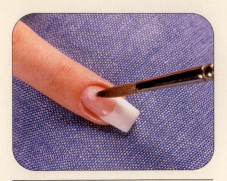

Figure 16-31 Complete refill area at cuticle with pink product ball.

10. **After all 10 smile lines are filled in, complete the pink refill** (Figure 16–31).

11. **Place a final product ball of clear to seal in the pink and white as one piece and build up the stress area** (optional).

12. **Follow steps 17–21 of the Acrylic Nail Procedure**

13. **Finish nails with one of the following:**
    ❖ Use a three-way buffer, filing all the nail surfaces to a glossy shine.
    ❖ Polish the nails with a high-gloss topcoat.
    ❖ Apply an acrylic sealer or a U.V. gel coating.

14. **Complete acrylic post-service procedure.**

PROCEDURE 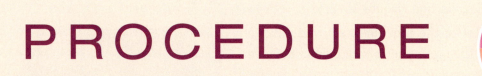 16-4

Acrylic Backfill (Without Using an Electric File)

Follow all pre-service steps.

Complete steps 1, 2, and 3 as described in Procedure 16–3.

4. **Flatten the stress area above, below, and on both sides of the new smile line area, using a coarse grit file.**

5. **Pick up a white acrylic product ball.** Recreate a new free edge with a curved smile line on top of the flattened nail surface.

6. **Pick up a pink acrylic product ball.** Place the ball above the smile line towards the cuticle. Press out product ball to re-establish the stress area dome. Be sure to amply cover the sidewall areas.

7. **Complete the refill service as described in Procedure 16–6.**

PROCEDURE

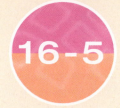

16-5

Acrylic Nail Application Over Bitten Nails

The procedure for applying acrylic nails over bitten nails is similar to the application of acrylic nails over forms. However, you must create a portion of the nail plate before applying the nail form.

1. **Complete acrylic application pre-service.**

2. **Remove polish.** Begin with your client's left hand, little finger, and work toward the thumb. Then repeat on the right hand.

3. **Clean nails.** Ask the client to dip nails in a fingerbowl filled with liquid soap. Then use a nail brush to clean the nails over a fingerbowl. Rinse nails briefly in clear water and dry thoroughly with a clean, disposable towel.

4. **Push back cuticle.** Use a cotton-tipped orangewood stick or a metal pusher to gently push back cuticle.

5. **Remove shine from natural nail surface.** Buff lightly over nail plate with medium/fine abrasive to remove the natural oil. Brush off filings.

6. **Apply nail antiseptic.** Apply nail antiseptic to nails with cotton-tipped orangewood stick, cotton, or spray. Begin with the little finger on the left hand and work toward the thumb.

7. **Apply primer.** Put on plastic gloves and a pair of safety glasses, and offer a pair of safety glasses to your client. Primer is meant for the nail plate only. People with bitten nails often have rough cuticles and damaged surrounding skin. Be very careful to avoid touching any of the client's skin with primer. Most primer bottles have self-contained brushes. These brushes hold too much primer and can cause primer burn. Use a separate primer brush to apply a dot of primer to the natural nail surface. Primer will spread evenly without moving the brush over the entire nail surface. Avoid overusing primer. Overly primed nails can become too slick and cause acrylic to lift. Do not use hair dryers or wave hands in the air. Allow primer to dry naturally to a chalky white appearance.

SANITATION CAUTION

Check primer for clarity on a regular basis to make sure it is not contaminated with bacteria. If bacteria are present, the primer will appear grainy and cloudy.

16

8. **Prepare acrylic liquid and powder.** Pour acrylic liquid and acrylic powder into separate small containers.

9. **Form acrylic ball.** Pick up a small ball of acrylic product of medium/dry consistency. Use white for the two-color method.

10. **Place ball of acrylic on skin.** Apply a small ball of acrylic product on the skin near bitten nail.

11. **Create nail plate.** Use the middle of your brush to dab and press to shape a nail plate or a base for the form on which the acrylic nail will be built. Do not place acrylic product beyond the sidewall line.

12. **Pull skin away.** Allow the acrylic to dry completely. You should be able to hear a click when you tap it with the end of a brush. Then gently pull the client's skin away at the free edge line. You will now have a free edge that is large enough to support a nail form.

13. **Position nail form.** Position nail form under newly created free edge.

14. **Place ball of acrylic.** Pick up ball of acrylic of medium consistency and place it on the nail form where the nail meets the nail form.

15. **Shape free edge.** Use the middle of your brush to dab and press the acrylic to shape an extension. Make the free edge extend only slightly beyond fingertip because people with bitten nails are not used to having long nails.

16. **Place second ball of acrylic.** Pick up a second ball of acrylic of medium consistency and place it next to the free edge line in center of nail. If you are using the two-color method, use pink powder.

17. **Shape second ball of acrylic.** Dab and press product to sidewalls and cuticle area, making sure the product is very thin around all edges.

18. **Apply acrylic beads.** Pick up small, wet beads of acrylic powder and place at cuticle area. Use the moisture in the brush to smooth these beads over cuticle and entire nail plate. If you are using a two-color method, use pink powder.

19. **Remove forms.** When nails are thoroughly dry, loosen forms and slide them off. Nails are dry when they make a clicking sound when lightly tapped.

20. **Shape nails.** Use coarse/medium abrasive to shape free edge and to remove imperfections.

16

21. **Buff nails.** Buff nails with block buffer until entire surface is smooth.

22. **Apply cuticle oil.** Rub cuticle oil into surrounding skin and nail surface.

23. **Apply hand cream and massage hand and arm.**

24. **Clean nails.** Ask the client to dip nails in a fingerbowl filled with liquid soap. Then use a nail brush to clean nails over fingerbowl. Rinse with water. Dry thoroughly with a clean, disposable towel. Your two-color acrylic nails are finished except for a brush-on sealer or a buffed shine.

25. **Apply polish.** Polish one-color acrylic nails.

26. **Complete acrylic application post-service.**

◆ ◆ ◆ ACRYLIC NAIL MAINTENANCE AND REMOVAL

Regular maintenance helps prevent acrylic nails from lifting or cracking. When acrylic nails lift, crack, or grow out with no maintenance, moisture and dirt can become trapped under the acrylic nail and fungus can begin to grow.

Acrylic Maintenance

There are two basic types of maintenance for acrylic nails—fills and crack repair.

Fills

Fills refer to the addition of acrylic to the new growth area of the nails. Acrylic nails should be filled in every two to three weeks, depending on how fast the nail grows. During fills, a defining of the contour of the nail should be performed (rebalancing). Without a rebalancing, the nail will begin to look unnatural and uneven as it grows longer. The new growth area near the cuticle will be noticeably lower than the rest of the nail. Use the following procedure for rebalancing.

16

PROCEDURE 16-6

Acrylic Nail Refills

1. **Complete acrylic application pre-service.**

2. **Remove old polish.**

3. **Smooth ledge between new growth and acrylic nail.** Use a medium/fine abrasive to smooth the ledge of acrylic in the new growth area so that it blends into the nail plate.

4. **Refine entire nail.** Hold an abrasive flat and glide it over entire nail to reshape and refine the nail and thin out the free edge.

5. **Buff nail.** Use a buffer block to buff acrylic and blend it into new growth area.

6. **Blend acrylic that has lifted.** Use a file to smooth out any acrylic that might have lifted.

7. **Clean nail.** Use a fingerbowl filled with warm water and liquid soap and a nail brush to gently wash nails. Do not soak nails.

8. **Push back cuticles.** Use a cotton-tipped orangewood stick to gently push back cuticle.

9. **Remove shine from natural nail surface.** Buff lightly over nail plate with medium/fine abrasive to remove the natural oil. Brush off filings.

10. **Apply nail antiseptic.** Apply nail antiseptic to nails with cotton-tipped orangewood stick, cotton, or spray.

11. **Apply primer.** Put on plastic gloves and a pair of safety glasses, and offer a pair of safety glasses to your client. Most primer bottles have self-contained brushes. These brushes hold too much primer and can cause primer burn. Use a separate primer brush to apply a dot of primer to the natural nail surface. Primer will spread evenly without moving the brush over the entire nail surface. Avoid overusing primer. Overly primed nails can become too slick and cause acrylic to lift. Do not use hair dryers or wave hands in the air. Allow primer to dry naturally to a chalky white appearance.

12. **Prepare acrylic liquid and powder.** Pour acrylic liquid and acrylic powder into separate small containers.

SAFETY CAUTION

Do not use a nipper to clip away loose acrylic. Nipping may perpetuate the lifting problem and can damage the nail plate. If lifting is excessive, soak off acrylic and start fresh with a new nail application.

16

13. **Place balls of acrylic.** Pick up one or more small balls of acrylic and place them on the new growth area. Be sure to use pink acrylic if you are using a two-color method.

14. **Shape balls of acrylic.** Use middle of brush to dab and press the acrylic until it blends into the existing sculptured nail.

15. **Place balls of acrylic.** Pick up one or more small wet balls of acrylic and place them at the base of the nail bed towards the cuticle.

16. **Shape beads of acrylic.** Use the moisture in the brush to smooth these beads over entire nail plate. Glide brush over nail to smooth out imperfections. Acrylic application near the cuticle, sidewall, and free edge should be extremely thin for a natural-looking nail. If you are using a two-color acrylic product, use the pink powder in this step.

17. **Shape nails.** Allow nails to dry thoroughly. Nails are dry when they make a clicking sound when lightly tapped. Use a coarse/medium grit abrasive to shape free edge and remove any imperfections. Use medium/fine abrasive to glide over nail with long sweeping strokes to further shape and perfect nail surface. Taper nail shape toward cuticle, nail tip, and sidewalls, making it thin at all edges. (After four or five weeks of growth, the white acrylic free edge created with the two-color method grows beyond the natural free edge. At this time, your client may want to start wearing polish, may ask you to file back the white free edge to create a one-color nail, or want you to do a backfill.)

18. **Buff nail.** Smooth entire surface of nail using a block buffer until it is smooth.

19. **Apply cuticle oil.** Rub cuticle oil into surrounding skin, cuticle, and nail surface using a cotton-tipped orangewood stick.

20. **Apply hand cream and massage hand and arm.**

21. **Clean nails.**

22. **Apply polish.**

23. **Complete acrylic application post-service.**

Crack Repair for Acrylic Nails

Acrylic **crack repair** is the addition of extra acrylic to fill the crack in an acrylic nail and reinforce the rest of the nail. Follow Procedure 16-7 for this maintenance technique.

PROCEDURE 16-7

Acrylic Nail Crack Repair

1. **Complete acrylic application pre-service.**
2. **Remove old polish.**
3. **File cracked acrylic.** File a "V" shape into the crack or file flush to remove crack.
4. **Clean nails.** Ask client to wash hands with liquid soap. Rinse nails briefly in clear water. Dry nails thoroughly with a clean, disposable towel.
5. **Apply nail antiseptic.** Apply nail antiseptic to nails using cotton-tipped orangewood stick, cotton, or spray.
6. **Apply primer.** If natural nail plate is exposed, put on plastic gloves and a pair of safety glasses and apply a dot of primer to the area.
7. **Apply nail form.** If the crack is large, apply a nail form for added support.
8. **Prepare acrylic liquid and powder.** Pour acrylic liquid and acrylic powder into separate small containers.
9. **Place balls of acrylic.** Pick up one or more small beads of acrylic and apply them to the cracked area. If you are using the two-color system, be sure to use the correct color acrylic.
10. **Shape balls of acrylic.** Dab and press the acrylic to fill crack. Be careful not to let acrylic seep under form or under existing nail.
11. **Place additional balls of acrylic.** Apply additional acrylic, if needed, to fill in crack or reinforce the rest of the nail. Shape acrylic and allow it to dry thoroughly.
12. **Remove form** (if used).
13. **Reshape nail.**
14. **Buff until smooth.**
15. **Clean nails.**
16. **Apply cuticle oil.**
17. **Apply hand cream and massage hand and arm.**
18. **Clean nails.**
19. **Apply polish.**
20. **Complete acrylic application post-service.**

PROCEDURE

Acrylic Removal

1. **Fill bowl with acetone.** Fill glass bowl with enough acetone to cover client's fingertips.

2. **Soak fingertips.** Soak client's fingertips for 15 minutes or as long as needed to remove acrylic product. Refer to the manufacturer's directions for acrylic removal.

3. **Remove acrylic.** Use a metal pusher or a new orangewood stick and gently push off softened acrylic nail. Repeat until all acrylic has been removed. Do not pry off acrylic with nippers, as this will damage the natural nail plate.

4. **Buff nails.** Gently buff natural nail with a fine block buffer to remove the acrylic residue.

5. **Condition cuticle.** Condition cuticle and surrounding skin with cuticle oil and hand lotion.

◆ ◆ ◆ ODORLESS ACRYLICS

Odorless acrylics have a completely different chemistry from traditional acrylics. The chemicals used do not evaporate as in traditional acrylics; therefore, you cannot smell them. The liquid monomer is much denser than traditional acrylics and will pick up 4–5 times the amount of powder. This ratio creates a snowy product ball on your brush. Multiple circular motions are needed to form the proper ratio. Lift your brush and tap gently to remove excess powder from the product ball. Once the product ball is placed on the nail it will slowly wet out to a firm, glossy ball. Use a dry brush, wiping frequently, to avoid the product sticking to the brush. A patting brush technique moves the product on the nail surface. Never rewet the brush. This will offset the powder-liquid ratio. As the surface self-levels, a light, brushing stroke contours the surface to perfection. The chemicals in the liquid react with those of the powder to become hard. This is similar to the way a microwave oven cooks food—from the inside out. As the inner layers become hard, the unused portion of the monomer rises to the top surface forming a tacky layer. Once dried, this layer can be removed using either acetone or a manufacturer-recommended cleaner.

The layer may also be filed off. As you file, stroke in one direction, down toward the free edge. Many nail technicians prefer odorless products for the following reasons.

1. **No odor:** No evaporation, no loss of product, cost effective.

2. **More time to sculpt:** Drying time is 3–5 minutes; product can be moved about more slowly. Odorless acrylics self-level resulting in less final shaping.

3. **Easier filing:** The tacky layer rolls off easily to reveal a perfectly domed, hard finished surface beneath. Due to the differences in their chemistries, they are not compatible with other acrylics. Do not mix products.

LIGHT-CURED ACRYLICS

Light-cured acrylics are similar to odorless acrylics with an added feature, **photo initiators**. These photo initiators trigger the chemicals to harden when exposed to a special ultraviolet (U.V.) lamp made for artificial light cure nail products. The chemicals in light-cured acrylics also do not evaporate, so they too are odorless. The entire procedure is exactly like that of an odorless acrylic except for the need of a U.V. lamp. Follow the manufacturer's guidelines. Each light-cured product uses a slightly different technique, but remains mostly as described in the preceding odorless section. Due to the differences in their chemistries they are not compatible with other acrylics. Do not mix products.

COLORED ACRYLICS

All acrylics are manufactured "clear." Then pigments are added to create the colors of pink, white, and natural. The more white added, the more opaque the color becomes. The less white added, the clearer the color remains. The newest colors available are mimicking the nail polish industry. Every color of the rainbow is available. Nail artistry on the acrylic nail is limited only to your imagination. Some technicians also use colors to go beyond the traditional pink and white French manicure combinations. One word of caution: with the nail bed surface completely covered with an opaque color, you cannot see the health of the nail beneath. Use colored acrylics wisely. Floral patterns and designs with sparse coverings allow for a visual check of the nail bed and result in a healthier client.

DIPPING METHODS

Many acrylic products available on the market utilize a brush-on liquid and a tub of "dip-in" or "sprinkle-on" powder. Most of these do not use an acrylic liquid monomer. This method uses a **cyanoacrylate** (si-ah-no-ah-

16

KRILL-ate) monomer ester. Cyanoacrylate is a very fast-setting glue. Apply the glue to the nail surface with or without the use of a tip extension. The powder is then applied over the glue. The glue hardens as the powder is absorbed into the glue. Some systems require an activator to complete the hardening process. Once dry, the overlay is filed and shaped to a finished nail and polished. Follow normal pre- and post-service procedures for all types of artificial nail systems.

BUSINESS TIP

Celebrate the Holidays

Taking advantage of gift-giving holidays like Christmas, Chanukah, St. Valentine's Day, Secretary's Day, and Mother's Day brings you a 20 to 50 percent temporary surge in retail sales. To make money during the holidays, you must do two things: decorate festively to encourage clients to consider shopping for presents, and offer a wide range of gifts that customers can conveniently buy while they're at their appointments. Try creating two or three festive packages with different product combinations and sizes, priced from $5.00 to $15.00. People buy these for stocking stuffers or to give as office or church/synagogue gifts. Also, don't forget to offer gift certificates in any denomination.

acrylic nails	A nail enhancement created by combining acrylic liquid with acrylic powder, and applied directly to the natural nail.
backfill	A maintenance procedure performed every four to six weeks on acrylic nails to remove the grown out free-edge area and replace the smile line.
catalyst	The substance that creates a chemical reaction between acrylic liquid and acrylic powder, combining them to form the acylic used for nail enhancements.
cyanoacrylate	A very fast setting glue used with brush-on or dip-in acrylic powder.
fills	The addition of acrylic to the new growth area of the nails. This procedure should take place every two to three weeks.
odorless acrylics	Acrylics that are much different from traditional acrylics in that they do not evaporate, have no smell, and are much denser, giving the nail technician more time to sculpt.
photo initiators	A feature of light-cured acrylics that triggers the chemicals to harden when exposed to a special U.V. lamp.
polymer	Substance formed by combining many small molecules (monomers), usually in long, chain-like structures.
polymerization	Chemical reaction that creates polymers; also called curing or hardening.
reaction	A transformation that occurs in a reactor, changing liquid monomer into a polymer.
rebalancing	Redefining the contour of the nail during a fill procedure to keep the nail looking natural.

review questions

1. Describe the origin of acrylic nail chemistry and what makes it work.

2. List the supplies needed for acrylic nail application.

3. Describe the procedures for application of acrylic nails over forms, over tips, on natural nails, and on bitten nails.

4. Describe the safety precautions for applying primer.

5. Describe the proper procedure for maintaining healthy acrylic nails.

6. How does the procedure for acrylic nail application over bitten nails differ from other acrylic nail procedures?

7. Describe how to perform regular maintenance on acrylic nails.

8. Describe the proper procedure for the removal of the acrylic product.

9. Explain how the application of odorless and light-cured acrylics differs from the application of traditional acrylics.

10. How does the dipping method of using acrylics differ from all other methods?

16

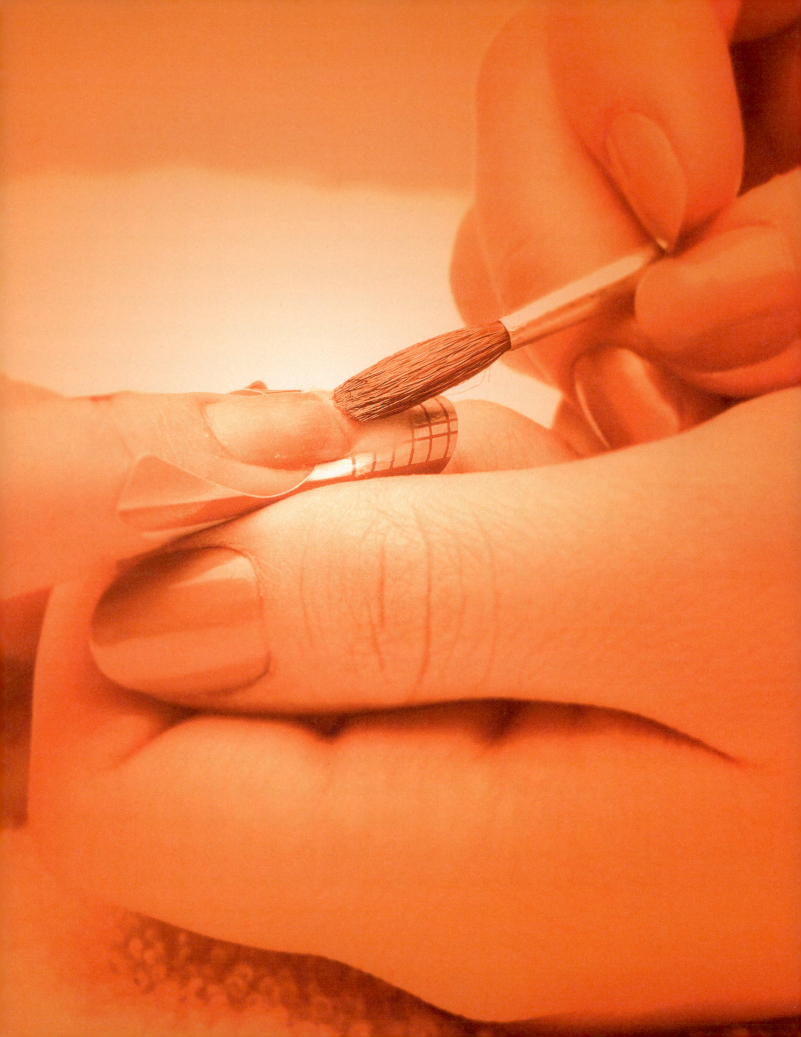

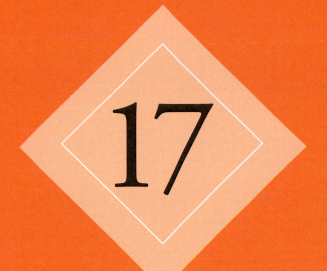

17

GELS

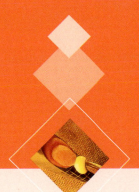

Author: Lin Halpern

CHAPTER OUTLINE

Light-cured Gel on Tips or Natural Nails

No-light Gels • No-light Gels and Fiberglass/Silk Wrap

Gel Maintenance and Removal

PROCEDURES

17-1 Light-cured Gel Application • 17-2 Light-cured Gel Over Forms

17-3 No-light Gel Application

17-4 Combining No-light Gels and Fiberglass or Silk Wrap

Learning Objectives

After you have completed this chapter, you should be able to:

1 Describe the chemistry difference between U.V. gel and a no-light gel.

2 Identify the supplies needed for gel application.

3 Demonstrate the proper procedures for applying light-cured gels using forms, over tips, and to natural nails.

4 Demonstrate the proper procedures for applying no-light gels over tips and to natural nails.

5 Explain how both kinds of gels are removed.

Key Terms

Page number indicates where in the chapter the term is used.

activator-cured
pg. 321

halogen bulb
pg. 313

light-cured gel
pg. 313

no-light gel
pg. 313

ultraviolet bulb
pg. 313

water-cured
pg. 321

This chapter introduces **light-cured gels** and **no-light gels** as an alternative method for an artificial nail service.

U.V. (light-cured) Gels: The important connection between what the ultraviolet nail lamp does for the U.V. gel was once a mystery. The manufacturers of U.V. gel products were not electricians and the electricians were not chemists. Finally, the two have joined forces, creating the perfect combination. Light-cured gel chemistry begins with the same raw materials as acrylic chemistry. The manufacturing process changes to produce a *urethane acrylate ester* (YOUR-a-thane ah-KRILL-ate ES-ter). Gels can be easy to apply when mastered, easy to file, easy to maintain, and odor-free. When working with natural nail overlays, tip extension overlays, or building with the use of a form, U.V. gels can have a strong bond to the natural nail plate. The nail plate is gently prepared and a series of gel layers is applied. Each layer requires a short exposure under a U.V. nail lamp to cure. The U.V. gel and nail plate bond together as one piece.

No-Light Gels: These "gels" are not gels in the manner explained above, but are thicker glues made of *cyanoacrylate* (si-ah-no-ah-KRILL-ate). Derived from similar raw materials, no-light gel glue can be applied either by itself, over a silk or fiberglass wrap, or in conjunction with acrylic powders. Glues from thin to thick dry at different rates of speed. An accelerator can be used to speed up the process. Follow the manufacturer's instructions carefully when using any of these products alone or in combinations.

Gels are available in colors that need no polish. These nails look as if they have already been polished and stay the same color until the gel itself is removed. Polish may be worn over colored gels. When polish is removed, the gel color will remain the same. Colored gels are a great base for nail art.

LIGHT-CURED GEL ON TIPS OR NATURAL NAILS

Supplies

In addition to the materials in your basic manicuring set-up, you will need the following items:

Light-cured Gel

Gels are usually packaged in small pots or squeeze tubes.

Curing Light

A box that has an **ultraviolet** or **halogen bulb** to cure or harden the gel nail. The type of light and the shape of the box varies from manufacturer to manufacturer. It is advisable to use the lamp from the same manufacturer as the gel you are using.

Brush

Some nail technicians prefer to use a synthetic brush with small, flat, square bristles to hold and spread the gel.

Primer

Use if recommended by the gel manufacturer.

Block Buffer

Nail Tips

Nail Prep

Sanitizes and/or dehydrates the nail.

Adhesive (Glue)

There are many types of glue for securing nail tips to short, natural nails. Select a container best suited for the type of work you are doing. Choose a small size (4–6 gms maximum). Glue has a shelf life of up to 6 months depending on usage. Be sure to close cap securely, set upright, and store at room temperature between 60–85°F.

Files and Buffers (Abrasives)

Select medium (180) grit for natural nail preparation and initial shaping. Choose a medium/fine (240) grit for smoothing, and a fine block buffer with a grit of 350 or more for final buffing.

Clean Terry Cloth Towel/Disposable Paper Towel

To present a professional work surface, provide a new terry cloth or paper towel for each client.

Gel Application Pre-service

1. **Complete the pre-service sanitation procedure on pages 41–43.**

2. **Prepare your workstation with everything you need at your fingertips.** Always have enough supplies to prevent running out while servicing a client.

3. **Greet your client with a smile.** Then ask her to wash her hands with soap provided at your wash station. At the same time, wash your hands and be sure to provide clean, disposable towels for drying the hands thoroughly.

4. **If this is your client's first appointment, a client health/record form should be prepared.** Mark the date of the service. This is important in the scheduling of future appointments. Record any skin or nail disorders, allergies, and medications being taken. If the client is a nail biter or does heavy work in a daily routine, write a brief notation alerting you of possible abusive activity to new gels. Add specific information about the service you will perform, e.g., gel overlay without polish, if polish is preferred, or write down the color chosen.) This will speed things along with each visit.

5. **If this is a return visit, do client consultation, using health/record form to record responses and observations.** Check for nail disorders and decide if it is safe and appropriate to perform a service on this client. If the client should not receive a service, explain your reasons and refer him or her to a doctor.

PROCEDURE 17-1

Light-cured Gel Application

1. **Remove polish.** Begin with your client's left hand, little finger, and work toward the thumb. Then repeat on the right hand.

2. **Clean nails.** Ask the client to dip nails in a fingerbowl filled with liquid soap. Then use a nail brush to clean nails over fingerbowl. Rinse nails briefly in clear water. Dry hands thoroughly with a clean, disposable towel.

3. **Apply nail antiseptic.** Apply nail antiseptic to nails. Begin with the little finger on the left hand and work toward the thumb (Figure 17–1).

4. **Push back cuticles.** Use a cotton-tipped orangewood stick or a metal pusher to gently push back the cuticles.

5. **Buff nails to remove shine.** Buff lightly over nail plate with a medium/fine abrasive to remove the natural oil (Figure 17–2). Brush off filings.

6. **Apply tips if desired.** If your client requires tips, apply them according to the procedure described in Chapter 14. Be sure to shorten and shape tip prior to application of the gel. During the procedure the gel overlaps the tip's edge to seal and protect it. During the filing process, the seal can be broken, allowing dirt particles to enter or the gel to peel. Be careful not to break that seal. For a pink and white French manicure look, select white tips with a cut-out smile line (Figure 17–3).

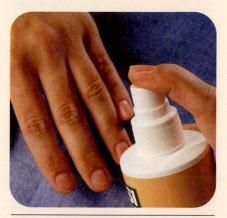

Figure 17–1 Apply antiseptic to nails and hands.

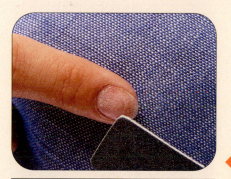

Figure 17–2 Remove shine from natural nail using vertical strokes.

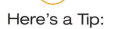

Here's a Tip:

The procedure recommended for applying and curing gel varies from one manufacturer to another. Some systems recommend applying gel to four nails on one hand and curing, and then repeating this procedure on the other hand before applying and curing gel on the thumbnails. Other manufacturers provide light sources that cure only one finger at a time. Be sure to follow the instructions recommended by the manufacturer of the system you are using.

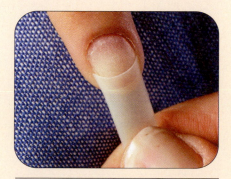

Figure 17–3 Select tip for proper fit, trim, and shape prior to gel application.

17

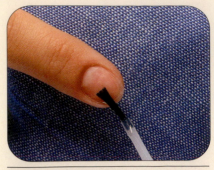

Figure 17-4 Apply primer to the natural nail and let dry to a chalky white.

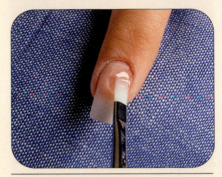

Figure 17-5 Apply gel #1 or base coat gel.

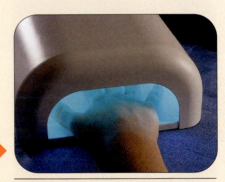

Figure 17-6 Cure gel in lamp.

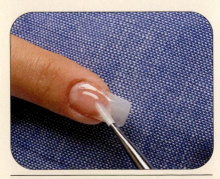

Figure 17-7 Apply gel #2 or building gel.

7. **Nail prep.** Follow manufacturer's instructions for nail preparation. Most gel systems do not require the application of a primer. A base coat gel or bonder is used to assure proper bonding to the natural nail and/or tip overlay (Figure 17–4).

8. **Apply gel #1, or base coat, gel.** Firmly brush gel onto entire nail surface including free edge. Keep gel from touching cuticle or sidewalls. If necessary, remove with a new orangewood stick. (Remember, orangewood sticks are not sanitizable.) Apply to client's left hand from pinky to pointer (Figure 17–5).

9. **Cure gel.** Place the hand in the lamp for the manufacturer's suggested cure time (Figure 17–6).

10. **Repeat steps 8 and 9 on the right hand.** Then repeat same steps for both thumbs.

11. **Apply gel #2, or building gel, to first hand.** Pick up or dispense a generous amount of gel down the center from cuticle to free edge over the cured, sticky first layer. As you drag the gel across the first layer, the tacky surface will pull the gel off the brush or out of the tube. Apply this line of gel on four nails on the client's left hand, from pinky to pointer (Figure 17–7).

12. **Cure gel.** Place the hand in the lamp for 20 seconds. This will "freeze" the gel in place, yet leave it ready for additional thinner layers.

13. **Repeat steps 11 and 12 on the right hand.**

14. **Repeat steps 11 and 12 for both thumbs.**

15. **Pick up or dispense a slightly smaller amount of gel.** Starting from cuticle, stroke down one side of the gel line and repeat down the other side toward the free edge using light, polish-style strokes. Wrap gel around the entire free edge to seal and protect the natural nail or tip's free edge. Apply to four nails on client's left hand, from pinky to pointer (Figure 17–8).

16. **Cure gel.** Place the hand in the lamp for the manufacturer's suggested cure time.

17. **Repeat steps 15 and 16 on the right hand.**

18. **Repeat steps 15 and 16 for both thumbs.**

19. **Remove tacky residue.** Wipe entire nail surfaces with cleaner as per manufacturer's directions. The cleanser is usually acetone based or alcohol (Figure 17–9).

20. **Check nail contours.** Gel nails are very easily filed. Using 180 grit abrasive, refine the surface contour. Gently file the side-

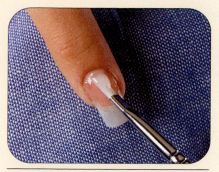

Figure 17–8 Dispense a smaller amount of gel.

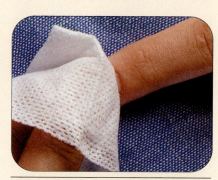

Figure 17–9 Remove tacky residue with a cleaner.

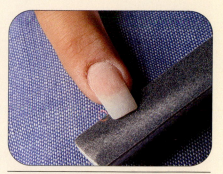

Figure 17–10 File, shape and contour entire surface.

walls and free edge to even out the gel (Figure 17–10). Bevel down, stroking file at a 45-degree angle from top center dome to free edge. Check the free edge thickness. Even out imperfections with gentle file strokes.

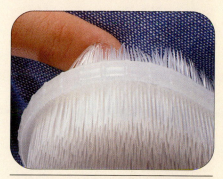

Figure 17–11 Remove dust filings with a nylon manicure brush.

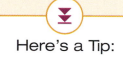

Here's a Tip:

During the procedure keep brush and gel away from light to prevent hardening of gel.

21. **Buff and dust.** Vigorously buff entire nail surface to a smooth finish. Dust off nail filings using a nylon manicure brush (Figure 17–11).

22. **Apply top coat gel.** Pick up or dispense a small amount of gel. Starting from cuticle, stroke down, using polish-style strokes, covering the entire nail surface. Be sure to wrap gel around the entire free edge to seal and protect the natural nail or tip's free edge.

23. **Repeat steps 16 and 19.**

24. **Apply cuticle oil.** Rub cuticle oil into surrounding skin and nail surface (Figure 17–12).

25. **Apply hand and lotion and massage hand and arm.**

26. **Clean nails.** Ask the client to dip nails into a fingerbowl filled with liquid soap. Then use nail brush to clean nails over fingerbowl. Rinse with water and dry thoroughly with a clean, disposable towel.

27. **Apply polish** if desired (Figure 17–13).

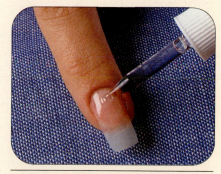

Figure 17–12 Apply cuticle oil.

17

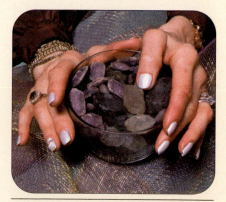

Figure 17–13 Apply polish.

Gel Application Post-service

Your light-cured gel service is complete. Follow the post-service procedure described below.

1. **Make another appointment.** Schedule another appointment with your client to maintain the service she has just received or to perform another service.

2. **Suggest retail products.** Suggest that your client buy products necessary to maintain her nails throughout the week. Polish, lotion, top coat, etc. are valuable maintenance tools for her to have.

3. **Clean up around your table.** Take the time to restore the basic set-up of your table.

4. **Discard used materials.** Place all used materials in the plastic bag at the side of the table. Empty the bag frequently when you are doing gel nails.

5. **Sanitize table and implements.** Perform the complete pre-service sanitation procedure. In most states, this procedure calls for 20 minutes of proper sanitation before implements can be used on the next client.

PROCEDURE

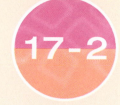

17-2

Light-cured Gel Over Forms

Clients who want to strengthen and lengthen their natural nails with a light-weight artificial nail may choose gel nails over forms.

1. **Complete gel application pre-service.** Place light-cured gel supplies, including nail forms, on your manicuring table.

2. **Apply nail forms.** Fit forms onto all ten fingers just as you would for acrylic nails over forms. Remember to sanitize reusable forms or use disposable ones.

3. **Apply gel to natural nail.** Apply gel first to the natural nail only, not the nail form (Figure 17–14).

4. **Cure gel** (Figure 17–15).

5. **Create a free edge.** Apply gel to the nail form to create a free edge.

6. **Cure gel.**

7. **Apply gel to entire nail.** Apply gel to entire nail—both the natural nail and the free edge.

8. **Cure gel.**

9. **Remove forms.**

10. **Shape free edge.**

11. **Apply gel to entire nail without form** (Figure 17–16)**.**

12. **Cure gel.**

13. **Remove tacky residue.** Wipe entire nail surfaces with cleaner as per manufacturer's directions. The cleanser is usually acetone based or alcohol.

14. **Check nail contours.** Gel nails are very easily filed. Using 180-grit abrasive, redefine the surface contour. Gently file the sidewalls and free edge to even out the gel. Bevel down, stroking file at a 45-degree angle, from top center dome to free edge. Check the free edge thickness. Even out imperfections with a gentle file stroke.

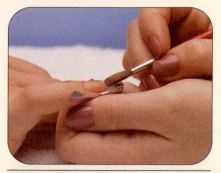

Figure 17–14 Apply gel to natural nail in form

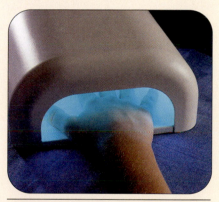

Figure 17–15 Cure gel.

17

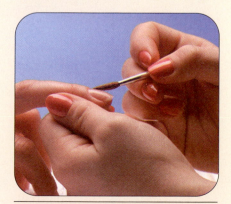

Figure 17–16 Apply gel to entire nail without form.

15. **Buff and dust.** Vigorously buff entire nail surface to a smooth finish. Dust off nail filings using a nylon manicure brush.

16. **Apply top coat gel.** Pick up or dispense a small amount of gel. Starting from cuticle, stroke down, using polish-style strokes, covering the entire nail surface. Be sure to wrap gel around the entire free edge to seal and protect the natural nail or the tip's free edge.

17. **Repeat steps 12 and 13.**

18. **Apply cuticle oil.** Rub cuticle oil into surrounding skin and nail surface.

19. **Apply hand lotion and massage hand and arm.**

20. **Clean nails.** Ask client to dip nails into a fingerbowl filled with liquid soap. Then use a nail brush to clean nails over fingerbowl. Rinse with water and dry thoroughly with a clean, disposable towel.

21. **Apply polish** if desired.

22. **Complete gel application post-service.**

◆ ◆ NO-LIGHT GELS

A no-light gel is a thicker viscosity cyanoacrylate monomer. Its generic trade name is super glue (thick glue). This gel-like material can be applied with a brush, like nail polish, or with the bottle itself to spread a thin coat of gel onto the entire nail, including the tip of the free edge. To harden the "gel" layer, a droplet of activator is dispensed atop the "gel." It is brushed on, sprayed on, or the gel is water-cured. Once the two chemistries unite, the gel hardens. This system does not require an ultraviolet lamp to cure or harden. It is a **no-light gel** system. Following is a generic procedure designed to show how no-light gels are applied. For actual application you will need to follow the manufacturer's instructions carefully.

Supplies

In addition to the materials in your basic manicuring set-up, you will need the following items.

Activator (of choice)

Block Buffer

Nail Tips

Adhesive

PROCEDURE 17-3

No-light Gel Application

1. **Complete gel application pre-service.**

2. **Remove polish.** Begin with your client's left hand, little finger, and work toward the thumb. Then repeat on the right hand.

3. **Clean nails.** Ask the client to dip nails in a fingerbowl filled with liquid soap. Then use a nail brush to clean nails over fingerbowl. Rinse nails briefly in clear water.

4. **Push back cuticles.** Use a cotton-tipped orangewood stick or a metal pusher to gently push back cuticles.

5. **Buff nails to remove shine.** Buff lightly over nail plate with a medium/fine abrasive to remove the natural oil. Brush off filings.

6. **Apply nail antiseptic.** Apply nail antiseptic to nails. Begin with the little finger on the left hand and work toward the thumb.

7. **Apply tips if desired.** If your client wants tips, apply them according to the procedure described in Chapter 14.

8. **Apply gel.** Use brush to paint on gel or use bottle to spread a thin coat of gel onto entire nail. Apply gel to the five nails of one hand. Do not brush on cuticle because gel will lift.

Here's a Tip:

Some gels run and must be applied and cured one finger at a time. Be guided by manufacturer's instructions.

9. **Cure gel with activator or water.** **Activator-Cured:** Spray or brush gel activator (also called glue dry or adhesive dryer) onto nail plate. If you use a spray, hold it at least 8 inches away from the client's nails to reduce the chance of having your client experience a heat reaction from the activator. **Water-Cured:** Immerse nails in lukewarm water for 2–5 minutes, depending on manufacturer's directions.

17

10. **Repeat steps 8 and 9 on the right hand.**

11. **Apply second coat of gel and cure if necessary.** With no-light gels, a second application of gel may not be necessary. Follow your manufacturer's directions for correct application.

12. **Shape and refine nails.** Shape and refine the entire surface of the nail with a medium/fine abrasive. Use a light touch to remove any imperfections.

13. **Buff nail.** Buff nail with a block buffer to shine.

14. **Apply cuticle oil.** Rub cuticle oil into surrounding skin and nail surface.

15. **Apply hand cream and massage hand and arm.**

16. **Clean nails.** Ask client to dip nails in a fingerbowl filled with liquid soap. Then use a nail brush to clean nails over fingerbowl. Rinse with water and dry thoroughly with a clean, disposable towel.

17. **Apply polish.**

18. **Complete gel application post-service.**

NO-LIGHT GELS AND FIBERGLASS/SILK WRAP

This procedure combines two systems. The use of a fiberglass or silk layering system combined with glue has strengthened natural nails for the past 25 years. Recent advancements indicate that using no-light gels, alternately layered with fiberglass or silk, works as a harmonious system. Layering no-light gel and fiberglass or silk in a sandwich effect creates a strong, woven combination for a nail enhancement. Between the first coat and the second coat of gel, a layer of wrap is applied.

17

PROCEDURE

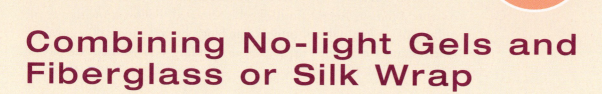

17-4

Combining No-light Gels and Fiberglass or Silk Wrap

1. **Pre-cut fiberglass or silk sections in no greater than 1/4"-wide and 1/2"-long strips.** Adjust and trim length of strips accordingly to size of the client's nail beds. Avoid excess overhanging material.

2. **Place a section of fiberglass or silk material diagonally across wet gel.** Use a new orangewood stick to carefully position it in place. Place the first strip from the upper left corner to lower right corner of the nail, slightly above the stress area. Position the second strip from the upper right corner to lower left corner of nail, forming an "X."

3. **Activate and follow with the second coat of gel.** Activate and finish as you would in the no-light gel procedure.

◆◆◆ GEL MAINTENANCE AND REMOVAL

17

Gel Maintenance

Both light-cured and no-light gels should be maintained every two to three weeks, depending on how fast the client's nails grow. Use a medium abrasive file and buff entire nail to remove shine. Eliminate regrowth ledge by gliding file over ledge area. Hold file flat at ledge, not at an angle, because this can make a groove and damage the natural nail plate. Shape nail and blend it into the natural nail. Continue buffing until there is no line between hardened gel and natural nail plate. Be careful not to damage the natural nail plate by buffing too roughly. When the nail is smooth, follow the procedure for the application of gel on natural nails.

Gel Removal

Read and follow manufacturer's recommended procedure to remove gel nails. U.V. gel may only be buffed off layer by layer. U.V. gel is impervious to acetone and will not soak off. No-light gels using cyanoacrylate can be soaked off. Soak client's nails in a small bowl filled with acetone for 15–25 minutes, without lifting hands from bowl. Using a new orangewood stick or a metal pusher, gently scrape from cuticle to free edge to slide off the softened product. Repeat until all gel is removed. Follow up with a gentle buffing of the natural nail using a fine block buffer. This will remove the glue residue. Condition cuticle and surrounding skin with cuticle oil and lotion or follow with a manicure.

BUSINESS TIP

Teen Time

Take advantage of teenagers' interests in good grooming by introducing them to professional nail care. Ideal lures include a 20 percent discount on all prom and graduation nail services. Contact local schools to see when these events take place; then spread the word by advertising the promotion in high school newspapers six to eight weeks ahead of time. Another option is to hold a "back-to-school night." Decorate the salon in fun colors, provide refreshments, and invite teens to pay a $10.00 registration fee for a night of nail education and fashion manicures, plus a take-home bag of trial-sized products. Many technicians report success with discounted nail extensions offered to the cheerleading squad, sports manicures to the volleyball team, or even a "good grade" discount for any teen earning a 3.0 or higher grade point average.

chapter glossary

activator-cured	A method of curing a no-light gel by spraying or brushing gel activator onto the nail plate.
halogen bulb	A bulb used to harden some nail gels.
light-cured gel	A type of gel used with artificial nails that hardens when exposed to an ultraviolet or halogen light source.
no-light gel	A type of gel used with artificial nails that hardens when a gel activator is sprayed or brushed on, or when they are soaked in water.
ultraviolet bulb	A bulb used to harden some nail gels that contains special rays of the spectrum beyond the violet rays.
water-cured	A method of curing a no-light gel by immersing nails in lukewarm water for several minutes.

review questions

1. Describe the chemistry difference between U.V. gel and a no-light gel.

2. Identify the supplies needed for gel application.

3. Demonstrate the proper procedures for applying light-cured gels using forms, over tips, and natural nails.

4. Demonstrate the proper procedures for applying no-light gel over tips and natural nails.

5. Explain how both kinds of gels are removed.

17

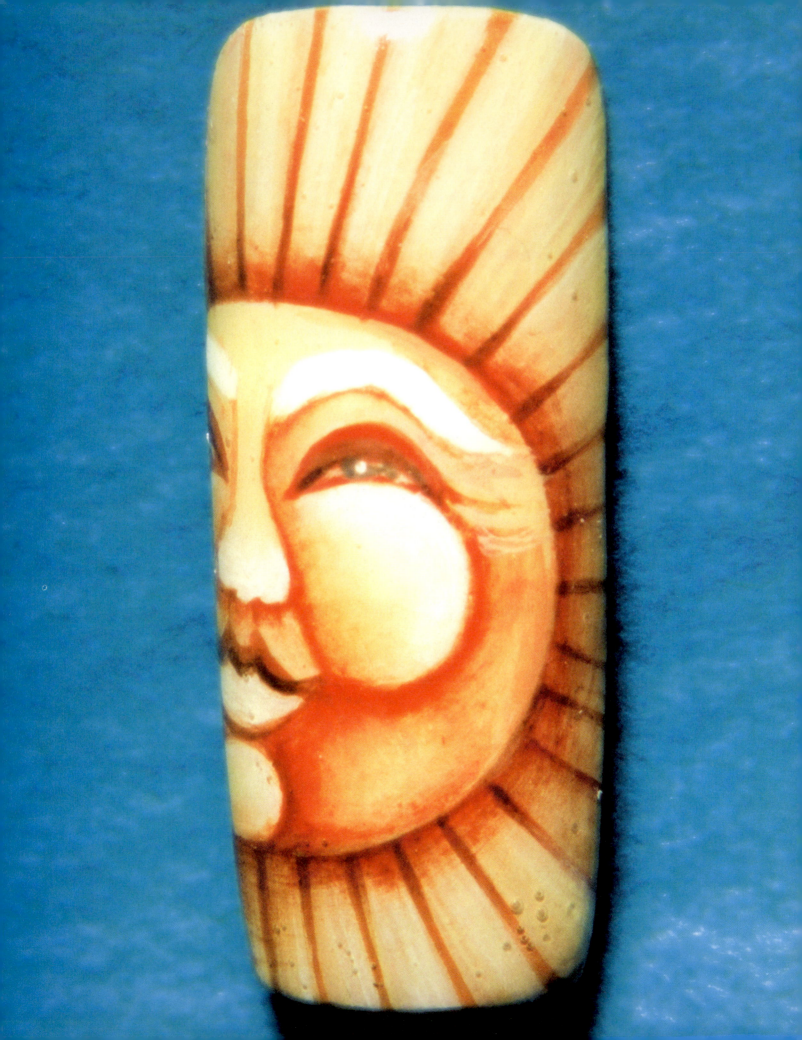

18

THE CREATIVE TOUCH

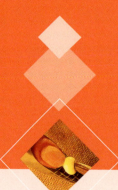

Author: Rebecca Moran

CHAPTER OUTLINE

The Basics and Foundation of Nail Art • **Creating Nail Art**

Gold Leafing • **Freehand Painting**

Using an Airbrush for Nail Color and Nail Art

Getting Started and Finished • **Two-color Fade** • **Traditional French Manicure**

PROCEDURES

18-1 Gold Leaf Application • **18-2 Airbrushing**

18-3 Two-color Fade Application

18-4 Traditional French Manicure Application

Learning Objectives

After you have completed this chapter, you should be able to:

1 **Describe three different nail art supplies.**

2 **Describe techniques for using these supplies.**

3 **Demonstrate one nail art application.**

4 **Describe the use of the color wheel.**

5 **Describe the basic nail art brushes and their uses.**

6 **Describe airbrush equipment.**

7 **Demonstrate proper airbrush techniques.**

8 **Describe the two-color fade.**

Key Terms

Page number indicates where in the chapter the term is used.

air hose
pg. 342

color fade (color blend)
pg. 340

color wheel
pg. 331

complementary colors
pg. 331

floating the bead
pg. 330

fluid nozzle (tip)
pg. 341

foiling
pg. 332

freehand painting (flat nail art)
pg. 336

French manicure
pg. 340

gems
pg. 332

gravity-fed
pg. 341

internal mix
pg. 341

leafing (gold leafing)
pg. 334

mask knife
pg. 340

mask paper
pg. 340

nail art
pg. 329

needle
pg. 341

position
pg. 338

pressure
pg. 338

pull
pg. 338

primary colors
pg. 331

secondary colors
pg. 331

stencil
pg. 340

striping tape
pg. 333

tertiary colors
pg. 331

tip
pg. 341

well (small color cup or reservoir)
pg. 341

Nail art offers endless opportunities to express your creativity and your client's unique personality. There are numerous tools and supplies with which you can custom design, along with an endless palette of artistic creations. Your imagination and your client's preferences are your only limitations. This has fast become one of the most popular add-on services salons are offering. Nail art gives you and your client the flexibility of originating designs ranging from conservative, office-appropriate art forms to the more flamboyant holiday and expressive specialty art forms. There are very few limitations outside of proper sanitation and professionalism. This is one of those perks you get from being a nail technician, where you can really have fun with your job (Figure 18–1).

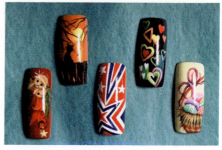

Figure 18–1 Nail art is the most creative part of a nail technician's job.

◆ ◆ ◆ THE BASICS AND FOUNDATION OF NAIL ART

The Rules

With so many forms of **nail art** to choose from, even the most artistically challenged can produce impressive works of art. There are only a few basic rules to follow to achieve success in this specialty.

1. The first rule is to be open-minded. Never look at a piece of artwork or an art product with the thought that you could never possibly do that. There are no circumstances in which that would be true. Nail art product line manufacturers would not be successful in this industry if they produced procedures so complicated that only a select few can master them. You will be surprised at how easy most of these services are, given ample patience and practice.

2. The second rule is to expose yourself to all avenues of art services. Select those that you are most comfortable with at first, then as you become more confident, add to your repertoire.

3. The third rule is to always listen to your client. As outstanding as your artwork may be, if it does not fit her lifestyle or comfort zone, she will never be satisfied or as excited about it as you are.

4. The final rule is to always remember, as many artists of all specialties and formats have said for years, that there is no such thing as a mistake in art, only creative opportunities. Ralph Waldo Emerson once wrote, "Every artist was first an amateur." Both of these phrases are very applicable to nail artists. You must practice, practice more, and practice again before you become comfortably proficient in the arena of nail art. But with patience and perseverance, it is very rewarding.

18

The Basics

There are many common threads between forms of nail art. The more common are as follows:

1. Ample time must be scheduled for these services. Introduce your client to your services, and explain the time requirements for those she is most interested in, as some art services are relatively quick while others can be time consuming. This keeps you on schedule and gives the client a realistic idea of the amount of time she will be spending with you, a professional courtesy for you both.

2. Have a display of your nail art designs, tastefully suited to your clientele and salon atmosphere. Seeing it in advance takes much of the apprehensiveness out of it for a new art client, and the expected results are very clear to both of you. A display will also generate interest in your art services.

3. Be competitively priced. For the services that are more mechanical, such as foiling, be sure that you are priced appropriately for your area and clientele. Always base your prices on the cost of materials, time investment, and general availability, but be sure that a common service to your area is priced competitively. For more specialized art service, such as freehand designs, price your work based on the time investment, cost of materials, and your level of expertise. You are a professional. Be sure to price your services reflectively, and be prepared to render artwork deserving of the fee.

4. Invest in good quality tools. They will need replacement far less often when properly maintained, and will give you a higher quality result. Brushes and air compressors are examples of tools worth the investment. This will be discussed later in this chapter.

5. Dedicate a pair of small scissors, such as stork shears, to be used solely for nail art purposes. The art products can be dulling and sticky, all of which may ruin or contaminate your silk and fiberglass wrap products. It will make everything much easier on you all the way around.

6. Let a polished nail dry completely before applying some types of nail art, unless specifically directed to do otherwise, as in hand painted nail art, more commonly known as flat nail art. When certain forms of dimensional art are applied to an unstable surface it takes longer to dry and harden, and it is quite likely to yield an undesired result. Additionally, always allow nail art to dry completely before sealing it, for the same reasons. When sealing nail art, be very careful not to touch the brush of the sealer to the surface of the nail, as it too can damage your art. Take the brush, load it with a generous bead of sealer, and drop the bead on the nail surface. With the brush, gently guide the bead over the entire surface of the nail until it is completely covered. This is referred to as **floating the bead**, as the brush basically floats on the surface of the sealer, directing its flow, but never coming in contact with the nail surface itself. Mastering this technique will

18

save you a great deal of time and frustration, not to mention already completed artwork.

Nail art is an exciting and creative part of a nail technician's job. It turns nails into small canvases on which you can paint pictures; create designs; make collages with gems, foils, leafing, and tapes; or express your client's creative side. In this chapter, you will gain a basic working knowledge of the most common forms of nail art products, tools, supplies, and procedures. However, there is always more to learn. Exploration of these options and continuing education are highly recommended. This is especially the case in freehand art and airbrushing, as it is often more beneficial and impressive to see something done hands-on and in person.

Color Theory

Before you can expect to successfully produce appealing nail art, it is imperative that you have a working knowledge of colors and how they relate, blend, clash, and complement one another. In many art supply stores you can easily obtain laminated color guides called **color wheels**. The color wheel illustrates and identifies the **primary colors**, **secondary colors**, **tertiary colors**, and **complementary colors** (Figure 18–2). Knowing the classifications of color will aid you in selecting both a polish and paint palette for your artwork that are pleasing to the eye and professional looking. It is a must-know when selecting paints for freehand nail art and airbrushing.

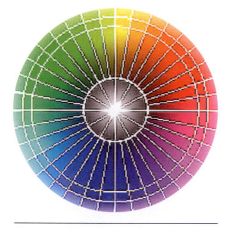

Figure 18-2 The color wheel

1. **Primary colors** are pure pigment colors that cannot be obtained from mixing any other colors together. They are the pure colors from which all other colors are made with varying amounts of black and white added to many. Primary colors are *red, yellow,* and *blue.*

2. **Secondary colors** are the colors directly resulting from mixing equal parts of two primary colors together. They also sit opposite the primary colors on the color wheel, and are the complementary colors of the primary colors. Secondary colors are *orange* (1:1 red and yellow), *green* (1:1 yellow and blue), and *violet* (1:1 blue and red).

3. **Tertiary colors** are the colors directly resulting from mixing equal parts of one primary color and one of its nearest secondary colors. The tertiary colors are *red-orange, red-violet, blue-violet, blue-green, yellow-green,* and *yellow-orange.* Some also refer to tertiary colors as intermediate colors.

4. **Complementary colors** are those colors located directly opposite each other on the color wheel. When complementary colors are mixed together in equal parts they produce a neutral, muddy brown, and when mixed in unequal parts they produce a neutral color dominated by the color of the greatest proportion, giving an overall sense of harmony. However, when these colors are applied side by side, they enhance each other. Thus making each other stand out and are boldly exciting to the eye.

Black is not actually considered to be a color, but is defined as the presence of all colors equally and the absence of light. *White* is also not considered to be a color; it is defined as the absence of all color. Colors located beside each other on the color wheel (analogous colors) blend well together and are beautiful when airbrushing a fade. These are colors that share the same primary color but differ in the second ingredient, resulting in various shades of the same color group.

◆ ◆ CREATING NAIL ART

Gems

Tiny rhinestones are popular nail art accents. They come in different sizes, colors, and shapes. **Gems** add sparkle, dimension, and texture to any design. To apply the gem, apply a dab of topcoat or nail art sealer on the nail where the gem is to be adhered. Dampening the end of an orangewood stick with water or, if it is a very large gem, dampen it with nail art sealer, pick up the gem by touching the dampened stick to the colorful, shiny side of the gem and placing it on the nail in the prepared area. Tweezers also work well when handling larger gems. You may need to apply a small amount of pressure on the gem when placing it on the nail to imbed it a bit for better adhesion. Once the gem is applied, finish it with a generous coat of nail art sealer.

If you remove the gem using acetone, moderate pressure, and a little patience, you may be able to reuse the gem. If the shiny, reflective backing separates from the gem during the removal process, the gem is no longer usable, as it will no longer reflect its color.

Foiling

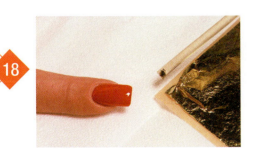

Figure 18-3 A dry nail ready for foiling

Foiling is one of the easiest and most cost-effective nail art techniques, yet it renders a stunning result and an almost endless creative opportunity and palette (Figure 18–3). Foil is available in a wide variety of colors and patterns, with gold, silver, and snakeskin among the most popular. It is most often sold in rolls, ranging from a few inches to several feet in length, but may also be found precut. While precuts are easy to handle and can be more convenient, they tend to be a bit more costly. To apply foil, you must first polish the nail and allow it to completely dry. The polish color will show through in spots, so it should be selected according to the color scheme and/or pattern to be used. Once the nail is dry, apply a very thin and even coat of **foil adhesive**. This is a special adhesive, just for foiling, that is generally tinted white or pink and when wet appears cloudy. When the adhesive is no longer visible and is clear, it is at a tacky stage and acts as double-sided sticky tape, sticking to the nail surface and pulling the foil from the cellophane. (Do not let it overdry or the foil will not stick to it.) If it is not allowed to completely reach the clear stage, however, it will be too wet and not only will the foil not stick to it, the nail polish will lift off the nail when you pull the cutting away from it. This is the trickiest part of the entire service. While the adhesive is processing, select the foil to be used and take small cuttings of each color. Usually between one and three colors are used per nail, and each strip is cut to a length of between one and two inches, depending on the number of colors being used. In the event that a patterned piece has been selected or entire coverage of one color is desired, the cuttings should be large enough for each nail to be serviced, and in corresponding quantities.

Once the adhesive has reached the clear, tacky stage, carefully hold the foil with your fingers, shiny, colored side facing up and away from the nail, dull, matted side (usually gold or gray) facing toward the nail surface. The first method is to quickly touch the back of the foil (the matted side) to the surface of the nail, pulling back away from it immediately. Continue doing the quick touch-and-remove (up-and-down) motion over the nail surface until the desired amount of the color has been deposited on the nail. As you do this, however, keep in mind that the foil is actually being removed from a clear sheet of cellophane and once the color is deposited, the foil will appear clear in that area, indicating that a covered part of the foil must come in contact with the nail surface next. If only the clear area touches the nail, it will remove the nail polish as it now sticks to the cellophane and comes up with the upward movement. In the second method, a more complete coverage is achieved, as the cut foil is gently laid on the surface of the nail and lightly burnished with your finger or an orangewood stick. When the desired amount of coverage has been achieved, slowly peel the cutting back from the nail. This method is very effective with pre-patterned foil, such as animal skin, floral, and holographic designs. Once the nails are foiled, you must seal the nail with the nail art sealer. As with all nail art, always *float the bead*, because the foil color may run or be scratched if the nail surface comes into contact with the brush of the sealer. As the nail art sealer dries, you will see an eye-catching crinkling effect appear in the foil. This service truly takes very little time and is very popular and lucrative.

Striping Tape

Striping tape comes in rolls or pages of various colors, widths, and lengths. Although the color selection is generous, gold, silver, and black have been the more popular colors for years. The tape has a tacky backing, and is only applied to a thoroughly dry, polished nail. If applying the nail tape over another design, the design must also be dry. You can have a pattern in mind when you start or you can use your imagination to create an original design every time.

◆◆ GOLD LEAFING

Leafing is a very fragile material of an extremely thin, unprotected foil-like consistency. It is commonly made available in sheets, although it is occasionally found in a loose form. Leafing comes in a variety of colors now, but it has always been available in gold and silver. The sheets of leafing are packaged in quantities ranging from 10 to 100 sheets per unit. It is most commonly known as **leafing** or **gold leafing**, but is also known as **nuggets** or **nugget sheets**. Because leafing is very fragile, you must handle it with great care. The sheets are packaged in bags or containers with sheets of thin tissue paper layered between the pages of leafing. When removing the sheets from the packaging, use tweezers or the paper used to separate the sheets. Leafing is very light weight, easily torn, and carried by the slightest air current, so keep the packages closed at all times and out of the reach of a draft or fan to avoid having little pieces of leafing floating all over the place.

The application of this form of art is quick and easy. With the nail prepared as usual, polished, and completely dry, apply a thin, even coat of foil adhesive. When the adhesive has reached the tacky stage by turning clear, apply the desired color(s) in small pieces or by the sheet, to the tacky area(s). For this, use tweezers or, for the smaller pieces, a slightly dampened orangewood stick. Rub gently with your finger, using a slight amount of pressure. If using a sheet you will get a more thin and even coverage. If using foil pieces, you will get a more textured appearance, giving the effect of nuggets. Once the application is completed, seal the finished nail by floating a bead of sealer over the entire nail. Leafing makes a great art form on its own, or acts as a complementary accent to any other form of art. For example, if you were to paint half of the nail red and the other half black, you could highlight the meeting point of the two colors with gold or silver leafing. As with all other forms of nail art, you should recommend that your client reapply top coat every three to four days to maintain a good seal and a high gloss finish.

18

PROCEDURE

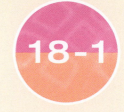

18-1

Gold Leaf Application

1. **Polish nails and let dry.**

2. **Apply adhesive on area you want covered with gold** (Figure 18–4).

3. **Using tweezers or a new orangewood stick, place bits of gold on nail and gently press onto wet adhesive.** Continue doing this until design is complete (Figures 18–5 and 18–6).

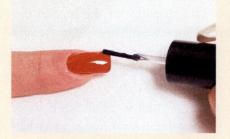

Figure 18-4 Apply adhesive.

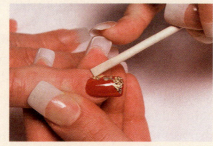

Figure 18-5 Apply gold leaf.

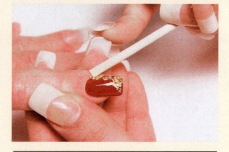

Figure 18-6 Complete design.

4. **Use an orangewood stick to press gold leaf flat onto nail** (Figure 18–7).

5. **Apply sealer over gold leaf to finish.** Let dry. If you are going to add striping tape or a gemstone, do it before applying the final coat of clear polish (Figure 18–8).

6. **A second or third coat of clear polish may be applied if needed to cover nail design.** Let each layer dry slightly before applying the next (Figure 18–9).

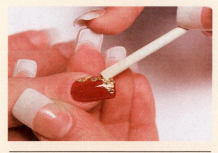

Figure 18-7 Press gold leaf flat.

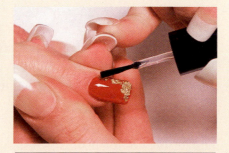

Figure 18-8 Apply clear polish.

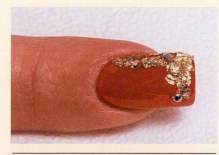

Figure 18-9 Finished nail with gold leaf.

Chapter 18 ● The Creative Touch

◆ ◆ FREEHAND PAINTING

Freehand painting, also referred to as **flat nail art**, is a very expressive form of nail art, with absolutely no limitations. With *imagination, education, knowledge, practice,* and *the right tools,* you can create absolutely anything. A working understanding of the theory of color is imperative, as well as having tools that work for you. Brushes and paints are the most critical tools for freehand art and proper selection of both is important. Quality and familiarity are necessary for the production of a satisfying, quality piece of finished art.

Brushes

Brushes come in many sizes, shapes, and qualities. There are a variety of bristle sources, resulting in a range of brushes from very soft to very firm, but use synthetic bristles for water-based paints (Figure 18–10). The smaller sizes of any brush are usually a better choice for painting nails. **Bristles** can be made of any one or combination of numerous sources. The filaments, which comprise the bristles, or actual brush itself, are bundled together and inserted into the ferrule. The anatomy of the bristles is a factor in the style, shape, and potential performance of the brush. The very end of the bristles, furthest away from the handle, is referred to as either the **tip**, **toe**, or **chisel edge**, depending on the style of the brush. Round brushes, for example, would have tips or toes, while flat and bright brushes have a chiseled edge. The midsection of the bristles is called the **belly** of the brush. This is the area of the brush that retains the most water and paint. The area of the brush where the bristles meet the **ferrule**, the metal on the brush, is called the **heel** of the brush, more specifically located on the end of the ferrule itself. The more common brushes for flat nail art are as follows.

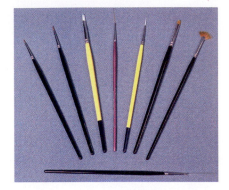

Figure 18-10 A selection of brushes

Round Brush

This is the most common and versatile style of brush. It has a tapered tip and large belly. It has a very good capacity for holding paint and water. Round brushes made of the softer hairs have a desirable point at the tip. Those made of the stiffer bristles do not form a point at the tip due to the filaments used. They are flexible and offer good blocking while still yielding the intricate details due to the fine point at the tip. This is a good brush to accomplish many different stroke patterns.

Liner Brush

This is a very versatile brush and possibly more common in the nail art industry than the aforementioned round brush. This is a very good detail brush, preferable for linework, outlining, and even lettering.

Flat Brush

This brush has a square tip with long bristles or hairs giving it added flexibility. It is also referred to as a shader brush. A flat brush holds a large amount of paint and water while offering the versatility of multiple strokes. When used flat on the painting surface it will give long, fluid strokes. When used on the tip, also referred to as the chiseled edge, with the handle straight up, it renders a fine line. This is also a brush very conducive to such techniques as double loading, blending, and shading.

Bright Brush

This is is a short, flat brush. The shortness of the bristles gives the brush a much stiffer motion, resulting in more texture in the painting and more control.

Fan Brush

This brush is another version of a flat brush, only the ferrule is modified in such a way that the bristles or hairs are spread out like a fan. This brush is most commonly used for blending and special effects. When used in a dry brush technique, the brush, being slightly loaded with paint at the tips and floated across the painting surface, gives an effect similar to that of airbrushing. It is a fairly common brush in nail artistry, and has many useful applications with a little practice.

Spotter Brush

This brush is also called a *detailer*. It is a short, round brush, having very little belly but a very fine point at the tip. It is another common brush to the nail art professional, offering maximum control for intricate, detailed work.

Striper Brush

This brush comes in various lengths. The striper brush is an extremely long, flat brush, having only a few filaments. It is incredibly efficient when creating long lines, striping effects, and animal prints. The shorter version of this brush, called the **stripette** or **short striper**, yields a similar effect. This brush is challenging to control to the beginner, but with relatively little practice it can be easily mastered and will soon become the nail art professional's best friend.

There are other brush styles, all having their own special effect to offer an artist. However, it is recommended to begin with a limited palette of colors and supply of brushes. This better enables the novice artist to master the basics first, avoiding the overwhelming confusion of extra tools. As your artistic abilities increase, add to your tool supply and expand your portfolio of designs. Having a good liner, striper, round, fan, flat, and detailer is more than enough to get started. Another useful tool, complimentary to the freehand artist, is a **marbleizer**, also known as a **stylus**. It comes in a variety of sizes, having a wooden handle in the center with a metal extension from each end with a ball tip. The ball tips range in size and are excellent for dotting small circles of color on a nail, creating polka dots, eyes, bubbles and much more. Additionally, they can be used to swirl drops of different colored paints or polish across the nail surface, giving a marbleized finish.

Strokes

Brush strokes are accomplished in a variety of ways, but they all come down to three basics: pressure, pull, and position. The **pressure** refers to the amount of force an artist applies to the brush while in the stroke motion. The more pressure applied, the larger the coverage area and the wider the stroke. As the amount of pressure is decreased, the width of the stroke decreases accordingly. When the pressure is removed in a gradual manner while pulling the brush across the paint surface, the stripe will have a tapered effect, coming to a point where the brush tip is actually lifted straight up and off the nail.

The second basic is the **pull**. The nail technician must learn to pull a brush, not push it. Pulling the brush across the paint surface gives a fluid movement. Pushing it will give a rough and spattered movement, difficult to control. It would be like writing with a calligraphy pen in an upward motion, difficult and messy at best.

The third basic is **position**. Position refers to how you hold the brush to the nail. This is done in one of two ways: in a straight up-and-down manner, with only the tip touching the paint surface, as with a spotter, or in such a manner that you are laying the bristles, in part or in their entirety, across the paint surface and pulling the brush across. The first position is for detailed work such as lettering, intricate details, and outlining. The second would be done when striping. Lay the brush, tip to heel, on the nail at the start point and pull it toward the ending point, giving a very fluid, uniform stripe. Lift it off, only after the belly has reached the ending point, by pulling up and away. Do not do this abruptly as it will result in a rough ending. When you combine the pressure, pull, and position with the style of the brush, and add a little pivot or curve, you will be amazed at how many different design strokes you can create from only a few brushes. Some of the most versatile strokes include the comma (polywog), "C," leaf, "S," ribbon, and teardrop (Figure 18–11).

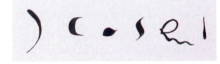

Figure 18–11 The most versatile strokes include the comma (polywog), "C," leaf, "S," ribbon, and teardrop.

Design Techniques

Animal Stripes

In the case of a zebra, paint or polish the entire nail in white and stripes with black paint (Figure 18–12). In the case of a tiger stripe, paint or polish the nail gold, bronze, or copper and paint stripes with black paint. Different color variations also work well and are quite popular, such as black on purple, blue, or pink. Using your liner or short striper brush, load the lower three-quarters of the brush with paint. Touch the tip of the brush to one side of the nail and lay the rest of the brush on the nail to the belly. Your stopping point should be in or around the center of the nail. Pull the brush across the nail to the center in a slightly wavy motion, lifting it further up and away from the nail as you pull near the stopping area. Continue this down one entire side, leaving ample room between strokes for an opposing stroke from the other side to meet at the center area. Having a tad more paint on the very tip of the brush adds to the width at the beginning point.

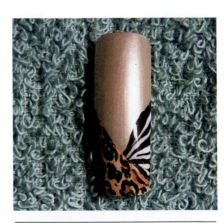

Figure 18–12 Animal stripes are quite popular.

Hearts

Hearts are much easier then they look (Figure 18–13). Simply place three dots on the prepared painting surface in the outline of an inverted triangle. Then connect the dots with a detailer as though you are drawing with a pencil, holding the brush straight up and down. In the middle of the two upper dots, bring the design down into a "v" shape, taking a rounded edge from the top dots to the outside of the design and down to the lower dot, joining all together in a "v" at the bottom. You are creating a small "v" above and within the boundaries of a much larger "v" connecting the two with semi circles at the top.

Flower Petals

Create these petals by loading a #2 flat brush or smaller with a darker color on one side and a lighter color on the other. This is *double loading*. Place the tip of the brush on the prepared nail. Lay the brush down to about half of its length on the nail. Pivot one side of the brush a one-quarter turn, applying increased pressure in the beginning and less toward the end of the movement. Then pull the brush to the end of the petal, which is actually toward the center on some flowers, lifting up and away as you approach the ending point. This stroke will give you a wide teardrop, creating a flower petal. By double loading, you automatically get a shaded/highlighted effect. One important detail of the double load is that the highlights stay on the same side of the flower, so the brush must begin in the same position, with the colors in the same location for each petal. Another type of flower petal is accomplished by using a 10/0 liner brush, laying the tip on the prepared painting surface, applying pressure, and pulling. As you pull up and away, move the brush in a slight "C" shape, narrowing the stroke at the end. This is called a *comma stroke*. Both of these strokes can yield several designs when placed singularly or grouped (Figure 18–14).

Leaves

A leaf is made the same way as a flower petal, with the narrower part of the stroke being the outermost part of the leaf. To add width and dimension to the leaf, double load a small, flat brush with two shades of green. Start with the flat brush on its chiseled edge, perpendicular to the nail. Press, one-quarter turn left or right, lift, and pull up. Look at nature and duplicate it.

Stems and Branches

These are easily and quickly incorporated into a design with a striper brush, liner brush, or flat brush. With a striper or liner, simply pull the brush, applying more pressure where width is desired and less where it is not. With a flat brush, lay in the stem or branch by using the chiseled edge of the brush only, pulling it into place. Experiment with combinations of lines, accented with flowers, dots, and hearts. You will be surprised at how many possible designs you can create. As always, continuing education and hands-on training are strongly recommended, especially in the beginning. Good luck and ENJOY.

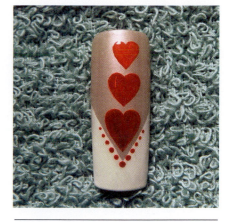

Figure 18-13 Hearts are easier than they look.

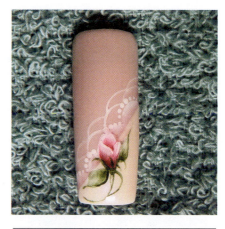

Figure 18-14 Flower petals

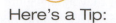

Here's a Tip:

To create a truly dimensional design, parts or all of the design will need to be undercoated. An undercoating of white or light gray paint will accent the richness of a color. Otherwise, the background color of the nail will interfere with some colors and keep them from showing up as the original tone or hue. This is called *neutralizing the canvas*.

Colored Acrylic Painting

The range of colored acrylic, clear acrylic with glitter or sparkle additives, and its variations, has opened a new door for the nail artist. Mastering acrylic application, color knowledge, and brush strokes put you at the threshold of design magic. "Painting" with acrylics can be as rewarding as any of the previously mentioned art forms. Experiment with your own designs or seek out manufacturers who make colored acrylics and their additives. There are also continuing education classes and videos available to help you reach your full potential.

USING AN AIRBRUSH FOR NAIL COLOR AND NAIL ART

Airbrushing nails has become a popular salon service. Many nail technicians are offering their clients an alternative to traditional nail color by airbrushing the nail color for their clients. Subtle color combinations may be achieved by airbrushing two or more colors on the nails at the same time. This technique is called a **color fade** or **color blend** (Figure 18–15). By airbrushing the nail color the nail technician may charge an additional price for the special nail color technique.

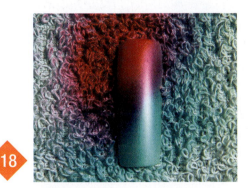

Figure 18–15 Two-color fade

One of the most popular techniques used in airbrushing is the **French manicure** (Figure 18–16). The airbrushed French manicure has no bumps or unevenness at the white tip. The application is very smooth and the white tip has a perfect shape every time. The airbrushed French manicure is accomplished as quickly as hand polishing, yet you may charge more for the airbrushed service.

The nail is a hard surface and has no ability to absorb like a fabric does—such as a T-shirt. It is impossible to draw with an airbrush on the nail—the paint will bead up and drip off the nail. You must use a *design tool*, like a **stencil** or **mask paper** (Figure 18–17). There are precut stencils and mask paper on the market that have designs already in them. You may custom-cut your own designs by using a **mask knife** on uncut stencil or mask paper (Figure 18–18). Place the material to be cut on a glass plate or self-healing mat and carefully cut your design out with the mask knife. Use the full edge of the knife, not just the point of the blade, or you will have an uneven and jagged cut.

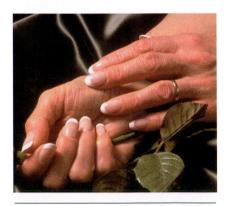

Figure 18–16 French manicure

18

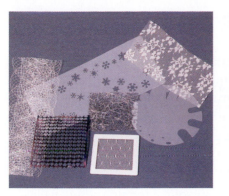

Figure 18-17 Stencils are made of plastic, paper, or fabric.

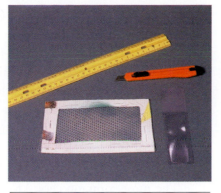

Figure 18-18 Customized mask stencil with paper and knife

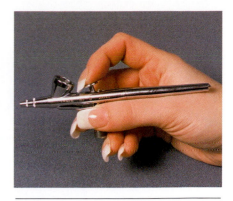

Figure 18-19 Double action airbrush

Airbrush Equipment and Operation

An airbrush looks like a small spray gun. It uses compressed air to force paint out of its tip, creating a fine mist of paint. There are many types of airbrushes available that are suitable for airbrushing fingernails. Some airbrushes are made with metal parts. Other airbrushes made of solvent-resistant resin are now available (Figure 18–19).

All airbrushes work on the same principle. They combine air and paint to form an atomized spray for painting. Airbrushes differ in the (1) type of trigger action, (2) location of air and paint mixing, (3) ease of use and maintenance. Each airbrush has a small cone-shaped **fluid nozzle**, also called a **tip**, that a tapered **needle** fits into (Figure 18–20). When the needle fits snugly in the fluid nozzle, no paint is released when the trigger is depressed. When the needle is drawn back, the airbrush begins to release paint. The further the needle is drawn back, the more paint is released. Control of the amount of paint released varies with different types of airbrushes.

There are many different makes of airbrush systems available on the market today. You want to avoid those that are designed for volume paint application; they are not economical or practical choices for airbrushing nails. Airbrushes that have a large siphon bottle attached below the body of the gun take too long to change colors and do not offer the features you will want as a nail airbrush artist.

Some airbrush systems are designed for **gravity-fed** paint (gravity pulls the paint into the airbrush), which mixes the paint with air inside the airbrush (**internal mix**). This type of airbrush usually has a **well** or **small color cup** for the paint to be placed in the airbrush. A well (also called a **reservoir**) is a hole in the top of the airbrush, where drops of paint are placed. If the airbrush has a color cup, it may be located on top of the airbrush or it may be attached to the side of the airbrush for the paint.

Even though we have narrowed the scope of airbrushes to choose from, there are still many differences in airbrushes available. When you purchase an airbrush, retain the manufacturer's airbrush diagram that comes with it for future reference. This diagram outlines the correct

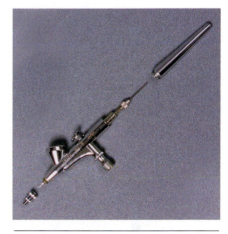

Figure 18-20 Parts of the airbrush: handle, shell/body, nozzle/tip, cap, needle

18

assembly of your airbrush as well as the order numbers for parts in case you lose or break something.

The **air hose** connects the airbrush to the compressor, which is the **air source**. Each airbrush has a unique size fitting; be sure that the size fitting on your hose will fit your airbrush. It is best if you buy them at the same time. The end of the hose that attaches to your compressor is usually a 1/4-inch thread, although there are a few air sources that have a different size fitting. If you find that you have a hose that does not attach to one or both pieces of equipment, adapters are available.

The most common choice for an air source for airbrushing nails is a small compressor. The compressor takes air from the room you are working in and compresses it. You may require an air pressure regulator attached to the compressor in order to control the air pressure being released into your air hose. Most airbrush nail technicians work at a pressure between 25 and 35 pounds per square inch (psi). You will require a moisture trap or moisture separator for your airbrush system since you are using air from the environment that you are working in. There is moisture or water in the air. When the compressed air from the compressor reaches the air hose, the moisture begins to accumulate in the air hose. The moisture will form water droplets which will eventually spit out from the airbrush. A moisture separator will prevent this from happening.

You will need airbrush paint, airbrush cleaner, and appropriate nail polishes to protect the airbrush paint on the nail. Check that the literature and product labeling clearly state that the products you are using are recommended for use on nails. Use the airbrush products per manufacturer's directions to ensure that you have the manufacturer's liability. If you are unsure about whether the airbrush product is recommended for use on nails, check with the manufacturer prior to use. Ask for a written document for your files if the labeling is not clear.

Consult your professional beauty or nail distributor to see the different types of equipment and airbrush products available. Many manufacturers offer complete systems for airbrushing nails, which include everything you need to get started. Your school may have different types or brands of equipment available for you to experiment with. Look for seminars that may permit you to rent the equipment before committing to a purchase.

◆ ◆ ◆ GETTING STARTED AND FINISHED

Set-up and Practice

When you begin practicing, you will need a table, good lighting, a comfortable chair, your airbrush equipment, and supplies. Prepare a number of nail tips to be airbrushed by mounting them to a surface and base coating them. Assemble your airbrush, hose, and compressor per the manufacturer's directions. Place your airbrush paints and airbrush polishes in an accessible tray, roll cart, drawer, or polish rack. Have your design and cleaning tools in a tray, drawer, or rollcart ready for use. Put your airbrush cleaner in a squirt bottle.

Set up a cleaning area for the airbrush off to the side of the work area. Either side is fine as long as it is comfortable for you. One recommended set-up is to have a separate roll-cart for all of your airbrushing equipment and supplies. You could also use one of the drawers that is at a comfortable height when you sit at your work table. Pull out the drawer and line it with terry or paper toweling. Inside the drawer, place your plastic tray or jar that you will spray your airbrush into when cleaning it. Regardless of what you are using—an open tray, bowl, or jar—generously line the inside with absorbent material to prevent your overspray from bouncing off the bottom surface of the container and spattering back out and all over. Place your cleaning brushes, airbrush cleaner bottle, and other cleaning items in the open drawer. Avoid spraying into your wastebasket—it looks unsanitary and unprofessional.

Begin practicing on absorbent paper. Some manufacturers suggest that when you start airbrushing for the day, place a few drops of cleaner into your airbrush and spray it out into your cleaning station. This wets the airbrush inside and your airbrush nail paints will move through the airbrush better. To become familiar with how your airbrush operates, start spraying onto the paper approximately two to three inches from the surface of the paper. The first thing most people notice, if you are spraying properly, is that you will not see the airbrush paint leave your airbrush. It will seem to appear magically on the paper in front of you.

To airbrush properly, you need to move your whole arm up and down, diagonally, or side to side in order to move the airbrush spray around on your surface. Do not move from the wrist! Your wrist must remain straight and relaxed. If you move from the wrist, you will find the airbrush color will be inconsistent in coverage and intensity. This will occur because the airbrush starts out far from the surface, moves closer as your wrist straightens out and then further away as your wrist completes the movement. If you find you are moving your wrist, grasp your wrist with your other hand while practicing and consciously move your whole arm. After awhile, your movements will correct themselves and you will be fine.

Practice spraying a consistent row of dots. When the dot appears where you expect it to, you have learned how to properly aim your airbrush. The next practice step is to draw lines. To draw crisp lines, you must have the airbrush nozzle very close to the paper. The further you pull the airbrush away from the paper the wider and softer the line will become. After experimenting with dots and lines, draw a grid on your paper by drawing horizontal and vertical lines overlapping each other. This will create rows of boxes. Place a dot in each of the boxes. You are now ready to practice the technique used for airbrushing nails.

When airbrushing nails, the distance from the nail will vary according to the type of airbrush you are using. Most people will use the

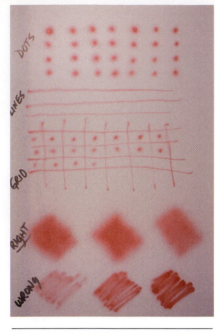

Figure 18-21 Practice on paper to achieve an even coating of color.

airbrush two to three inches from the nail surface. On your paper, spray a smooth, even box of color by moving your arm back and forth slowly. Develop even color with no lines by moving back and forth over the same area a few times. If you are seeing streaks or lines on the paper and not a smooth even box of color, the airbrush is either too close to the paper or you are releasing too much paint at a time. Practice this technique until you can achieve an even coating of color on the paper with no streaks (Figure 18–21).

Now you are ready to practice on nail tips. Place your base coaed nail tips about two to three inches apart on your practice surface. Lightly coat the nail with your airbrush color. Repeated passes over the nail will build up the airbrush nail color. When first learning, most people are impatient and want to see the color right away. If you are too close to the nail tip or release too much paint at one time on the nail surface, the airbrush paint will puddle and begin to run off the nail. (In Figure 18–22, the first nail is sprayed too quickly or too closely. The second nail tip has the correct, dry appearance.) When correctly applying airbrush nail color, the airbrush paint on the nail should appear dull, with a powdery look to it. If the airbrush paint is shiny or appears as droplets, wipe the nail tip off with a water dampened wipe and try again. The best way to apply airbrush nail color is to work on five nail tips at a time, as if you were working on a client's hand. Apply one dry layer of color to each nail tip. Usually three passes of the airbrush up and down over the nail tip will cover it with color lightly. Move to the next nail tip and repeat the procedure until you have airbrushed each nail tip once. Start with the first nail tip and repeat the procedure on each nail tip until you have reached your desired airbrushed nail color. When you have successfully completed applying the airbrushed nail color to the five nail tips, you are ready to move on to practicing a color fade or French manicure.

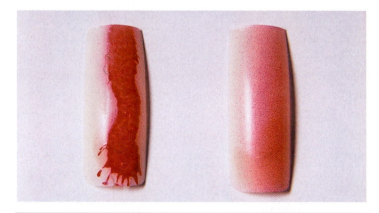

Figure 18-22 The nail tip at left shows what happens when paint is sprayed too close to the nail tip or too much paint is released on the surface. The paint will puddle and run off the nail. The nail on the right has the correct appearance, achieved by light passes of the airbrush to build up color.

PROCEDURE

Airbrushing

One of the benefits of adding airbrushing to your services is that you do not require live models to practice your skills. You should become proficient at airbrushing your nail tips prior to working on live models. When you are skilled at airbrushing on nail tips, you are ready to practice on a few close friends or relatives to become comfortable holding the client's hand and cleaning up the overspray when done.

1. **After completing your nail service and prior to the airbrush nail color service, have the client pay the bill, put on a coat, and dig in the pockets or purses for necessary items.**

2. **Ask the client to use a nail brush and cleanse the hands and nails of any dust or oils from the nail service.** Dry the nail and cuticle area thoroughly, checking for droplets of water or missed oils and dust that would interfere with the airbrush nail color application.

3. **Apply your base coat(s) to the nails.** Be sure to get complete coverage of the sides and free edges of the nails.

4. **Airbrush your client's nails just as you practiced on the nail tips.** Hold the client's hand in yours. Your hand should encircle each of your client's fingers as you spray it. Your hand catches the overspray as you work so it does not fall onto the other nails on your client's hand. Place your thumb on the finger just above the cuticle area. Most of the overspray lands on your thumb and little on the client's finger. This reduces cleanup on your client. Use a similar procedure when airbrushing toenails. The paint washes off your hands when you sanitize prior to your next client.

5. **Apply paint bonder or thin top coat to the dry airbrush nail paint.** Keep your polish brush parallel to the nail, guiding the liquid down the nail. Do not touch the nail surface with the bristles of the brush since this may scratch or drag the paint. Be sure to have enough bonder on the polish brush; a dry polish brush or bristle may also damage your paint. Apply sealer to all

ten nails. Be sure to saturate all the paint and to bumper the sides and free edge of the nails.

6. **Any airbrush paint that is not sealed to the nail may be washed away later.** By the same token, any sealer that gets on the surrounding skin will seal the overspray making it much harder to wash off later. Therefore, use extreme care when applying top coat or sealer. Allow the sealer to dry two to three minutes. Clean your airbrush and put it away at this time.

7. **Apply one or two more top coats or layers of recommended sealer.** Be sure to bumper the sides and free edge of the nails. While applying the protective glaze, instruct your client on proper home maintenance of airbrushed nail color or nail art. Allow client's nails to dry for ten minutes.

8. **Cleanse the fingers or toes per manufacturer's directions.** This may be accomplished at the nail table, pedicure station, or, with some airbrush skin cleaner products, at a sink. Have the client pat hands or feet on a towel to dry the skin, but avoid pressure on nails for another ten minutes. Use an orangewood stick or cotton-wrapped implement saturated with polish remover to remove any paint sealed to skin by top coat or protective nail glaze. Alcohol or cuticle oil is also often effective in loosening the paint, and both are less harsh to the skin.

9. **You may apply a quick-dry product if desired.** Use spray-on products instead of brush-on products for less risk of injury to the airbrushed nail service. Airbrushed nail color is usually surface dry in ten minutes and completely dry within a half hour since only clear nail polish is applied.

10. **Airbrushed nail color will last as well as traditional nail polish.** If you do not get these results, evaluate your airbrush nail paint and airbrush nail polishes. You may need to experiment with different brands or combinations of products for maximum durability. Follow manufacturer's directions.

11. **Airbrushed nail color is generally removed with regular nail polish remover (acetone will work quickest) unless manufacturer of your paint stipulates otherwise.** Many of the nail art sealers are very hard and durable, so it may take longer to remove them.

Airbrush nail color artists vary in their client skin cleaning procedures. Some nail technicians cleanse the airbrush paint on the skin after the paint bonder is applied and allowed to dry. Others send their clients home with a small container of airbrush paint skin cleanser for use at home after the color has dried. Many times soap and warm water are enough to remove unwanted paint on skin. Experiment with different procedures to find which one works best for you.

In order to offer airbrushed nail color successfully to every client you service, it is necessary to have your airbrush equipment and supplies ready to use at all times. Many people have airbrush systems that are in a box collecting dust. When an opportunity arises for them to use their airbrush equipment, they are not prepared and usually do not have the time in their schedule to set up their airbrush system. Having your airbrush system in a roll-cart by your side or set up at a nail table/pedicure station provides you with the ability to airbrush at a moment's notice, simply by plugging in or turning on your compressor.

◆ ◆ ◆ TWO-COLOR FADE

The nail color fade, or color blend, is another one of the most used airbrushed nail color services. It will appeal to every client that you service; the airbrush paint colors selected are key to the success of this design for each individual. A conservative client might prefer subtle, soft hues of similar colors while an outgoing client might choose bold colors that strongly contrast. This multi-color airbrush nail service justifies an additional charge for the nail color application. This technique may be used as the background for an airbrushed nail design or on its own as an airbrushed nail color service.

PROCEDURE 18-3

Two-color Fade Application

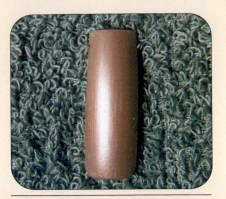

Figure 18-23 Apply base coat.

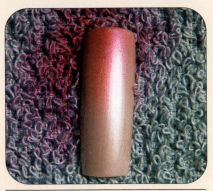

Figure 18-24 Create a soft edge for the second color to overlap.

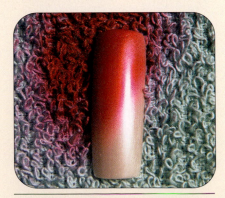

Figure 18-25 Continue applying paint until your desired color is released.

1. **Apply your base coat to the nail.** If the nail to be covered is a dark tone that may influence your nail color or if you are using a transparent airbrush nail paint, apply a crystalline, special effect, or white base coat (Figure 18–23).

2. **Complete the start-up procedure as recommended by the manufacturer.** Place your paint color into your gun and start feeding it in by spraying onto the surface next to your nails. When the airbrush paint is loaded into your airbrush and it is spraying correctly, you are ready to begin application on the nail. Apply a dry, even coat going back and forth diagonally over the top two-thirds of the nail, moving your whole arm. If you are working on more than one nail, apply this light, dry coat diagonally to all the nails. Apply more coats of the airbrush paint at the cuticle area, with fewer coats toward the center of the nail to create a soft edge for the second color to overlap (Figure 18–24).

Here's a Tip:

When using pearlescent or metallic paints, you will find the airbrush may clog more easily. (You should use pearlescent and metallic paints only after you have mastered opaque and transparent paints!) With the pearlescent paint, you may have to pull your hand a bit further away from the nail and release slightly more paint to get an even spray. Practice will make the adjustment smoother.

3. **Continue applying light, dry coats of paint diagonally until you have reached the desired color or opacity in the nail cuticle area fading towards the center** (Figure 18–25).

4. **Clean your airbrush gun of the first color paint.** Choose a color that is appropriate for your client—one that contrasts and creates a transition color. When airbrushing the second color, start at the bottom of the nail tip and move up two-thirds of

the nail (Figure 18–26). Apply more coats or passes of the airbrush over the free edge or nail tip, with fewer passes or coats of paint through the center of the nail. If the colors chosen mix when overlapped, you will begin to see a transition color start to develop.

5. **Continue to apply a dry, even coat going back and forth diagonally over the bottom two-thirds of the nail,** until you have achieved the desired color at the free edge of the nail (Figure 18–26). If a transition color does develop, you control how much of the color is on the nail by the amount the two paint colors overlap. Remember when working on your client, the airbrushed color fade on the right hand should be a mirror image of the color fade on the left hand. Many nail technicians prefer to have the colors travel from the outer corner of the nail (toward the pinkie finger) to the inner corner of the cuticle (toward the thumb), but each airbrush artist has his or her own style.

6. **After you have completed all nails, apply a thin top coat or sealer and let it dry for three minutes.** If you are not going to continue airbrushing, clean your airbrush at this time. Apply another coat of the protective sealer for durability. Instruct your client on home maintenance of the airbrushed nail color.

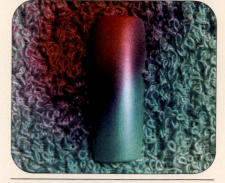

Figure 18–26 For the second color, start at the bottom of the nail tip and move up two-thirds of the nail.

The color fade demonstrates a technique one can accomplish only with an airbrush: the subtle change from one color to another with no bump, line, or demarcation in the nail color coating. The photo (Figure 18–27) shows a few possible variations of this design. The nail tip on the left is a subtle blend for the conservative client. It is a cognac nail color with a transparent gold shimmer splashed at the free edge. The center nail is a bit more daring: pearl red in the cuticle fading into a true pink nail tip. The nail tip on the right is the nail tip completed in the preceding procedure. This nail color selection is for a bold client who wants people to notice her nails!

Be aware that many metallic and pearlescent paints will not be visible until sealed. It is important to realize and remember that most paints (opaque, translucent, metallic, or pearlescent) look very different before and after sealing. Knowing your paints is very important. Also, always work from the lightest to the darkest color when possible.

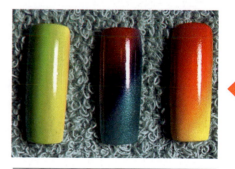

Figure 18–27 Three variations of the design.

18

◆◆◆ TRADITIONAL FRENCH MANICURE (WITH OPTIONAL LUNULA)

The French manicure is the reason why most nail technicians look into airbrushed nail color. The hand-polished French manicure cannot compare to the airbrushed version! The airbrushed French is easier, quicker, and more attractive than the hand-polished version. The airbrushed French manicure has a clean, sophisticated look yet retains a neutral color application that matches all clothing. Each airbrush nail technician has a favorite method of achieving the traditional French manicure, which is a skin-toned nail bed with a curved French white tip.

B·U·S·I·N·E·S·S TIP

The Artistic Touch

If you're like most nail technicians, you have a specific number of customers who are enthusiastic nail art fans. But that shouldn't stop you from selling the service to other segments of your clientele. The secret behind selling nail art is introducing the right design to the right client at the right time. An understated geometric design, or two similarly-toned blocks of neutral color may be just right for the more conservative client who normally wouldn't even consider nail art. Others who might not be interested in this service could find it difficult to resist a jack-o-lantern sitting on the pinkie near Halloween or a cupid on the index finger to celebrate Valentine's Day.

18

PROCEDURE

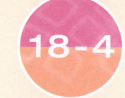

Traditional French Manicure Application

1. **Apply a clear base coat to the nail(s).** (You may use a French manicure polish to achieve the nail bed color if desired. Allow plenty of time for the nail polish to dry. If you choose not to airbrush the nail bed color, skip to step 4.) You can use a crystalline base coat to neutralize the color of the nail tip (Figure 18–28).

2. **Choose your French manicure airbrush paint.** Mist the French manicure color over the nail lightly. If you desire the color to be opaque, continue the passes of your airbrush over the nail until the desired color or opacity is achieved. If your client desires a transparent French manicure color, mist the opaque color lightly. Most airbrush paint colors may be made slightly transparent by adding a couple drops of distilled water.

3. **Optional:** Add a shimmer to your French manicure paint by misting a gold highlight or shimmer evenly over the French beige (Figure 18–29).

4. **French tip application with a stencil:** You will use a curved edge to cover the nail bed color and expose the nail tip to be sprayed white. This is an excellent method for a soft-edged French nail tip.

   ❖ You can cut a curved piece of paper, but there are many ready-made stencils on the market.

   ❖ Hold the stencil as close to the nail as possible, exposing the nail tip to be sprayed. Keep the stencil parallel to the nail to avoid scratching the paint on the nail. The self-adhesive masks are a bit more user-friendly for this service.

   ❖ When you have the stencil lined up, mist the nail tip white. Build the color slowly, to avoid getting the paint wet and runny. (Watch the edge of your stencil if it is plastic. The paint easily accumulates and may run down onto the nail.

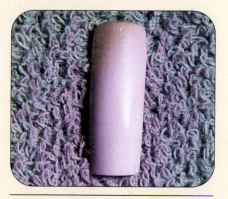

Figure 18-28 Apply base coat.

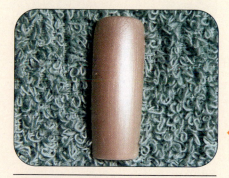

Figure 18-29 Add a shimmer to your French manicure by using a gold highlight.

18

Chapter 18 ● The Creative Touch

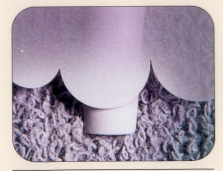

Figure 18-30 Mist paint over the stencil.

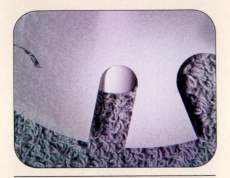

Figure 18-31 Add a lunula, or moon, with the stencil.

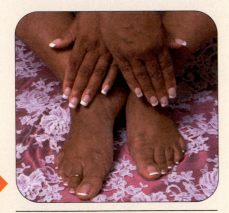

Figure 18-32 Finished French manicure

Dry the stencil with air from your airbrush without moving it, as it is difficult to line up the stencil in precisely the same position.)

❖ When working with stencils, mist paint, then blow air to dry the nail tip and stencil. Repeat the process until the nail tip is the desired color (Figure 18–30).

5. **If the nails you are working on are very curved, you may have to touch up the stenciled nails.** Using the stencil, roll the finger sideways and carefully line up the stencil with the white tip already sprayed. Mist the sides of the nail to match and complete the white tip. This is a less common necessity with the self-adhesive masks.

6. **Optional:** Adding a lunula or moon with a stencil creates the "real" look. Mist the lunula slightly lighter than nail tip color (Figure 18–31).

7. **After you have completed all nails, apply your nail paint bonder and let it dry for three minutes.** Apply the airbrush paint protective glaze for durability.

8. **This procedure is easily accomplished on toes.** Use your preferred method to apply the French manicure to the toes.

9. **Cleanse the toes with airbrush paint cleanser after they have been bonded and glazed** (Figure 18–32).

chapter glossary

air hose	The hose that connects an airbrush compressor (the air source) to the airbrush itself.
color fade (color blend)	An airbrushing technique applying subtle color combinations across the same nail at the same time.
color wheel	A color guide that illustrates and identifies the primary, secondary, tertiary, and complementary colors.
complementary colors	Colors located directly opposite each other on the color wheel.
floating the bead	A technique used to seal nail art where a bead of sealer is dropped onto the nail surface and the brush floats across the surface and completely covers it with sealer.
fluid nozzle (tip)	A small cone-shaped nozzle at the end of an airbrush that holds the needle that releases the paint.
foiling	One of the easiest and most cost-effective nail art techniques, it is applied after polish with a foil adhesive to create colors and patterns not available with polish.
freehand painting	Also referred to as flat nail art; a very expensive form of nail art using brushes and paint to create designs.
French manicure	An airbrushing technique that creates a natural looking nail with a smooth white tip at the free edge.
gems	Tiny jewels that add sparkle, dimension, and texture to any nail art.
gravity-fed	An airbrush system designed to pull the paint into the airbrush using gravity.
internal mix	Airbrush paint that is mixed with the air inside the actual airbrush.
leafing (gold leafing)	Also known as nuggets or nugget sheets; a thin, fragile foil-like material, available in gold, silver, and a variety of other colors used to create a quick and easy form of nail art.
mask knife	A one-sided knife used to cut designs out of mask paper or plastic to create nail art stencils.
mask paper	Paper that is used to create nail art design stencils.
nail art	An add-on service offered at many salons that applies creative and unique custom designs to the finished nail.
needle	The piece that fits into the fluid nozzle of an airbrush and controls the amount of paint released when the trigger is depressed.
position	The way a brush is held to create nail art; the brush can be positioned straight up-and-down or layed down with the bristles pulled across the paint surface.
pressure	The amount of force an artist applies to a brush while in the stroke motion when applying nail art.
primary colors	Pure pigment colors that cannot be obtained from mixing any other colors together.
pull	The flow of a brush across a painted nail surface, giving it a fluid movement and avoiding a rough, spattered look.
secondary colors	Colors directly resulting from mixing equal parts of two primary colors together; they are opposite primary colors on the color wheel.
stencil	Precut designs made of plastic, paper, or fabric, used to create nail art.

18

chapter glossary (continued)

striping tape	A tacky-backed tape available in an assortment of colors that is applied over nail polish or other nail art to create bolder designs.
tertiary colors	Colors directly resulting from mixing equal parts of one primary color and one of its nearest colors.
well	Also known as the small color cup or reservoir; a hole in the top of the airbrush where drips of paint are placed and stored.

review questions

1. Why should you develop nail art skills?

2. List the three basics of nail art.

3. What is the technique called for airbrushing two or more colors on the nail at the same time?

4. List four nail art services.

5. List four of the classifications of color on the color wheel.

6. How does the finished airbrushed French manicure differ from the traditional application?

7. Describe the parts of the airbrush and how they work together to release the paint.

8. Describe the best airbrush to use for nails.

9. What is the most common choice for an air source for airbrushing nails?

10. What is the most common air pressure used by nail technicians when airbrushing?

11. Describe the procedure for an airbrushed version of a French manicure.

part 5

THE BUSINESS OF NAIL TECHNOLOGY

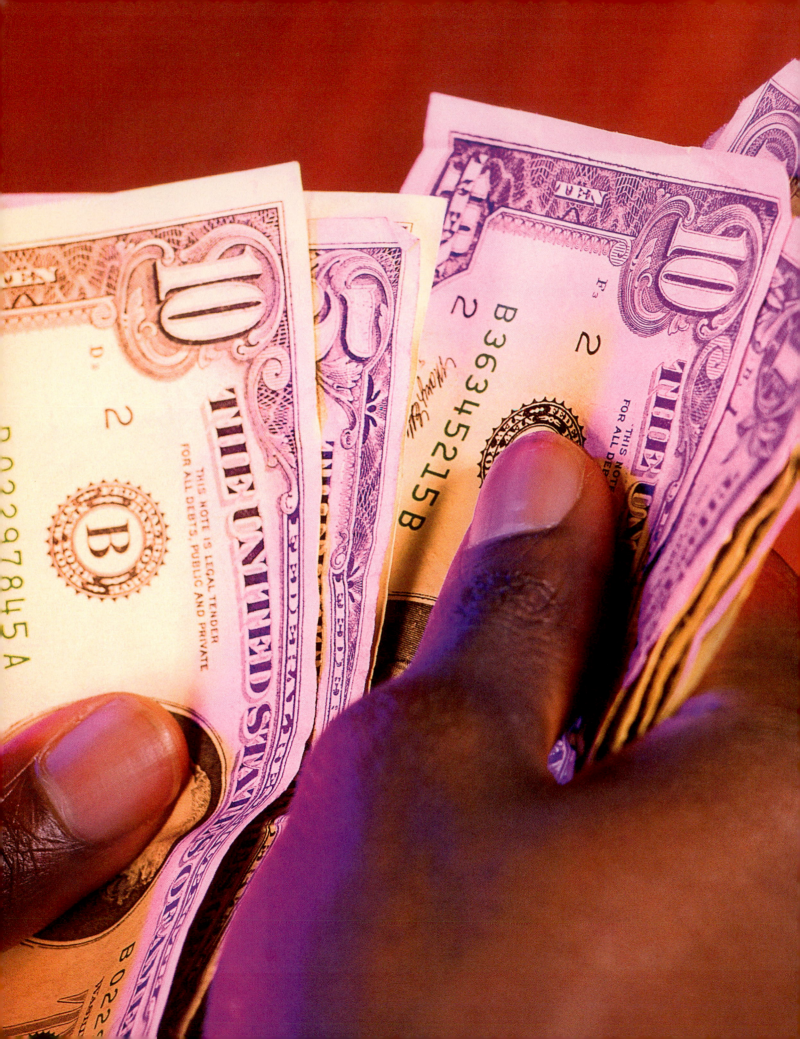

19

SALON BUSINESS

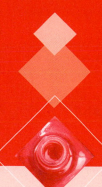

Author: LaCinda Headings

CHAPTER OUTLINE

Your Working Environment • Make Your Decision
Types of Compensation • Booth Rental and Salon Ownership
Interviewing with Success • Keeping Good Personal Records
Understanding Salon Business Records
Booking Appointments • Advertising Yourself
Collecting Payment for Services • Where to Go for Help

Learning Objectives

After you have completed this chapter, you should be able to:

1 Discuss the advantages and disadvantages of working in the four types of salons.

2 List ten questions you will need to ask before deciding what salon is right for you.

3 List eight questions that will help you determine if a salon has safe working conditions.

4 Explain the difference between income and expenses and give two examples of each.

5 List four types of salon compensation.

6 List the practical uses for business records that are required by local, state, and federal laws.

7 Explain the difference between an employee and a booth renter.

8 List seven questions a successful interviewer might ask.

9 List the types of information that a salon can gather by keeping accurate records.

10 Discuss the advantages of keeping proper service, inventory, and personal appointment records.

11 List the guidelines that should be followed in booking appointments.

12 List six sources of support for nail technicians.

Key Terms

Page number indicates where in the chapter the term is used.

booth rental
pg. 362

client service record
pg. 366

compensation
pg. 361

cover letter
pg. 364

expenses
pg. 365

full-service salon
pg. 359

income
pg. 365

interview
pg. 362

mentor
pg. 369

nails-only salon
pg. 359

resume
pg. 363

salon ownership
pg. 362

salon spa (day spa)
pg. 360

tanning salon
pg. 360

You are training to become part of a $6 billion nail care industry. If you want to be financially successful in this business, you must know more than how to give clients manicures, pedicures, or artificial nail services. You need to also be a well-rounded, good business person. From the moment you receive a job offer, you have to negotiate how much money you earn and how you are to be paid. When you develop a clientele, you will handle tips and, possibly, a commission.

If you someday decide to open your own salon, you will be responsible for the complicated business of renting or buying a shop, and paying expenses such as electricity, telephone, advertising, safety systems, employee salaries, and taxes. You may be an expert nail technician, but if you can't handle the business part of nail care, you will not make as much money as nail technicians who can.

Regardless of whether you work for someone else or for yourself, you need to understand the *business* of salon business. This chapter will prepare you for the real world by helping you understand how to put your best foot forward when looking for a job, the salon working environment, the importance of accurate financial and client record keeping, and where you can go for support.

◆ ◆ ◆ YOUR WORKING ENVIRONMENT

Good business sense begins with the decisions you make when looking for your first job. Should you work for a full-service salon, a nails-only salon, a tanning salon, or a spa? There are advantages and disadvantages to each choice.

The Full-service Salon

Unless they are large and very successful, **full-service salons** often employ only one nail technician. The arrangement is a convenient one for both the nail technician and the salon. You automatically get all of the nail-care business in the salon, and your services make it convenient for clients to have their nails done when they are there for hair-care or skin-care services.

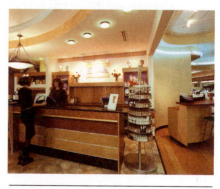

Figure 19-1 A full-service salon

On the other hand, at a full-service salon, there won't be other nail technicians with whom to share ideas and experience. There also won't be someone to fill in for you when you are sick or on vacation. If the salon is a traditional one, you may be limited in the variety of artificial nail services that you are allowed to perform (Figure 19–1).

The Nails-only Salon

In a **nails-only salon** you will work with several other nail technicians. In addition to having the opportunity to share ideas and experiences, you could increase your business by serving their clients when they are sick, on vacation, or retire. Also, the client is coming to this salon specifically for a nail service. There is no prompting them for your particular expertise (Figure 19–2).

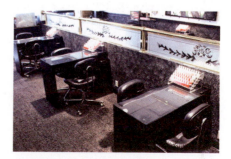

Figure 19-2 A nails-only salon

19

The client who patronizes a nails-only salon may take nail care more seriously than clients who have their nails done in full-service salons. Your clients may have special nail problems, or want more creative artificial nail services. If this is the case, you will gain valuable experience. A nails-only salon is a good place for a nail technician to establish a serious clientele. On the other hand, there could be competition for clients in a nails-only salon where there are many nail technicians.

The Tanning Salon

Some **tanning salons** also offer nail services. The opportunity for rapid growth is great in this type of salon. A tanning salon has clients coming in the door every fifteen to thirty minutes. If the salon is open from 8:00 A.M. to 8:00 P.M., there could be twenty-four to forty-eight tanners every day that you have the opportunity to present your services to and make your nail clients! Again, the disadvantage could be that you are the only nail technician so you have little opportunity to share new ideas. Continuing education is critical in this type of environment.

The Salon or Day Spa

A rapidly growing segment of salon industry is the **salon spa** or **day spa**. This type of salon features relaxing services such as body massage, hydrotherapy, and facials. Many spas have whirlpool pedicure thrones to pamper their clients. Natural nail care and low-odor products are important to the holistic atmosphere of a salon spa. This is a more controlled atmosphere and an excellent choice for someone who likes tranquil surroundings (Figure 19–3).

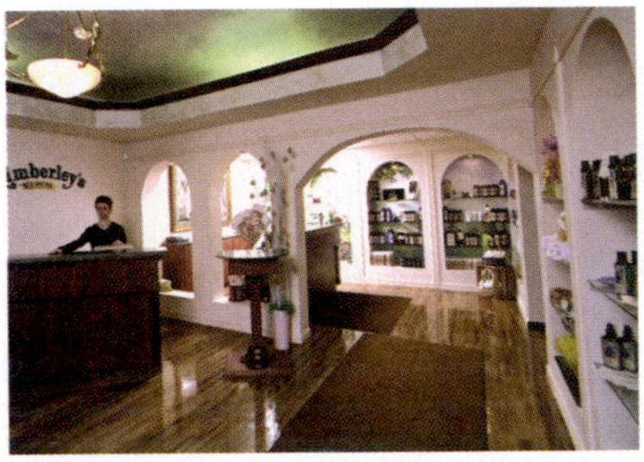

Figure 19-3 A day spa, offering relaxing body services as well as nail care

◆ ◆ ◆ MAKE YOUR DECISION

Before you make a decision about what salon is right for you, visit several. Observe the working environment and decide which feels comfortable to you.

You will want to consider the following factors in deciding on the salon that is right for you.

1. Will the salon provide additional training for you or encourage you to attend training outside the salon?

2. Will the salon help you build a clientele? Will they spend money on advertising? Will they refer customers to you?

3. Will you be considered an employee, or will you be a booth renter? What are the terms of the booth rental? Does your state allow this system?

4. If you are an employee, how will the salon pay you? Will you receive a weekly salary or salary plus commission? Will you receive a commission on retail products sold? Is there a regular salary review?

5. Will the salon provide nail-care products or will you have to bring your own?

6. Does the salon offer benefits such as medical, liability, life insurance, or paid sick days?

7. Are there fixed or flexible working hours?

8. What is the dress code?

9. Does the salon close for a regular vacation period, or does each employee take a separate vacation?

10. What is the salon's reputation? There is an advantage to working in a successful "upscale" salon where you can make good contacts and learn valuable tricks of the trade from your employer and coworkers.

11. Does the salon have safe working conditions?

    a. Does it have proper ventilation, like an exhaust system to the outside?

    b. Does it provide separate refrigerators for food and nail product storage?

    c. Are MSDSs on display or within easy access to employees?

    d. Are workstations well equipped and clean, with plastic disposal bags that can be closed?

    e. Are nail technicians required to wear dust masks?

    f. Are nail technicians required to wear safety glasses?

    g. Are aerosol cans used or are safe application methods used, such as pumps or brush-on products?

    h. Are salon workers ready for emergencies? Are the telephone numbers for poison control, the hospital, paramedics, the fire station, or the police posted in a visible place?

◆ ◆ ◆ TYPES OF COMPENSATION

As vast as your choices are in types of salons to work at, so are your choices of compensation. **Compensation** is payment for services rendered. There are many ways that salons can compensate you.

The following are common ways that salons compensate their employees.

❖ **Hourly wage:** The salon pays you for the hours you work in the salon.

❖ **Salary:** The salon pays you a set amount each pay period regardless of the number of hours worked.

❖ **Commission:** The salon pays you a percentage of the profit your services generate for the salon. This percentage varies from salon to salon.

❖ **Salary or hourly wage plus commission:** The salon guarantees you a base pay. The *base pay* can be based on hours worked or a salary. If your percentage of the profit you bring into the salon exceeds your base, the salon pays you commission plus your salary. Again, the percentage varies from salon to salon.

Receiving compensation makes you an employee of the salon. As an employee, the salon is required to withhold appropriate taxes from your paycheck. Most salons furnish supplies (unless you are a booth renter). They stock retail products and provide a receptionist for their employees if the salon is large enough to bear the expense.

◆ ◆ BOOTH RENTAL AND SALON OWNERSHIP

Some salons do not hire employees. Instead, they rent salon space to individuals. This is called **booth rental**. In a booth rental situation, the nail technician pays the salon a certain amount of money per week or month for space within the salon to work. In a very real sense, booth renters own their own business. Booth renters collect their own money, purchase their own supplies, and pay self-employment taxes. If you would like to be your own boss, but are not ready to open your own salon, booth renting may be a great option, providing your state has no regulations against this practice.

Another way to be your own boss is to enter the world of **salon ownership**. If you feel that you have something unique to offer other salon professionals and customers, opening or buying a salon might be for you. When you are opening your own salon, you have the opportunity to create a working environment that fits your personality. You may choose to open a high energy, cutting edge salon or you might decide to open a plush, pampering salon. Investing in a salon is not just deciding what atmosphere you want. Successfully opening a salon takes a lot of preparation and work. Proper preparation is not just important in applying nail enhancements— the more prepared you are for opening your salon the more chance you have of success.

Buying an established salon that has an existing clientele is another option. When selling, salon owners usually include their client list with the physical part of their business. If you do not already have a clientele, this can be a great opportunity. Be careful to look at all aspects of the business that is for sale. As with opening your own salon, it is still advisable to start with a business plan.

◆ ◆ INTERVIEWING WITH SUCCESS

If you decide to work as an employee, you will be expected to go through the interview process. An **interview** is a conversation between you and your potential employer where information is exchanged. That means that the interviewer is not the only person asking the questions. The interview is as much for you as it is for the owner. During an interview, you have a chance to get to know the salon owner/manager and see if you will fit into the salon culture (Figure 19–4).

Look Your Best

First impressions are lasting ones. Before you even open your mouth to introduce yourself, your *appearance* has made an impression. Doing your research about a salon will help you make a great first impression. If the salon is on the cutting edge and ultra trendy, you should dress the part by wearing the latest styles. But if the salon is more conservative, dress more conservatively. Remember, in an interview situation, it is better to be professionally dressed than to be too casual. First impressions come from more than just your clothes. Your nails should look impeccable (of course!) and your hair and make-up should convey that you are in the beauty business. Body language is important as well. Greet your interviewer with a firm handshake and a smile. Look him or her in the eye when answering questions. All these things add up to a great first impression (Figure 19–5).

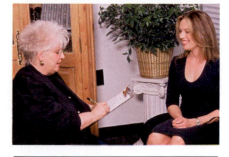

Figure 19-4 The interview is an exchange of information

Your Resume

Most salon owners will ask you for a resume before you come for an interview. A **resume** is a written summary of your work and academic experience as well as your qualifications for the job. Your resume makes an impression about who you are before you even meet your potential employer. Do your research and pick several salons that you would like to work at. Then find out who does the hiring at those salons and send them a resume. A resume consists of five main parts.

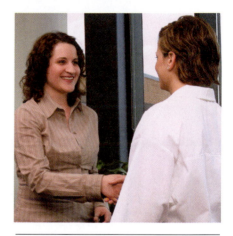

Figure 19-5 Body language is important.

1. **Personal information.** Your contact information. Include your name, address, and phone number where you can be reached for questions and to set up an interview.

2. **Your objective.** One sentence that briefly states your career goals. This sentence reflects your personality and passion for your new career.

3. **Your work experience.** A chronological recap of your past jobs. In this section, be sure to highlight the experience gained in previous jobs that would contribute to being a success in the salon business. Customer relations and sales experiences are valuable cross-over skills. Include clinic floor work performed while at school in this section. You are working on paying customers! Take care to account for all times in your work history. Some potential employers look for gaps in your work history to see how reliable you are. If you did take some time off from the work force, say to have a baby, list that time as "full-time mother." Highlight the experience you have gained from being a mother, such as organizational skills, that could be valuable in a salon.

4. **Education.** A listing of your academic background. Be sure to include any extra nail industry classes you have taken, such as manufacturer classes at your school, shows, or distributor classes. You can also

include offices held in school clubs such as Student Council that would show leadership abilities.

5. **References.** A list of people who your potential employer can contact and who can attest to your qualifications for the job. Include three to five references. Avoid using family members or friends unless you had working relationships with them in a previous job. Print your references on a separate sheet to avoid overcrowding your resume.

A resume should be typed or printed from a computer on heavy-weight stock paper. Use standard one-inch margins on all sides. Be sure to check for typographical errors. If you are typing the resume and have used correction tape or fluid, make a clean copy to avoid sending a resume that has been noticeably corrected. When sending a resume to a potential employer, include a cover letter. A **cover letter** is a letter to the salon owner that tells why you want to work in the salon, briefly describes your qualifications, and asks for an interview. It is a good idea to follow up with a phone call to see if they received your resume and ask if you can set up an interview.

The Interview

You sent your resume and the salon owner has called you to come in for an interview. The more prepared you are for your interview, the less nervous you will be. Prepare by going through this list of questions that a potential employer could ask during an interview and deciding how you would answer each question. The questions are always easier when you know the answers.

Following are questions the interviewer may ask you.

❖ Why did you choose this career?
❖ Why should I/we hire you?
❖ What interests you about our salon?
❖ Describe your problem-solving skills.
❖ What motivates you?
❖ What are your short-term and long-term goals?
❖ What are your strengths and weaknesses?

Remember that the interview is an exchange of information. You should be prepared with questions of your own so that you can have all the information you need to make an informed decision about working at the salon.

Following are questions for you to ask the interviewer.

❖ What kind of continuing education programs does your salon offer?
❖ What are your expectations of your employees?
❖ What nail services does your salon offer?
❖ What product lines do your nail technicians use and sell in the salon?
❖ Does the salon provide supplies needed for services?

- ❖ What kinds of sanitation procedures are used in the salon?
- ❖ What are the hours of the salon?
- ❖ What is the dress code?
- ❖ What is your compensation structure?
- ❖ Do you offer any benefits such as medical, sick days, and vacation pay?

It is a good idea to send a thank-you note to the owner after your interview. Besides being proper etiquette, it also lets the salon owner know that you have good follow-up skills.

KEEPING GOOD PERSONAL RECORDS

Although you may not be required to keep business records for your salon, you will want to develop a simple and efficient system for keeping track of your own income and expenses. You will also want to save all of your check stubs, cancelled checks, receipts, and invoices. Basically, **income** is the money you make and **expenses** are what you spend. Another valuable personal record is your appointment calendar. These are all important for your tax records, and will vary depending on what type of employment arrangement you have with the salon.

Income

To keep a correct, concise, and complete record of your income, you should create a form with room to list each source of income. It might include salary, commission from services, commission from retail products sold, and tips.

Expenses

Your tax-deductible expenses working in the salon could include equipment, supplies, magazines or books that explain techniques, comfortable shoes, uniforms (if required), and tuition for special courses on nail techniques. Consult your tax professional to learn more about exactly what expenses can be deducted from your tax liability.

Appointments

As a booth renter, you need to use a personal appointment calendar to help you arrange your work time. If you keep this calendar with you, you can plan each day's schedule before you arrive at the salon. You will know who your clients are, when each one will arrive, and the services you will perform. With this information, you can prepare all your supplies ahead of time, so you are more efficient. If you are an employee, your schedule is available through the receptionist or at the front desk.

19

◆◆ UNDERSTANDING SALON BUSINESS RECORDS

Most salons use the services of an accountant to help them keep accurate records that meet the requirements of local, state, and federal laws. These records are used to

1. determine income, expenses, and profit or loss.

2. prove the value of your clientele or the worth of the salon to prospective buyers.

3. get a bank loan.

4. compute income tax, social security, unemployment, and disability insurance, among others.

Businesses hold daily sales slips, the appointment book, and the petty cash book for at least one year. The payroll book, canceled checks, monthly and yearly records, and service and inventory records are usually held for at least seven years for tax purposes (Figure 19–6).

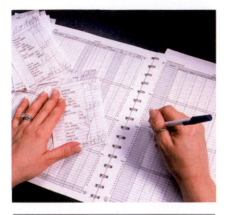

Figure 19-6 Keep accurate and neat business records.

Using Business Records

Accurate records will help you and your employer gather the following valuable information.

1. **Profit and loss comparisons with other weeks, months, or years.** As an example, over a period of time, you can see which are the slow months and which are the busiest in your business. This will allow you to cut expenses by not being overstocked during slow months, and being fully stocked during busy periods. You can also schedule vacations or renovations during the slow months and have a full staff and full service during the busy months.

2. **Changes in demands for services.** If the demand for a service is growing, your salon may choose to hire more nail technicians to service this growing demand.

3. **Inventory.** If you keep accurate records of inventory, you can cut costs by keeping the appropriate stock levels. This means that you are neither overstocked nor running short of supplies needed for services. Daily inventory records also help you quickly detect any loss of stock from theft.

4. **Net income.** Net income refers to all the income you make less all the expenses. Accurate net income records can help you establish the net worth of the business at the end of the year.

5. **Materials and supply levels.** Records will help you compare the use of materials and supplies with the services rendered to make sure that neither too much nor too little is being used.

Keeping Client Records

A **client service record** lists services rendered and merchandise sold to each client. All service records should contain the name and address of the client, date, amount charged, product used, results obtained, and client's preferences and tastes. Some salons use a card file system or a memorandum book to keep service records. Others are fully computerized and maintain those records electronically. With the service record for each client should be any release statements that he or she has signed. Service records are especially valuable if another nail technician has to fill in for a client's usual nail technician. If the client's usual service is explained in detail on the card, it can be done accurately and efficiently. Also, keep a record of service challenges and the solutions tried.

The client health/record form lists clients' personal information, such as what types of jobs they have, what hobbies they enjoy, and what medications they take. It is a good idea to start your day by reading the records of clients scheduled for services during the day. Your clients will be happy to know you remembered the things that are important to them. See Chapter 9 for a complete discussion of client records.

Computerization

In this age of instant information, more and more salons are incorporating computers into their salon business. Computerization of salon records allows you to access information at the touch of a button. There are computer programs designed specifically for the beauty industry that help keep track of all salon records. These programs can schedule appointments, generate mailing lists, and control inventory. Some programs can even tell you when your clients could be out of the home care products that they purchased. A computer is a valuable tool to use in the salon business (Figure 19–7).

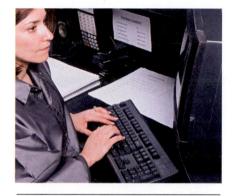

Figure 19-7 A computer is a very valuable tool in the salon.

◆ ◆ ● BOOKING APPOINTMENTS

The system used in your salon will determine whether you book appointments with clients or they are booked by a receptionist. Keeping a proper record of appointments will cut down on the confusion, annoyance, and stress of overbooking and help prevent clients from arriving at the wrong time and having to wait.

Regardless of who books the appointments, the following guidelines should be followed (Figure 19–8).

1. Always have a supply of appointment books, pencils, erasers, pens, a calendar, and a message pad or access to the computer.

2. Be prompt. Whether you are answering the phone or acknowledging your client's presence at the counter, try not to keep him or her waiting.

3. Identify both yourself and the salon by name when you answer the telephone.

4. Be pleasant. Let clients know you are pleased to talk with them. When talking with your client, smile! Even when you are on the phone, the person on the other end can hear your smile.

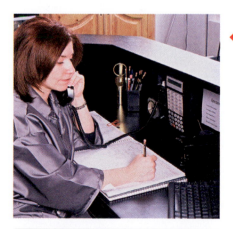

Figure 19-8 Keep an accurate record of appointments.

5. Make sure to take the following information when a client calls to make an appointment: client's name and phone number, type of service to be performed, date, and time of appointment. Repeat the information to the client to be sure you are correct, then block out the amount of time needed to perform the service in the appointment book or in the computer.

6. Speak clearly. Do not mumble or shout. Use correct English and avoid slang.

7. Be tactful and courteous when speaking. Refer to clients by their last name.

8. If you are busy enough to have appointments made in advance, it is a good practice to call your clients the night before the appointment to remind them and confirm the time. This will reduce your number of no-shows.

9. Always ask your clients at the end of their appointment if they wish to reschedule.

ADVERTISING YOURSELF

The first thing you might want to do when you begin a job in the salon is to make a list of every service you offer. Write a brief description of the service, length of time needed to perform it, and the cost of the service.

A copy of your service list should be kept near the appointment book so there will be no confusion among your clients about these facts. Give your coworkers a copy of your list of services and encourage them to offer your services to their clients.

COLLECTING PAYMENT FOR SERVICES

In some salons, the nail technician collects payments from clients. In others, the receptionist handles all payments. In either case, you will probably be required to prepare a ticket detailing the services you have performed for that client. The ticket should include the client's name, the date, the service provided, and the cost. The ticket will make it clear to clients what they are paying for and provide an accurate record of the transaction.

Do not offer reduced prices to "special" clients. This can lead to a difficult situation if your other clients are denied a price reduction.

WHERE TO GO FOR HELP

As with any new career, unfamiliar territory lies ahead. There are many places you can go for support.

19

❖ Trade magazines have helpful articles and resources for nail technicians who want to stay current in the industry.

❖ Professional organizations provide education and membership privileges, such as group insurance and discounts.

❖ Product distributors and their sales consultants can work with you to design promotions and grow your business. They are also a great source of continuing education.

❖ Manufacturers provide technical hotlines that can help you troubleshoot product challenges.

❖ The World Wide Web is a valuable resource for everything. With a computer and access to the Internet, salons can research products, obtain an MSDS, and chat with other nail technicians from all over the world. There are sites targeted to the nail professional as well as general business resources. There are also chat groups, mailing lists, and bulletin boards dedicated to helping nail technicians.

❖ Mentors can be a big help when starting out in a new career. A **mentor** is an experienced colleague that is a trusted teacher or adviser. Mentors can help perfect your technique, give business advice, and provide emotional support. Mentors realize that if they help others they can elevate the professionalism of the entire industry. Understand that some nail technicians will view you as their competition, so find someone who is willing to share their "secrets of success" with you. Some new nail technicians are lucky enough to find their mentor in the salon they go to work in. Places to look for mentors are classes, shows, and the Internet. Your school may have a network of mentors already in place.

B U S I N E S S TIP

Common Courtesy

No one likes to be kept waiting—and that includes your clients. When a customer comes through the door, make an effort to greet her right away. If you happen to be with another client when your next customer arrives, offer her a beverage and give her an estimate of when you will be with her. Furthermore, if you are running more than fifteen minutes late for the entire day, call each of your clients and alert them. This allows them to push back their appointments or rebook. Incorporating these simple, courteous gestures shows the client that her time is important and you value her business. Everyone likes to go places where they are treated well. To make your salon a place that people like to go, practice common courtesy.

chapter glossary

booth rental	A business opportunity where salons rent space to individual nail technicians. A weekly or monthly rental fee is paid to the salon, and the nail technician is responsible for his or her own business expenses.
client service record	A record that lists the services rendered, products used, charges, and merchandise sold to each client.
compensation	Any payment made for services rendered.
cover letter	A letter to the salon owner or manager that accompanies a resume to briefly describe why you are interested in a position, how you qualify, and to request an interview.
expenses	The costs of supplies, equipment, rent, etc. to run a business.
full-service salon	A salon that provides a variety of health and beauty services from nail care to skin care to hair care.
income	The money taken in for providing a service.
interview	A formal conversation between you and a potential employer where information is exchanged to decide whether you are right for a position in a salon and whether the salon is right for you.
mentor	An experienced colleague that becomes a trusted teacher or advisor and helps you perfect your career.
nails-only salon	A salon that employs several nail technicians specifically for nail services.
resume	A written summary of your work and academic experience and qualifications for a job.
salon ownership	Complete financial investment in a salon by opening a new salon or buying an existing salon.
salon spa (day spa)	A salon that offers many relaxing services such as body massage, hydrotherapy, and facials. These salons often feature pedicure and manicure services and promote natural nail care.
tanning salon	A salon that offers primarily tanning services, but often employs a nail technician to provide an added service to its clients.

19

review questions

1. What are the advantages and disadvantages of working in the four types of salons?

2. What are ten questions that will help you determine if a salon is right for you?

3. What are eight questions that will help you determine if a salon has safe working conditions?

4. Explain the difference between income and expenses and give two examples of each.

5. List four types of salon compensation.

6. List four practical uses for business records that are required by local, state, and federal laws.

7. Explain the difference between an employee and a booth renter.

8. List seven questions a successful interviewer might ask.

9. List five types of information that a salon can gather by keeping accurate business records.

10. Discuss the advantages of keeping proper service, inventory, and personal appointment records.

11. List nine guidelines that should be followed in booking appointments.

12. List six sources of support for nail technicians.

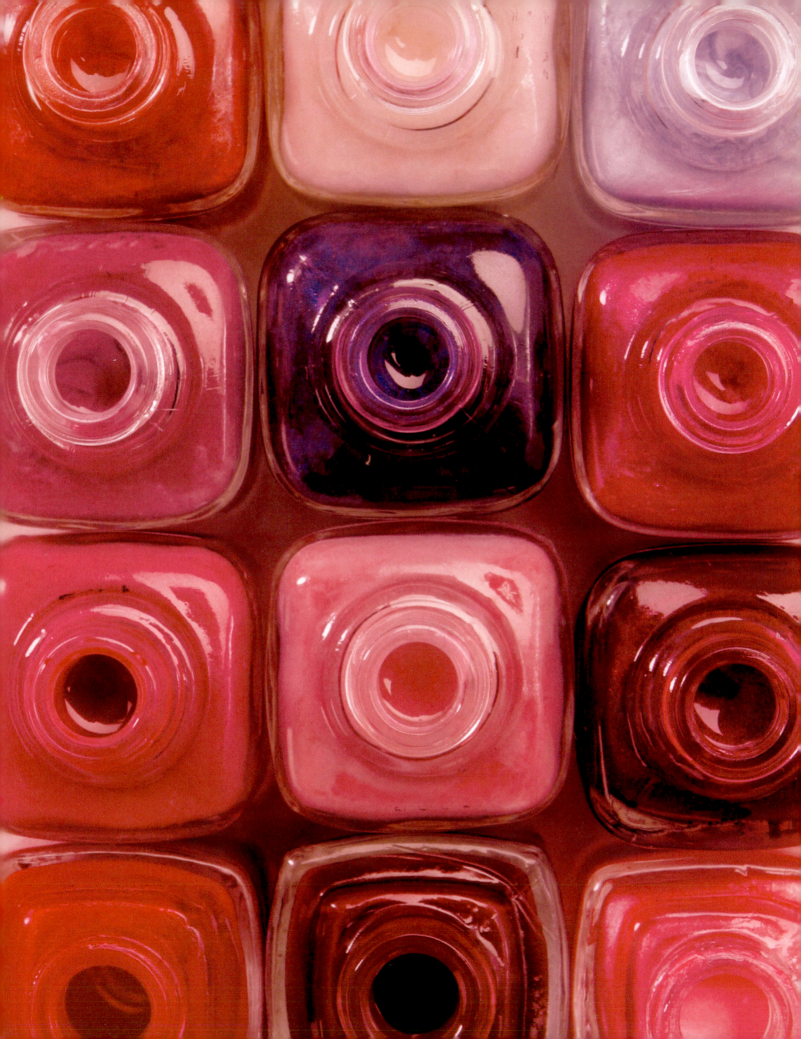

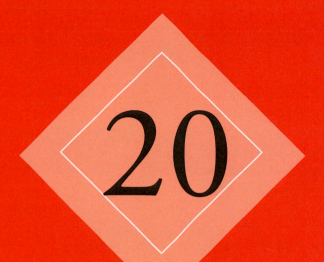

20

SELLING NAIL PRODUCTS AND SERVICES

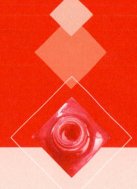

Author: LaCinda Headings

CHAPTER OUTLINE

Know Your Products and Services
Know What Your Client Needs and Wants
Marketing • Present Your Products and Services
Answer Questions and Objections • Close the Sale
Tracking Your Success

Learning Objectives

After you have completed this chapter, you should be able to:

1. List the five basic principles of selling products and services.

2. Explain the difference between product or service features and benefits and list examples of each.

3. List three methods of marketing in the salon with examples of each.

4. Describe the least expensive, most effective form of advertising.

5. Discuss how to set prices for products and services.

6. List monthly events and give examples of promotional tie-ins to each.

7. Discuss ways to fill open time slots in your daily schedule.

8. Calculate client retention rates.

Key Terms

Page number indicates where in the chapter the term is used.

advertising
pg. 378

benefits
pg. 376

business card
pg. 378

client retention rate
pg. 384

feature
pg. 375

level system
pg. 378

marketing
pg. 377

promotions
pg. 379

salon literature
pg. 378

salon menu
pg. 378

word of mouth advertising
pg. 378

yellow pages
pg. 379

If you want to be a successful nail technician, you need to be a good salesperson too. You are responsible for selling both nail services and the products that will help your clients maintain those services. You will be successful if you understand that customers buy products and services based on two things. First, they buy solutions to their problems. Secondly, they buy a product because of how it makes them look and feel.

The five basic steps in meeting your clients' needs and selling your products and services are described in this chapter. The basic steps to selling include:

1. Know your products and services.

2. Know what your client needs and wants.

3. Present your products and services.

4. Answer your client's questions and objections properly.

5. Close the sale.

The beauty industry markets solutions to problems and the feeling people get when they know they look good. You have the products and services at your fingertips to give your clients that feeling. Knowing how to sell those products and services is the key to your success. In this chapter, you will learn about setting prices for and marketing your products and services, basic principles of selling, and tracking your success.

KNOW YOUR PRODUCTS AND SERVICES

In the nail salon, products and services are very closely related. When you perform a nail service for your client, you select the products that are best for that person. Then you use them to perform a service that meets your client's needs and wants.

When you have finished with the nail service, you sell your client the products needed to maintain the service between visits to the salon.

There are two ways to know your products and services. One way is to know the features, and the other way is to know the benefits.

Features

A **feature** is a specific fact about a product or service that describes it. Read labels, product bulletins, and industry literature to learn the features of your nail products. You look for information such as the ingredients your products contain, safety precautions you should follow when using them, how to apply them, and how to maintain them. Features of nail services include the procedures and how long they take to perform, the chemicals used, how much the services cost, what effect they have on the clients' nails, and how often they need maintenance (Figure 20–1).

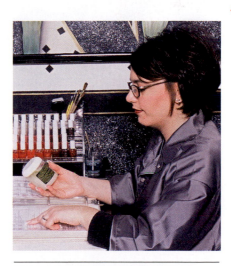

Figure 20–1 Read all about your retail products.

The features of colored gel nails over tips include the fact that they are durable, lightweight, and come in a variety of colors. Light-cured gels take about 30 minutes to perform, use acrylic-based gel with a special light source, will not harm healthy nails, and need maintenance every two to three weeks.

Benefits

The **benefits** of a product or service are what it will do for your client or how it will fulfill your client's needs and wants. The benefits of colored gel nails over tips are long, beautiful nails that save you both time and money. They give you nails that always look freshly polished, are lightweight and comfortable to wear, and require maintenance every two to three weeks instead of once a week.

You will be a good salesperson when you can turn the features of your products and services into benefits that meet the needs and desires of your clients.

◆ ◆ ◆ KNOW WHAT YOUR CLIENT NEEDS AND WANTS

It is important to know your clients' nail needs if you want to sell them nail products and services that meet those needs. You can discover some of those needs during the client consultation (see Chapter 9).

As you observe your client and communicate with him or her, you will want to answer questions such as these.

1. **Does your client have special nail problems?** Clients with nail problems will need special nail services. Does your client have short bitten nails or nails that crack and tear easily? These clients may need services that strengthen or overlay their natural nails.

2. **What is your client's lifestyle?** The kind of life your client leads will determine what type of nail services they need. A business person may want nails that have a well-groomed look and are short and polished in a pale conservative color. A jewelry or cosmetics salesperson may want long, acrylic nails. A gardener or pianist might need short, natural-looking nails. A quilter might need short nails but want them polished in the latest fashion color. Be sure you give your clients the services and products that suit their activities and image (Figure 20–2).

3. **Is your client preparing for a special occasion?** A client who is going to a wedding might want nails that are the same color as the dress she is wearing or a fancy French manicure. A client who is going on a job interview will probably want nails that look natural but well groomed. If your client is wearing a witch's costume to a Halloween party, she might want extra long acrylic nails painted black and covered in nail art.

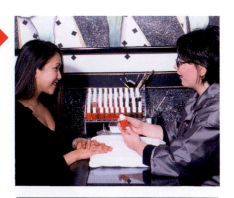

Figure 20-2 Determine which services or products best suit your clients by discussing their lifestyles with them.

20

4. **What products do you use on your nails at home?** Almost every woman uses polishes, polish removers, lotions, and other nail care products at home. Knowing what they use and do not use will allow you to suggest professional products that will fulfill their needs and better maintain the services you provide. For instance, if you apply a wrap to the nail, you will want your client to use a non-acetone remover that will not break down the surface of the wrap service.

◆ ◆ ◆ MARKETING

Marketing describes the commercial processes involved in promoting, selling, and distributing a product or service. Successful salons and nail technicians never stop marketing themselves. Methods of marketing in the salon include salon literature, outside advertising, ongoing promotions, salon newsletters, and birthday cards with a special "Thank You" inside.

Setting Prices for Your Products and Services

To begin marketing your products and services, you must set the prices you are going to charge for them. Many salons will have prices set for you, but if you are renting space or the salon does not have set prices for the products and services you offer, you will need to decide what to charge your clients. The general rule for pricing professional products sold in the salon is to double the salon cost of those products. For example, if you buy a product from your distributor for $2.00, you would resell it to your client for $4.00. Most manufacturers have a suggested retail price list on which you can base those prices. Selling home care products in the salon helps both your clients and you (Figure 20–3). They will have the products they need to maintain their service at home and you and the salon will make more money.

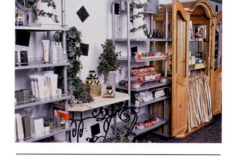

Figure 20-3 An attractive retail display should be in full view of your clients.

Base your service prices on both your market and the cost of doing that service. If you are working in an upscale salon and using top-of-the-line products, charge more for your service than if you are working in an economy salon and using less expensive products. Check to see what similar salons in your area are charging for the same services. When you are starting out you may want your prices to be comparable. If your prices are too low in a high-end market, your services will be perceived as inferior. On the other hand, if your prices are too high in a lower-budget market, you could price yourself out of business. Keep this in mind, but do not base your prices solely on the market and forget to factor in your overhead.

What do you do when your prices are not high enough to cover your overhead and make a profit? The answer is to raise your prices. Many salon professionals fear raising their prices for fear of losing clients. Think about this: most companies offer "cost-of-living" pay increases on a yearly basis to their workers. Your cost of living and doing business goes up constantly and you need to pass that increase on to your clients. Opportune times to raise your prices are when your product costs increase or when you have attended continuing education classes and have more expertise. Some salons build employee raises into their pricing structure by having a **level system**. In a level system, new nail technicians charge a lower price. With experience and achievements in the salon, the salon promotes the nail technician to a higher level and higher price structure. For example, a Level 1 Technician charges $40 for a full set, a Level 2 Technician charges $42, and a Level 3 Technician charges $45.

Marketing with Salon Literature

Business cards and salon menus are examples of **salon literature**. **Business cards** are an advertisement of your business and your salon image. They promote your business. Your cards should contain enough information to let clients know what you do, where you do it, and how they can contact you. They should include the salon's name and your name, along with the salon's address and phone number. Give several of your business cards to all new or potential clients. You can even use your cards to record your client's next appointment or the products you have recommended for them. A **salon menu** is a listing of your services, just like a menu at a restaurant. It includes a brief description of each service, the time it takes, and the price you charge for those services. It may also feature what products the salon carries for home care (Figure 20–4).

Marketing through Advertising

Advertising is the act of calling public attention to your product or service. To be effective when advertising, do not just advertise who you are and where you work. Advertise what makes you special. Why should clients come to you instead of going to someone else? Are you quick and efficient, enabling clients to get in and out over their lunch hour? Or do you take pride in providing a relaxing and pampering service? Do you specialize in nail art or natural looking nails? Advertising what makes you special will attract clients that will stay with you. They know before setting foot in your salon that the services you provide are the services they will find valuable.

Newspaper, radio, and TV are commonly the mediums that come to mind when thinking about advertising. These are effective when used properly, but can be very costly. The least expensive and most effective form of advertising for the salon professional is **word of mouth advertising**. Clients who enjoy your services recommend you to their friends. Capitalize on this by asking your clients for referrals. Advertising a referral program will give your clients an incentive to refer their friends to you. Give them a stack of your business cards. Be sure to have your clients write their name on the cards they give away so that you know who referred the new client. When you collect a certain amount of referral cards passed out by a client, reward her with an "add-on" product or service. For example, you could give your clients nail art or a paraffin dip after their manicure or pedicure for every customer they send you. The cost of the nail art or the paraffin is minimal compared to the profit you make from gaining a new client! You could take it a step further and offer a complimentary fill-in

Figure 20-4 A salon menu is a listing of the services you offer.

20

service for every five new clients an existing client sends your way. Be careful not to do all of these things for the same referring client, as it will become very expensive for you.

Yellow pages are another great place to advertise. When people move into a new area, they use the yellow pages to find the goods and services they need. To be most effective with the yellow pages, purchase advertising space in addition to listing your business in the alphabetical listing. Most consumers looking for a new salon will look at the advertisements and would not find you unless they knew the name of your salon and could look it up. Consider listing your business under several categories to increase the chances of new customers finding you in the yellow pages. Beauty salons, spas, nail salons, and manicuring are some of the possible categories listed in most yellow pages.

Marketing with Promotions

Promotions are events designed to promote a specific product or service. Salons run promotions to introduce new services or products and to increase the purchases of existing services or products. There are many kinds of promotions that can be used in the salon. Product give-aways are examples of promotions used to attract new clients and help build your business. Consider running a two-for-one promotion for new customers. In this promotion, the clients get half price, but now you have two clients that will be booking services with you instead of just one! To promote your maintenance products, you could run a promotion where the customer gets a "value added" on the maintenance product, when they purchase a *new service*. For instance, you may offer the 12-oz. scented lotion your client wants to buy, for the price of the 8-oz. size when a spa manicure or pedicure is booked.

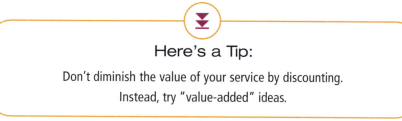

Here's a Tip:

Don't diminish the value of your service by discounting.
Instead, try "value-added" ideas.

It is common to tie promotions to holidays or events throughout the year. You can do this by creating and using a yearly promotional calendar. Here is a list of monthly events and ideas to center a promotion around and a promotional idea for each one.

January	New Year's – A book of coupons to use throughout the new year.
February	Valentines Day – Two-for-one sweetheart deals.
March	First Day of Spring – Pedicure specials.
April	Prom Season – Nail art and polish to match your dress.
May	Mother's Day – Gift certificates for any service plus complimentary paraffin.

June	Weddings – Bridesmaid party discounts and added value, the groom is complimentary.
July	Independence Day – Beat-the-heat service specials like a pedicure with a cool mint masque.
August/ September	Back to School – Promote larger sizes of maintenance products for the college bound.
October	Breast Cancer Awareness Month – Organize a fundraiser among your clients.
November/ December	Holidays – Promote gift certificates, baskets, and stocking stuffers.

Target Advertising

If you know what kind of client you want to attract, you can market directly to them. If you want to attract a young clientele, advertise in high school or college newspapers. If you want to attract the businessperson, consider advertising in local business publications. Direct mailing and the "Welcome Wagon" are great ways to target those customers who live in your zip code.

◆ ◆ ◆ PRESENT YOUR PRODUCTS AND SERVICES

There are two powerful opportunities to sell your products and services to your clients. One way is while you are performing the service. The other way is to have the products and services displayed attractively near your workstation.

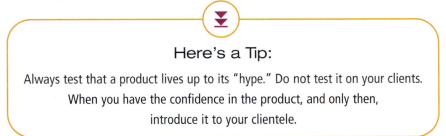

Here's a Tip:

Always test that a product lives up to its "hype." Do not test it on your clients. When you have the confidence in the product, and only then, introduce it to your clientele.

Sell While You Work

When you are performing a service, tell your clients what you are doing, what products you are using, and why. If one of the procedures, such as nail filing and polish touch-up, can be done by your clients, suggest the type of abrasive and polish they should buy and tell them how to use the products.

While you are giving one service to a client, discuss other services and the features, benefits, and costs of each. If you are giving an acrylic nail service, mention that you offer a buff-and-polish service that would freshen the polish between fills, or discuss the benefits of a pedicure. Your clients may want to try other services in the future.

BUSINESS TIP

Marketing Fun

If you want to introduce a new product that you might need to charge for (e.g., U.V. top coat), have clients bring in their wedding/baby pictures. Offer the top coat complimentary for the first time for anyone who brings in pictures. This gives the client the opportunity to try the product and have fun at the same time by sharing with you and/or other clients.

Display a List of Your Services

The menu of services your salon offers should be displayed prominently in the reception area. If not, have your service list displayed near your station. The card should be attractive and clear. It should list your services and the cost of each. You may put in other information you think would be helpful to your clients, such as length of time for each service, its features, and its benefits.

Display Your Products

Display the nail products sold by your salon attractively and in view of your clients when they are having a service performed. Have written promotional materials about the products within easy reach of your clients so they can take information with them. Also, have free samples of nail products, when possible, and encourage your clients to take some and try them. Have tester bottles of your products available so your clients can touch and smell them.

Do not pass up the opportunity to sell your clients polish, top coat, hand cream, polish remover, cuticle oil, and other products they will need to maintain their nail services between visits to the salon. Using only professional salon items throughout the salon assures your clients you have confidence in those products. For instance, putting a professional hand wash in the bathroom promotes your professional image and says, "I think this is a great product." Also, if this product is in your inventory for sale, this is an ideal opportunity for your client to try and buy.

◆◆ ANSWER QUESTIONS AND OBJECTIONS

Be ready to answer any questions or objections your clients have about your products and service (Figure 20–5).

Questions

Clients may want to know what brand of polish has the most unusual colors, how nail art is done and what materials are used, or how long a

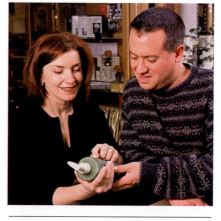

Figure 20-5 Be ready to answer a client's questions about your products.

service takes. They may want to know the advantages and disadvantages of a service or what they should do when their nail breaks. Be as knowledgeable as you can about your products and services, but don't be afraid to say you don't know the answer and will find it for your client. The knowledge you exhibit establishes trust between you and your client. This is important when you make recommendations.

Objections

Do not be afraid of client objections to a product or service. A client may object to the price, length of time a service takes, the results of a service, or the frequent maintenance of a particular service. Answer the objection honestly and pleasantly, describing the advantages of the product or service and weighing them against the disadvantages. When a client has valid objections to a product or service, suggest another option that will serve his or her needs better.

◆ ◆ ◆ CLOSE THE SALE

When a client decides to buy a product or service, you have closed the sale. There are three basic steps to closing a sale for nail products and services: suggestion selling, wrap-up, and scheduling another appointment (Figure 20–6).

Suggestion Selling

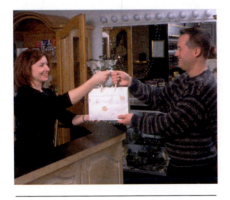

Figure 20-6 When a client decides to buy a product or service, you have closed the sale.

Suggestion selling occurs when you suggest products or services for your client to buy. You will be successful at suggestion selling when you can match your products and services with your client's needs and wants. After performing a service, you should try to sell your clients the products needed to maintain their nails until their next appointment. Giving your clients the opportunity to purchase the products you have suggested, from your salon, means that they will not have to look for them elsewhere. Plus, you will know that they are using quality, professional products that will not harm your craftsmanship.

You might suggest that a client buy an additional service before leaving. As an example, for clients with rough hands, suggest they get a paraffin waxing treatment to soften them.

Wrap-up

After the client has decided what to buy, you can close the sale by saying, "Should I wrap this up for you?" or "Will this be cash or charge?"

Scheduling Another Appointment

Before a client leaves the salon, schedule another appointment for maintenance of the service you just performed or for another service. Confirm future appointments by giving each client the salon appointment card or your business card with the date and time of the next appointment. Advance scheduling is a good way to build a steady, happy clientele.

BUSINESS TIP

Easy Home Care Sales

Grouping products together into pre-made packages is a natural way to sell retail around the holiday time, but what about creating such kits for everyday home use? It's a great way to push products, plus clients love the convenience of having all the essentials at their fingertips. Don't know where to start? Gather together the components for your best-selling service—such as the ever-popular French manicure, the natural manicure, or the pedicure—for home use. The trick is to anticipate what clients will need in order to care for their specific type of manicure or pedicure between visits, then assemble those items in different home care kits—one for every type of nail service.

TRACKING YOUR SUCCESS

Take a look at successful nail technicians and you will discover that they all have something in common. Successful nail technicians are those who have full books and a regular clientele. Knowing how to achieve those two things will insure your success.

Filling Your Books

Of course, you know that the more appointments you have during the day, the more money you will make. Your objective is to be scheduled every hour of your workday. When you start out in the salon, you will probably not have a full book, unless you are fortunate enough to be taking over someone else's established clientele. There will probably be some gaps in your day. One way to fill that time is to add on services for clients that are already at your table. When you notice an empty block of time on your appointment book, look at the appointments you do have. Think about what additional services you could suggest to those clients that would fill that time. Another way to fill time in your appointment book is to pre-book your client's maintenance appointments. You may want to consider giving them a *standing appointment time*. A standing appointment is an appointment that occurs the same day and time. Some of your standing appointments will come in every week, some every other week. Clients that have standing appointments are less likely to forget their appointments because they have scheduled a time that is convenient for them on a regular basis. If you still have open times in your day, use that time to do things that will get clients in the door and into your chair. Send out appointment reminders. Call to confirm appointments for the next day. If you work in a full-service salon, offer sample services to clients getting other services. Work on marketing ideas to attract new clients.

Client Retention

It is more expensive to attract new clients than it is to use the clients you already service to fill your books. Your **client retention rate** measures how many of your clients are existing clients. To figure your retention rate, count how many clients you saw during the week. How many of those were regular clients? Divide the amount of regular clients you had by the total amount of clients you saw and you will see what your percentage of retention is. For example, if you had 20 regular clients out of 30 total clients, you would have a retention rate of 67 percent (20 / 30 = .67). Strive to turn all of your new customers into your regular clients. If you re-book those 10 new customers, your retention rate will go up. The higher your retention rate is, the fuller your books are. The fuller your books are, the more money you make!

Setting Goals

Your success in the nail business is totally up to you. You can determine how much money you want to make and set goals to make it happen. Be careful: setting a goal of a full book and a high income in one year could be overwhelming when you are starting out with an empty book. Start by breaking your goal down into daily, weekly, and monthly goals. Your daily goal could be to get three new customers in your chair. Your weekly goal could be to increase your client retention rate by 5 percent each week. Your monthly goal could be to increase the amount of services each of your clients receives. By achieving those smaller daily, weekly, monthly goals, you can easily achieve your ultimate goal of a full book and a high income.

20

advertising	The act of calling public attention to your product or service, but letting potential clients know what makes you special.
benefits	The usefulness of a product or service in providing what your client wants; how a product or service will fulfill your client's needs.
business card	A small card containing your name; the salon's name, address, and phone number; and your expertise used to advertise your business and image.
client retention rate	A measurement of how many of your clients are existing clients versus how many are new.
feature	A specific fact about a product or service that describes it and makes it appropriate for a client.
level system	A compensation system based on paying technicians and charging clients according to the technician's experience and achievements. The more experience, the higher the pay for the technician and the higher the charges to the client.
marketing	The commercial processes involved in promoting, selling, and distributing a product or service.
promotions	Marketing strategies using events or give-aways to promote specific services or products.
salon literature	Marketing pieces like business cards and salon menus used to promote business for a salon.
salon menu	A listing of services and products a salon offers. It should include a brief description of each service, along with the time it takes to complete and costs.
word of mouth advertising	A referral system where satisfied clients recommend your services to friends, you offer business cards to friends for an incentive, or you reward clients with free services for sending in new clients.
yellow pages	Commercial pages found in local telephone books used to advertise salon services and products as well as provide immediate access to your phone number and address.

review questions

1. What are the five basic principles of selling products and services?

2. What is the difference between a product or service feature and a benefit? List examples of each.

3. What are three methods of marketing in the salon? Give examples of each.

4. Discuss how to set prices for products and services.

5. What is the least expensive, most effective form of advertising?

6. List several monthly events and give examples of promotions for each.

7. What are three ways to fill open time slots in your daily schedule?

8. Calculate the client retention rate of a nail technician that has 23 regular clients out 35 total clients for the week.

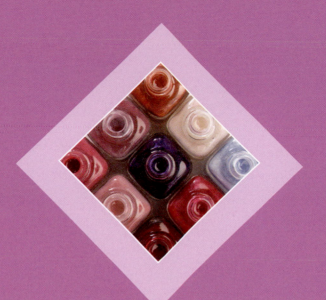

GLOSSARY

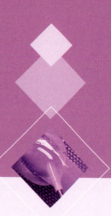

abrasive A rough surface used to shape or smooth the nail and remove the shine.

Acquired Immune Deficiency Syndrome (AIDS) A disease that can lie dormant for many years, caused by the HIV virus that attacks and usually destroys the body's immune system.

acrylic A substance that is mixed with liquid and applied to an artificial nail tip to strengthen the natural nail and the tip.

activator-cured A method of curing a no-light gel by spraying or brushing gel activator onto the nail plate.

adhesion A chemical reaction resulting in two surfaces sticking together.

adhesive An agent that causes two surfaces to stick together.

adipose Fatty connective tissue that gives smoothness and shape to the body.

advertising The act of calling public attention to your product or service, and letting potential clients know what makes you special.

air hose The hose that connects an airbrush compressor (the air source) to the airbrush itself.

albinism A congenital absence of melanin pigment in the body, including the skin, hair, and eyes.

allergic sensitizer A substance that causes serious allergic reactions due to prolonged or repeated exposure.

analysis The information-gathering section of the client consultation when the nail technician asks the client questions and analyzes the nails and skin of the client.

antiseptics Sanitizers that help prevent skin infections by reducing the number of pathogens in an opening in the skin.

aromatherapy The use of aromatic fragrances to induce relaxation; therapy through aroma.

arrector pili muscles Minute involuntary muscle fibers in the skin at the base of the hair follicles that cause goose bumps.

asepsis Blood that is free of disease-producing bacteria.

bacilli The most common, rod-shaped bacteria that produces such diseases as tetanus, influenza, typhoid, tuberculosis, and diphtheria.

backfill A maintenance procedure performed every four to six weeks on acrylic nails to remove the grown out free-edge area and replace the smile line.

bacteria (plural of bacterium). Small, one-celled microorganisms that can only be seen through a microscope.

bactericides Disinfectants that kill harmful bacteria.

Basal layer Formerly known as the stratum germinativum, it is the deepest layer of the epidermis, laying on the corneum. From this layer, all other cells of the epidermis arise.

bed epithelium The thin layer of tissue that attaches the nail to the nail bed.

benefits The usefulness of a product or service in providing what your client wants; how a product or service will fulfill your client's needs.

bevel To slope the free edge of the nail surface to smooth any rough edges.

birthmark (nevus) A malformation of the skin due to abnormal pigmentation or dilated capillaries. The condition may be inherited.

bit The replaceable part of the electric file, usually carbide or diamond, that does the actual filing of the nail. It comes in different shapes and sizes for various nail styles and techniques. Sample shapes include barrel, cone, flat-tipped cone, football, and bullet.

blood The nutritive fluid that flows through the circulatory system to supply oxygen and nutrients to cells and tissues, and to remove carbon dioxide and waste from them.

blood-vascular system The group of structures, including the heart, arteries, veins, and capillaries, that distributes blood throughout the body.

booth rental A business opportunity where salons rent space to individual nail technicians. A weekly or monthly rental fee is paid to the salon, and the nail technician is responsible for his or her own business expenses.

breathing zone The invisible sphere of air, about the size of a beach ball, that sits directly in front of your mouth.

bruised nails A condition in which a clot of blood forms under the nail plate, usually due to an injury, characterized by a dark maroon or black spot.

buffer block A lightweight, rectangular block that is abrasive and used to buff nails.

bulla A large blister containing watery fluid.

business card A small card containing your name; the salon's name, address, and phone number; and your expertise used to advertise your business and image.

calluses (Tyloma) Superficial, thickened patches of epidermis resulting from excessive friction to areas like the hands and feet.

carpal tunnel syndrome The most common cumulative trauma disorder (CTD), affecting the hands and wrists.

carrier oil A base oil used in aromatherapy that is added to an essential oil to dilute the concentration of the essential oil. The carrier oil adds slippage and makes the massage easier to perform.

catalyst Any substance having the power to speed up a chemical reaction.

cells Basic units of all living things; tiny masses of protoplasm capable of performing all the fundamental functions of life.

chamois buffer An implement that holds a disposable chamois, used to add shine to the nail and to smooth out corrugations or wavy ridges on nails.

chemical Relating to chemistry; any substance of chemical composition.

chemical change Alteration in the chemical composition of a substance in which a new substance, with properties different from the original, is formed.

chemical reaction A chemical change in a molecule, usually as a result of heat or light.

chloasma Brown spots on the skin, especially the face and hands; also called liver spots or moth patches.

cilia Hairlike projections on bacilli and spirilla that move in a whiplike motion to propel the bacteria in liquid.

circulatory (vascular) system The system that controls the steady circulation of blood through the body by means of the heart and blood vessels.

client consultation A conversation between a nail technician and a new client to collect information on the client's general health, the health of the client's nails and skin, his or her lifestyle and needs, and the nail services the nail technician can perform.

client retention rate A measurement of how many of your clients are existing clients versus how many are new.

client service record A record that lists the services rendered, products used, charges, and merchandise sold to each client.

coatings Products, including nail polish, top coats, artificial enhancements, and adhesives, that cover the nail plate with a hard film.

cocci Round, pus-producing bacteria that appear singly or in groups.

color fade (color blend) An airbrushing technique using subtle color combinations across the same nail at the same time.

color wheel A color guide that illustrates and identifies the primary, secondary, tertiary, and complimentary colors.

compensation Any payment made for services rendered.

complimentary colors Colors located directly opposite each other on the color wheel.

concentric Perfectly balanced and centered bits that spin inside the drill motor chuck to make sure the file rotates smoothly and hits the nail evenly.

contagious Having a disease that is easily transmitted from one person to another.

contaminant A substance that causes contamination.

contaminated Made impure by contact; tainted or polluted.

corrosive A substance that has the power to eat away or destroy another substance.

cover letter A letter to the salon owner or manager that accompanies a resume to briefly describe why you are interested in a position, how you qualify, and to request an interview.

cross-linker A monomer that joins together different polymer chains.

crust An accumulation of serum and pus mixed with epidermal flakes; e.g., a scab on a sore.

cumulative trauma disorder (CTD) Also known as repetitive motion disorder; an occupational disability that can cause pain and crippling if not treated.

curette A small, spoon-shaped instrument used for cleaning debris from the edges of nail margins.

cuticle (eponychium) The crescent of toughened skin, around the base of the fingernails and toenails, that partially overlaps the lunula.

cuticle nippers An instrument used for manicures and pedicures to trim dead and flaky skin from around the nail bed.

cyanoacrylate A very fast setting glue used with brush-on or dip-in acrylic powder.

cyst A semisolid or fluid lump above and below the skin surface.

decontamination Elimination of contaminants, including pathogens, from any surface. Three types of decontamination include sterilization, sanitation, and disinfection.

dermatitis An abnormal inflammation of the skin. Different types include contact dermatitis, irritant contact dermatitis, and allergic contact dermatitis.

dermatology The study of healthy skin and skin disorders.

dermis The underlying or inner layer of the skin, located below the epidermis; also refers to the derma, corium, cutis, or "true skin."

diamond nail file A metal file with diamond dust, available in different grits, that is the same shape as other nail files. It can be easily sanitized and kept in disinfectant solutions.

digestive system Organs, including the mouth, stomach, intestines, salivary, and gastric glands, that change food into nutrients, for use by body cells, and wastes.

diplococci Cocci that grows in pairs and can cause pneumonia.

discolored nails A condition in which the nails turn a variety of colors, including yellow, blue, blue-grey, green, red, and purple. Discoloration can be caused by poor blood circulation, a heart condition, or topical or oral medications.

disinfectants Substances that destroy pathogens on implements and other nonliving surfaces; not safe for use on hands or nails.

disinfection Process used to destroy contaminants on implements an other nonliving surfaces; a higher level of decontamination than sanitation.

disinfection containers Glass, metal, or plastic jars or containers used to disinfect implements.

eczema The generic term used to describe a chronic, long-lasting, inflammatory skin disorder of unknown cause.

effleurage A light, continuous-stroking massage movement applied with fingers (digital) and palms (palmar) in a slow and rhythmic manner.

eggshell nails A condition, caused by improper diet, internal disease, medication, or nervous disorders, in which the nails become thin, white, and curved over the free edge.

elasticity The tissue's ability to return to normal and regain its original shape when a stress that is placed on it is removed.

elastic tissue Tissue found in the papillary layer of the dermis, composed primarily of elastin, that gives skin its ability to return to its original shape after it has been stretched.

elements The simplest forms of basic matter; substances that cannot be broken down into simpler forms without loss of identity.

endocrine system Group of specialized glands that affect the growth, development, sexual activity, and health of the entire body.

energy Internal or inherent power or capacity for performing work.

epidermis The outermost protective covering of the skin. It contains no blood vessels, but does include many small nerve endings. It consists of four layers.

eponychium (cuticle) The crescent of toughened skin, around the base of the fingernails and toenails, that partially overlaps the lunula.

essential oils Oils used in aromatherapy that are extracted, by various forms of distillations, from various parts of plants, including seeds, bark, roots, leaves, woods, and resin.

ethics The sense of right and wrong when interacting with clients, employers, and coworkers. Honesty, fairness, courtesy, and respect for the feelings and rights of others are the essential values in professional ethics.

evaporate To change from liquid to vapor form.

excoriation A sore or abrasion caused by scratching or scraping off the superficial layer of the skin.

excretory system Group of organs, including the kidneys, liver, skin, intestines, and lungs that purify the body by the elimination of waste.

expenses The costs of supplies, equipment, rent, etc. to run a business.

fabric wraps Nail wraps made of silk, linen, or fiberglass.

feature A specific fact about a product or service that describes it and makes it appropriate for a client.

fiberglass A very thin synthetic mesh with a loose weave used for nail wraps because it is especially strong and durable.

fills The addition of acrylic to the new growth area of the nails. This procedure should take place every two to three weeks.

fissure A crack in the skin that penetrates the dermis; e.g., chapped hands or lips.

flagella Hairlike projections on bacilli and spirilla that move in a whiplike motion to propel the bacteria in liquid.

floating the bead A technique used to seal nail art where a bead of sealer is dropped onto the nail surface and the brush floats across the surface and completely covers it with sealer.

fluid nozzle (tip) A small cone-shaped nozzle at the end of an airbrush that holds the needle that releases the paint.

flutes Long, slender cuts or grooves found in carbide file bits.

foiling One of the easiest and most cost effective nail art techniques, it is applied after polish with a foil adhesive to create colors and patterns not available with polish.

foot files (paddles) Large sanding files used to remove dry, flaky skin and smooth callus from the foot.

formaldehyde A suspected human cancer-causing agent found in formalin.

freehand painting Also referred to as flat nail art; a very expensive form of nail art using brushes and paint to create designs.

French manicure An airbrushing technique that creates a natural looking nail with a smooth white tip at the free edge.

friction blisters Localized reactions of the skin to friction from an external source. The middle layer of skin fills with a straw-colored fluid, creating the blisters.

friction movement Firm pressure applied to the bottom of the foot using thumb compression to work from side to side and toward the heel.

full-service salon A salon that provides a variety of health and beauty services from nail care to skin care to hair care.

fungi The general term used to describe plantlike parasites that can spread easily from nail to nail.

fungicides Disinfectants that destroy fungus.

furrows (corrugations) Long ridges that run either lengthwise or across the nail that create ridges or grooves in the nail. Furrows are caused by psoriasis, poor circulation, and frostbite.

gas A state of matter different from a liquid or solid because of its low molecular density; should not be confused with vapor, as it does not evaporate in the air as vapor.

gems Tiny jewels that add sparkle, dimension, and texture to any nail art.

germs Disease-causing bacteria.

gravity-fed An airbrush system designed to pull the paint into the airbrush using gravity.

grit The amount of abrasive material used on files and bits. The smaller the number, the larger amount of grits used; for example, if the grit is 240, it takes 240 pieces of grit to cover a 1" square; therefore, the grit is finer than a grit of 100.

halogen bulb A bulb used to harden some nail gels.

hand manipulation The process of skillfully treating, working, or operating with the hands.

hangnails (agnails) A common condition, caused by dry cuticles or cuticles that have been cut too close to the nail, in which the cuticle around the nail splits.

herpes simplex A viral infection commonly seen as a fever blister or cold sore.

histamines Chemicals in the blood that enlarge the vessels around an injury so that blood can get to a site quickly and help remove any irritating substance.

hospital-level disinfectant Disinfectant that must kill harmful bacteria and pathogenic viruses, destroy fungus, and pass special EPA registration tests.

hypodermis (fatty layer) Also known as the subcutis; the deepest layer of the skin, characterized by closely-packed fat cells.

hyponychium The toughened skin that lies underneath the distal edge of the nail, where it seals the nail's free edge to the normal skin.

immunity The ability of the body to resist disease and destroy microorganisms when they have entered the body. Immunity can be natural, naturally acquired, or artificially acquired.

immunocompromised Having an impaired or injured immune system; unable to fight off disease.

implements Tools that must be sanitized or disposed of after use with each client. Implements are usually small enough to be sanitized in a disinfection container.

income The money taken in for providing a service.

infection Contamination that occurs when body tissue is invaded by disease-causing microorganisms such as bacteria, viruses, and fungi.

inflammation A condition responding to body injury, irritation, or infection, characterized by redness, heat, pain, and swelling.

initiator A special ingredient in a monomer molecule that triggers a boost of energy used to create a monomer chain (polymer).

integumentary system Group of organs that make up the skin and its various accessory organs, such as oil and sweat glands, hair, and nails.

internal mix Airbrush paint that is mixed with the air inside the actual airbrush.

interview A formal conversation between you and a potential employer where information is exchanged to decide whether you are right for a position in a salon and whether the salon is right for you.

keratin The principal fiber protein found in hair and nails.

keratinization The microscopically visible changes, as well as the biochemical changes, that occur within the cells of the skin as they progress upward to the outer layer of the epidermis.

lacquer A solution of nitrocellulose in a volatile solvent used on nails and hair to add shine.

leafing (gold leafing) Also known as nuggets or nugget sheets; a thin, fragile foil-like material, available in gold, silver, and a variety of other colors used to create a quick and easy form of nail art.

lentigines (freckles) Small brown or yellow spots found on the skin.

leucoderma A general term for abnormal lack of pigmentation.

leukonychia A condition, caused by air bubbles, a bruise, or other injury to the nail, in which white spots appear on the nail.

level system A compensation system based on paying technicians and charging clients according to the technician's experience and achievements. The more experience, the higher the pay for the technician and the higher the charges to the client.

light-cured gel A type of gel used with artificial nails that hardens when exposed to an ultraviolet or halogen light source.

linen A closely woven, heavy material used for nail wraps because it stays opaque, even after the adhesive has been applied.

liquid nail wrap A thick polish made of tiny fibers designed to strengthen and preserve the natural nail as it grows.

local exhaust A device used to capture salon vapors and dust and expel them from a technician's breathing zone through an exhaust vent.

lunula The white, half-moon-shaped area of the matrix bed, found at the root of the nail.

lymph A slightly yellow, watery fluid that is made form the plasma of blood.

lymph-vascular (lymphatic) system A bodily system, including the lymph vessels, lacteals, and lymph nodes, that allows lymph to flow through and circulate back into the bloodstream.

macule Small, discolored spot or patch on the surface of the skin. Some macules are safe and some are not.

marketing The commercial processes involved in promoting, selling, and distributing a product or service.

mask knife A one-sided knife used to cut designs out of mask paper or plastic to create nail art stencils.

mask paper Paper that is used to create nail art design stencils.

massage A method of manipulation of the body by rubbing, pinching, kneading, and tapping for therapeutic purposes.

massage oils Blends of therapeutic oils used to lubricate, moisturize, and invigorate the skin during a massage or pedicure.

Material Safety Data Sheet (MSDS) A document supplied by product manufacturers, and available to anyone who uses the product, that contains basic safety and handling information about a product.

matrix bed The part of the nail extending from under the proximal nail groove, where it can be seen as a white, moon-shaped area under the nail plate.

matter A substance that occupies space; has physical and chemical properties; and exists in either solid, liquid, or gas form.

melanin The tiny grain of pigment in the epidermis that determines natural skin color and protects the sensitive cells against strong light rays.

melanoma Cancer of the pigment-producing cells of the skin. If left untreated, it will spread throughout the body and cause death.

melanonychia A condition, present in all dark-skinned races and extremely rare in caucasians, in which a black band of pigment cells grows from the proximal matrix bed toward the free edge of the nail.

mentor An experienced colleague that becomes a trusted teacher or advisor and helps you perfect your career.

metabolism The complex chemical process that takes place in living organisms whereby the cells are nourished and supplied with the energy needed to carry on their activities.

microorganisms Any living things that are too small to be seen by the eye.

mild abrasives Substances such as tin oxide, talc, silica, and kaolin used for smoothing or sanding the nails and skin.

mitosis Cell reproduction in which cells grow and split in half to form two identical cells. These two cells grow and split again, forming four cells. This process continues to repeat itself, creating millions of cells.

mold (fungus) A growth that starts with a yellowish-green color and darkens to black. It is usually caused by darkness and

moisture that has seeped under the edge of an artificial nail, but can also affect a natural nail.

molecule The smallest possible unit of any substance that retains its original characteristics.

monomers Individual molecules that join together to make a polymer.

motor nerves Nerves that carry impulses from nerve centers to muscles.

muscular system The parts of the body that cover, shape, and support the skeletal system.

myology The study of the structure, functions, and diseases of the muscles.

nail adhesive A glue or bonding agent used to secure a nail tip to the natural nail.

nail art An add-on service offered at many salons that applies creative and unique custom designs to the finished nail.

nail bed The portion of skin on which the body of the nail rests.

nail disorder Any condition of the nail caused by injury to the nail or disease or imbalance in the body.

nail folds Folds of normal skin that surround the nail plate, forming grooves and a wall to help determine the shape of the nail plate.

nail plate Formed by the matrix cells, it is the visible and functional body of the nail module.

nail rasp A metal file with an angled edge that can cut or file in only one direction.

nail tip An artificial nail made of plastic, nylon, or acetate that is adhered to the natural nail to add length.

nail wraps Nail-size pieces of cloth or paper that are bonded to the top of the nail plate with nail adhesive; often used to repair or strengthen natural nails or nail tips.

nails-only salon A salon that employs several nail technicians specifically for nail services.

natural barrier The protective barrier furnished by the eponychium tissue, protecting against bacteria and other invaders.

needle The piece that fits into the fluid nozzle of an airbrush that controls the amount of paint released when the trigger is depressed.

nerves Long, white cords made up of masses of neurons and held together by connective tissue that carry messages to various parts of the body from the central nervous system.

nervous system The bodily system that controls and coordinates the functions of all other systems of the body.

neurology The branch of medicine that deals with the nervous system and its disorders.

neuron (nerve cell) The basic structural unit of the nervous system, consisting of a cell body, dendrites, an axon, and an axon terminal. The neuron receives and sends messages to other neurons, glands, and muscles.

no-light gel A type of gel used with artificial nails that hardens when a gel activator is sprayed or brushed on, or when they are soaked in water.

nonpathogenic Non-disease-causing; not harmful.

objective symptoms Symptoms that are visible to the nail technician, such a pimples, pustules, or inflammation.

odorless acrylics Acrylics that are much different from traditional acrylics in that they do not evaporate, have no smell, and are much denser, giving the nail technician more time to sculpt.

onychatrophia (atrophy) A condition, caused by injury to the nail matrix or by internal disease, in which the nail wastes away, loses its shine, shrinks, and falls off.

onychauxis (hypertrophy) A condition, caused by internal imbalance, local infection, injury, or heredity, is the abnormal overgrowth of nails and thickening of the nail plate.

onychia An inflammation of the entire nail unit or a portion of the nail, characterized by red and swollen tissue, and possibly pus. The condition is usually caused by the entry of bacteria, fungi, or foreign materials through an opening in the skin.

onychocryptosis (ingrown nails) A common disorder in which the nail grows into the sides of the tissue around the nail. It can be a result of the matrix bed being folded or involuted deep into the soft tissues, penetrating the tissue, and creating a portal of entry for bacteria.

onychodermal band (solehorn) A combination build up of bed epithelium and hyponychial tissue found at the distal end of the nail. The grayish band of tissue helps attach the nail plate to the underlying tissues.

onychogryphosis (ram's horn nail) This disorder is characterized by a brownish, thick, hard-to-cut nail plate that is curved into the shape of a ram's horn because one side of the nail grew faster than the other. This condition is the result of an injury to the matrix bed, long-term neglect of the nails, or can be inherited.

onycholysis A condition in which the nail loosens from the nail bed, usually beginning at the free edge and continuing to the lunula, but does not come off. It can be caused by an internal disorder, trauma, infection, certain drug treatments, or an allergic reaction to certain nail products.

onychomadesis A condition, characterized by a shedding of the nail plate from the matrix bed, that occurs when the matrix bed stops producing nail plate for one to two weeks. It is caused by a localized infection, minor injury to the matrix bed, severe systemic illness, and, in some cases, chemotherapy or x-ray treatments for cancer.

onychomycosis (tinea unguium) An infectious disease of the nails caused by a fungus.

onychophagy Medical term for nails that have been bitten enough to become deformed.

onychophosis Growth of horny epithelium in the nail bed.

onychophyma Swelling of the nail.

onychoptosis A condition in which part or all of the nail sheds periodically and falls off the finger. It can be caused by syphilis, high fever, system upsets, a reaction to prescription drugs, or trauma.

onychorrhexis A condition, caused by injury to the fingers; excessive use of cuticle solvents and nail polish removers; or careless, rough filing, in which split or brittle nails have a series of lengthwise ridges.

onychosis (onychopathy) The technical term applied to nail disease.

onyx The technical term for nail of the fingers or toes.

organs Structures in the body, composed of specialized tissues, that perform specific functions.

osteology The scientific study of bones, their structure, and function.

oval nail A nail shape that is square with slightly rounded corners. This shape is attractive for most women's hands. The length of the nail can vary.

overexposure Dangerously prolonged, repeated, or long-term contact with certain chemicals.

paper wraps Temporary nail wraps made of very thin paper that dissolves in acetone and non-acetone remover.

papillae Small cone-shaped projections that extend upward into the epidermis from the dermis. Some contain looped capillaries, others contain small blood vessels, and yet others contain the melanin pigment.

papillary layer The outer layer of the dermis, directly beneath the epidermis.

papule Small pimple that does not contain fluid, but can develop pus.

parasite A tiny, multi-celled animal or plant organism that lives off living matter without providing any benefit to its host.

paronychia An infection of the tissue around the nail. Characteristics include redness, swelling, and tenderness of that tissue. In the later stages of this condition, the nail bed will thicken and discolor, and the nail plate will become crumbly and malformed.

pathogenic Disease-causing; disease-producing; harmful.

pathogens Any disease-causing microorganisms.

pedicure Standard service performed by nail technicians that includes care and massage of feet and trimming, shaping, and polishing toenails.

petrissage kneading movement A kneading movement in massage performed by lifting, squeezing, and pressing the tissue.

phenolics Highly effective, concentrated liquid disinfectants used in salons; can be destructive to certain materials and is very expensive.

photo initiators A feature of light-cured acrylics that triggers the chemicals to harden when exposed to a special U.V. lamp.

physically changed A substance that is changed in form or appearance only, without chemically altering it to create a new substance.

pigmented nevus (mole) Raised tan or brownish "tumor" on the skin, varying in size, shape, and surface. Some may have hair growing from them.

pledgets Small, fiber-free squares often used and by nail technicians to remove polish because the cotton fibers from the squares do not adhere to the nails, which can interfere with the polish application.

plicatured nail A deformity, caused by an injury to the matrix bed or can be inherited, in which the surface of the nail is flat, while the edge(s) of the plate are folded at a 90° or more angle. This condition is most often seen as the cause of ingrown nails.

pointed nail A nail shape suited to thin hands with narrow nail beds. The shape is tapered and somewhat longer; however, these nails are often weak and may break easily.

polymerizations Chemical reactions that create polymers; also called curing or hardening.

polymers Substances formed by combining many small molecules (monomers), usually in long, chain-like structures.

position The way a brush is held to create nail art; the brush can be positioned straight up-and-down or layed down with the bristles pulled across the paint surface.

pressure The amount of force an artist applies to a brush while in the stroke motion when applying nail art.

primary colors Pure pigment colors that cannot be obtained from mixing any other colors together.

primers Substances that improve adhesion.

promotions Marketing strategies using events or give-aways to promote specific services or products.

psoriasis A generalized disease, characterized by red patches, and scales, that produces mild to severe effects on the skin.

pterygium Forward growth of the cuticle, abnormally adhering the skin to the nail plate.

pull The flow of a brush across a painted nail surface giving it a fluid movement and avoiding a rough, spattered look.

pulmonary circulation Blood circulation from the heart to the lungs, to be purified, and back to the heart.

pumice powder A hardened volcanic substance, white or gray in color, used for smoothing and polishing.

pustule Lump on the skin with an inflamed base and a head containing pus.

pyogenic granuloma A severe inflammation of the nail in which a lump of red vascular tissue grows up from the nail bed to the nail plate. It is commonly caused by injury or infection.

quaternary ammonium compounds (quats) Safe and fast-acting salon disinfectants commonly used to clean implements, tables, and counter tops.

rebalancing Redefining the contour of the nail during a fill procedure to keep the nail looking natural.

recommendations The second section of the client consultation process when the nail technician discusses the benefits and results of recommended services.

reflex An automatic, involuntary response to a stimulus that involves the transmission of an impulse from a sensory receptor along an afferent nerve to the spinal cord, and a responsive impulse along an efferent neuron to a muscle, causing a reaction.

repair patch A piece of fabric cut to completely cover a crack or break in the nail during a four-week fabric wrap maintenance procedure.

respiratory system The system situated within the chest cavity, consisting of the nose, pharynx, larynx, trachea, bronchi, and lungs, that enables breathing.

resume A written summary of your work, academic experience, and qualifications for a job.

reticular layer The deeper layer of the dermis, containing cells, vessels, glands, nerve endings, and follicles, that supplies the skin with oxygen and nutrients.

revolutions per minute (RPMs) The number of times a bit rotates in one minute. In nail technology, how fast an electric drill goes.

rickettsia Organisms carried by fleas, ticks, and lice that are much smaller than bacteria, but larger than viruses and cause typhus and Rocky Mountain spotted fever.

rings of fire Ridges in the nail caused by using a barrel bit at the wrong angle near the cuticle, where the barrel's flat edge actually digs into the natural nail bed.

round nail A nail shape that is slightly tapered and extends just a bit past the tip of the finger. This natural looking shape is common for male clients.

salon conduct The proper way to behave when you are working with your clients, employer, and coworkers.

salon literature Marketing pieces like business cards and salon menus used to promote business for a salon.

salon menu A listing of services and products a salon offers. It should include a brief description of each service, along with the time it takes to complete and costs.

salon spa (day spa) A salon that offers many relaxing services such as body massage, hydrotherapy, and facials. These salons often feature pedicure and manicure services and promote natural nail care.

sanitization (sanitizing) The lowest level of decontamination possible used to reduce the number of contaminations on a surface or implement.

saturated Soaked or completely penetrated; absorbed all that a substance can possibly hold.

scales Dead skin produced during the shedding of the epidermis; e.g., severe dandruff.

scar A light-colored, slightly raised mark on the skin formed after an injury or lesion of the skin has healed.

scrubs Slightly abrasive products containing softening agents or oils to penetrate dry, flaky skin and callus that need to be removed during a pedicure.

sebaceous glands (oil glands) Oil glands of the skin, connected to the hair follicles, that secrete sebum.

secondary colors Colors directly resulting from mixing equal parts of two primary colors together; they are opposite primary colors on the color wheel.

secretory nerves Nerves of the sweat and oil glands that regulate perspiration and sebum excretion.

sensitization A greatly increased or exaggerated sensitivity to certain chemicals or products.

sensory nerves Nerves that carry impulses from sense organs to the brain to experience sensations like touch, cold, heat, pain, and pressure.

sepsis The presence in the blood or other tissues of pathogenic microorganisms or their toxins.

silk A thin, natural material with a tight weave, that is sometimes used for nail wraps; becomes transparent when adhesive is applied.

simple polymer chains The result of long chains of monomers that are attached from head to tail.

skeletal system The physical foundation or framework for the body.

soaks Products containing gentle soaps, moisturizers, and deep penetrating, surface-active ingredients, used in the pedicure bath to soften the skin of the foot.

solute The dissolved substance in a solution.

solvent A substance, usually liquid, that dissolves another substance without any change in chemical composition.

specialized ligaments Ligaments located at the proximal portion of the matrix bed and around the edges of the nail bed that anchor the matrix and the nail bed to the underlying bone.

spirilla Spiral or corkscrew-shaped bacteria that can cause such diseases as syphilis.

square nail A nail shape that is completely straight across with no rounding at the edges. The length of the nail can vary.

squoval nail A nail shape that extends slightly past the tip of the finger with the free edge rounded off.

stain An abnormal discoloration that remains after moles, freckles, or liver spots disappear, or after certain diseases.

staphylococci Cocci that grows in clusters and are found in local infections such as abscesses, pustules, and boils.

stencil Precut designs made of plastic, paper, or fabric, used to create nail art.

sterilization A difficult, multi-step process used to destroy all living organisms on an object or surface.

stratum corneum (horny layer) The outer layer of the epidermis composed of dead epithelial cells that continually shed and replace themselves.

stratum granulosum The granular layer of the epidermis where the process of keratinization is most active.

stratum lucidum The clear, transparent layer of the epidermis under the stratum corneum. It is most prominent on the palms of the hands and the soles of the feet.

streptococci Cocci that grows in chains and can cause such diseases and infections as strep throat, blood poisoning, and rheumatic fever.

stress strip A strip of fabric, 1/8″ long, applied during a four-week fabric wrap maintenance, to repair or strengthen a weak point in a nail.

striping tape A tacky-backed tape available in an assortment of colors that is applied over nail polish or other nail art to create bolder designs.

styptic powder An agent used to contract the skin to stop minor bleeding that may occur during a manicure.

subcutaneous tissue Fatty tissue known as adipose that gives smoothness and shape to the body. It contains stored fat to be burned for energy and acts as a protective cushion for the outer skin.

subjective symptoms Symptoms that can be felt by the client, such as itching, burning, or pain.

sudoriferous glands (sweat glands) Small, convoluted tubules that secrete sweat; found in the subcutaneous tissue and ending at the opening of the pores.

systemic (general) circulation Blood circulation from the heart throughout the body and then back to the heart.

systems Groups of bodily organs acting together to perform one or more functions, namely for the welfare of the entire body.

tactile corpuscles Small epidermal structures with nerve endings that are sensitive to touch and pressure.

tan Darkening of the skin caused by exposure to the ultraviolet rays of the sun.

tanning salon A salon that offers primarily tanning services, but often employs a nail technician to provide an added service to its clients.

tapotement A massage movement using a short, quick hacking, slapping, or tapping technique.

tertiary colors Colors directly resulting from mixing equal parts of one primary color and one of its nearest color.

tile-shaped nails A condition, caused by abnormal curvature of the matrix bed, in which there is an increased transverse curvature throughout the nail plate.

tip cutter An implement similar to a nail clipper used exclusively to trim artificial tips.

tip well cutting An alternative method of achieving the perfect smile lines using white tips or traditional tips with no tip blending.

tissues Collections of similar cells within the body, characterized by appearance, that perform particular functions.

torque Also known as horsepower; the amount of resistance (measured in pounds-per-square-inch) in a file as the bit turns.

toenail nippers Professional instruments with curved or straight jaws used for cutting toenails.

toxins Poisonous substances produced by some microorganisms.

trumpet (pincer) nail A condition, seen more often on toes than on fingers, caused by a bone spur on the top of the underlying bone or has been inherited. As the nail grows toward the end of the toe or finger, the edges of the nail plate curl inward, eventually forming the shape of a trumpet or cone.

tubercle A solid lump larger than a papule, varying in size from a pea to a hickory nut.

tumor An abnormal cell mass that varies in size, shape, and color. Nodules are small tumors.

ulcer An open lesion on the skin or mucous membrane of the body. Ulcers are accompanied by pus and loss of skin depth.

ultraviolet bulb A bulb used to harden some nail gels that contains special rays of the spectrum beyond the violet rays.

ultraviolet (U.V.) light Invisible rays of the color spectrum that are beyond the violet rays; shortest and least penetrating of the light rays.

vapor The gaseous state that is formed when liquid is heated and evaporates into the air.

vesicle A blister containing clear fluid. Poison ivy is an example of a condition that produces vesicles.

viricides Disinfectants that kill pathogenic viruses.

virus Pathogenic (disease-causing) agents, much smaller than bacteria, that enter a healthy cell, grow to maturity, and reproduce, often destroying the cell.

vitiligo An acquired form of leucoderma that affects the skin or hair. People with vitiligo must be protected from the sun.

warts (papilloma, verruca, and plantar wart) Non-cancerous viral infections of the skin caused by a specific human papillomavirus (HPV) that multiply within the nuclei of the cells that produce skin.

water-cured A method of curing a no-light gel by immersing nails in lukewarm water for several minutes.

well Also known as the small color cup or reservoir; a hole in the top of the airbrush where drips of paint are placed and stored.

wet sanitizers Covered receptacles large enough to hold a disinfectant solution in which objects to be sanitized can be completely immersed.

wheals (hives) Swollen, itchy bumps on the skin that last for several hours; often caused by insect bites or by allergic reactions.

word of mouth advertising A referral system where satisfied clients recommend your services to friends, you offer business cards to friends for an incentive, or you reward clients with free services for sending in new clients.

yeasts Substances containing minute cells of fungi used to promote fermentation; a high source of vitamin B.

yellow pages Commercial pages found in local telephone books

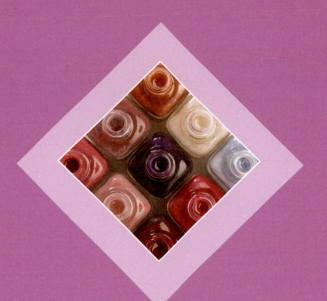

ANSWERS TO REVIEW QUESTIONS

CHAPTER 1

1. What is salon conduct?

   Salon conduct is the way you act when working with clients, your employer, and coworkers in the salon.

2. Give ten examples of professional salon conduct toward clients.

   Examples of professional salon conduct toward clients are: 1) being on time; 2) being prepared; 3) planning your day; 4) arranging appointments carefully; 5) keeping clients informed of schedule changes; 6) being courteous; 7) performing all tasks willingly and efficiently; 8) communicating with clients; 9) never complaining or arguing with a client; 10) using good judgment; 11) never chewing gum, smoking, or eating where you can be seen by clients. (Only 10 are needed.)

3. Explain why a salon might lose clients if nail technicians do not exhibit professional salon conduct.

   A salon might lose clients if nail technicians do not exhibit professional salon conduct because clients want to be treated with courtesy. If you are late, or you seem disorganized or uncaring, clients might feel uncomfortable. Clients should not feel that their appointments inconvenience you. Chewing gum, smoking, or eating in front of clients can annoy them. Smoking can also be potentially dangerous around chemicals and is against the law in many states.

4. Give ten examples of professional salon conduct toward employers and coworkers.

   Examples of professional salon conduct toward employers and coworkers are: 1) being willing to learn; 2) communicating; 3) giving credit to others; 4) respecting the opinions of coworkers; 5) taking the initiative; 6) using good judgment; 7) leaving personal problems at home; 8) never borrowing money from employers or coworkers; 9) promoting the salon; 10) developing your ability to sell.

5. Define professional ethics.

   Professional ethics is the sense of right and wrong when you interact with your clients, employer, and coworkers. The essential values in professional ethics are honesty, fairness, courtesy, and respect for the feelings and rights of others.

6. Give seven examples of professional ethics toward clients.

   Examples of professional ethics toward clients are: 1) suggesting services that meet clients' needs; 2) keeping your word and fulfilling all obligations; 3) treating all clients equally; 4) following state regulations for sanitation and safety; 5) being loyal; 6) not criticizing others; 7) not abandoning clients.

7. Give five examples of professional ethics toward employers and coworkers.

   Five examples of professional ethics toward employers and coworkers are: 1) being honest; 2) fulfilling obligations; 3) respecting the talents of your employer and coworkers; 4) not inviting criticism of coworkers; 5) never gossiping or starting rumors among coworkers.

8. Describe the type of appearance you should have as a professional nail technician.

   As a nail technician one should be clean and neat, have fresh breath and healthy teeth, wear clean clothes that are appropriate for the salon, and pay attention to hair, skin, and nails.

9. Explain why a salon might lose clients if it employs nail technicians who have an unprofessional appearance.

   A salon might lose clients if it employs nail technicians who have an unprofessional appearance because, as a member of the beauty industry, a nail technician should be pleasant to be around. If you are not clean and pleasant smelling, clients may object to having you touch them while performing nail services.

CHAPTER 2

1. What are bacteria? What do bacteria look like?

   Bacteria are microscopic organisms that live almost everywhere. They can be round, grow in chains, or look like the spiral of a corkscrew.

2. Are all bacteria harmful? Give examples to explain your answer.

   No, at least 70 percent of all bacteria are nonpathogenic or nondisease-producing. Many bacteria aid in the digestion of food and make oxygen.

3. What are the three main groups of pathogenic bacteria? Describe them.

   The three main groups of pathogenic bacteria are cocci, bacilli, and spirilla. Cocci grow in clusters, chains, or pairs; bacilli are the most common and are rod-shaped; spirilla are spiral or corkscrew-shaped.

4. Why can bacteria reproduce so quickly?

   They grow to maturity and then divide into two bacterium. The newly formed cells begin to grow and divide almost immediately.

5. Give examples of common infections caused by viruses.

   Hepatitis, chicken pox, influenza, colds, measles, and mumps are the most common examples.

6. Is it likely that salon services can cause AIDS?

   The chance of transmitting HIV in the salon is near zero! It is virtually impossible.

7. Describe the appearance of bacterial infection on the nail plate?

   Bacterial infections often appear as greenish yellow spots on the nail plate beneath the enhancement.

8. Do molds and mildew grow on or under the nail plate?

   No, molds and mildew do not infect the fingernail.

9. What is immunity? Name three types of immunity.

   Immunity is the ability of the body to resist disease and destroy microorganisms when they have entered the body. Immunity can be natural, naturally acquired, or artificially acquired.

10. Name five common sources of infection in the salon.

    Five common sources of infection in the salon include: 1) contaminated manicuring tools and equipment; 2) clients' nails, hands, and feet; 3) your clients', coworkers', and your own mouth, nose, and eyes; 4) open wounds or sores on you or your client; 5) objects throughout the entire salon, such as trash cans and doorknobs.

CHAPTER 3

1. What is the difference between disinfection and sanitation?

   Sanitation is the lowest form of decontamination. It is designed to significantly lower the number of pathogens on a surface. Disinfection is a much higher level of decontamination that kills all pathogens, except bacterial spores.

2. Disinfection is almost identical to _____ except disinfection does not kill bacterial spores.

   Sterilization.

3. What is an antiseptic?

   An antiseptic reduces the number of pathogens in a cut and the immune system kills what is left.

4. What is the best type of disinfectant to use in a salon?

   EPA registered, hospital-level disinfectants are perfect for salons.

5. What are the two most commonly used types of disinfectants?

   Quats and phenolics

6. Once implements are properly _____, they must be stored where they will remain free from _____.

   Disinfected, contamination

7. Formaldehyde is a strong _____ _____.
   Allergic sensitizer.

8. What must you use to remove implements from disinfectant containers?

   Rubber gloves or tongs.

9. Describe Universal Sanitation in your own words.

   Universal Sanitation means you do everything that is required to sanitize and disinfect the salon and your implements. No short cuts!

CHAPTER 4

1. List five early warning signs of chemical overexposure.

   Rash and other skin irritation, lightheadedness, insomnia, runny nose, sore throat, watery eyes, tingling toes, fatigue, irritability, sluggishness, breathing problems.

2. What does MSDS stand for?
   Material Safety Data Sheet

3. Name four simple and inexpensive things you can do to reduce vapors in the salon.

   To reduce vapors in the salon: 1) keep all products tightly sealed when not in use; 2) use a covered dappen dish or pump to limit the vapors in the air. 3) avoid using pressurized sprays; they create finer mists and are difficult to control; 4) empty your waste container often; it is one of the best sources of vapors.

4. Define breathing zone.

   Your breathing zone is an invisible sphere about the size of a beach ball that sits directly in front of your mouth.

5. Describe how a local exhaust system works. Why is it best?

   Local exhaust uses a moveable exhaust vent, hose, or tube to capture vapors, dusts, and mists. Specially designed blowers pull contaminants from the breathing zone down the exhaust tube and expel them from the building. They are best because they work. They don't try to do the impossible...clean the air and return it to the salon. That isn't possible in the salon environment.

6. What is the best and least expensive way to prevent excessive inhalation of dusts?

   Use a dust mask. It filters air as the air goes into your mouth.

7. Why should products be stored away from heat and pilot lights?

   Excessive heat will ruin them and some are more flammable than gasoline.

ANSWERS

8. Why should smoking not be allowed in the salon?

Many salon products are more flammable than gasoline.

9. What is CTD? Explain how this happens.

CTD is cumulative trauma disorder. It is caused by repetitive motions which can damage sensitive nerves, especially in the hands.

10. List seven symptoms of CTD.

Pain, numbness, aching, stiffness, tingling, weakness, and swelling.

CHAPTER 5

1. Nail plates are mostly protein made from chemicals called _____ _____.

Amino acids

2. Define molecules.

A molecule is a chemical in its simplest form.

3. What are catalysts and why are they important to nail chemistry?

Catalysts are chemicals that speed up chemical reactions. They make enhancements and overlays harden much more quickly.

4. A _____ is anything that dissolves another substance called a _____.

Solvent, solute

5. True or False? Primers can eat the nail plate. Explain your answer.

False, no enhancement product will dissolve or eat the nail plate. Heavy abrasives and overfiling strip the nail plate away and make it thin.

6. Define monomers.

The individual molecules that join to make the polymer are called monomers.

7. What are the two main differences between irritations and allergic reactions?

Allergic reactions become worse with each exposure, irritations do not. Also, irritations are temporary and allergic reactions can last a lifetime.

8. What six things can you avoid or do to ensure that clients never suffer from a product allergy?

To avoid product allergies: 1) *never* smooth the enhancement surface with more liquid monomer; 2) *never* use monomer to "clean up" the edges, under the nail or sidewalls; 3) *never* touch any monomer liquids, gels, or adhesives to the skin; 4) *never* touch the hairs of the brush with your fingers; 5) *never* mix your own special product blends; 6) *always* follow instructions —exactly!

9. Only _____ and _____ skin contact can cause a client to become allergic to products.

Prolonged, repeated

10. In your own words explain what Paracelsus discovered about toxic substances. How can you use this knowledge to work safely?

Paracelsus said that everything can be poisonous if we overexpose ourselves. So, learning to prevent overexposure would make a nail technician's job safe.

CHAPTER 6

1. How can an understanding of anatomy and physiology help you become a better nail technician?

An understanding of anatomy and physiology can help you become a better nail technician by giving you a scientific background for many of the nail service you provide. It will help you decide which services are better for clients' nail or skin conditions and how to adjust and control the service for best results.

2. What is the purpose of cells within the human body?

Cells are the basic functional units of all living things. Cells carry on all life processes and reproduce new cells, enabling the body to replace worn or injured tissues.

3. What is cell metabolism?

Cell metabolism is a complex chemical process in which cells are nourished and supplied with the elements necessary to carry on their many activities.

4. Name the five types of body tissue and explain the function of each.

Five types of body tissues are: 1) connective tissue, which supports, protects, and binds the body tissues together; 2) muscular tissue, which contracts and moves various parts of the body; 3) nerve tissue, which carries messages to and from the brain and coordinates all body functions; 4) epithelial tissue, which is a protective covering on body surfaces; 5) liquid tissue, which carries food, wastes, and hormones by means of blood and lymph.

5. What are the five most important organs of the body? Explain the function of each.

The five most important organs of the body are: 1) the brain, which controls the body; 2) the lungs, which supply oxygen to the blood; 3) the liver, which removes toxic products of digestion; 4) the kidneys, which excrete water and other waste products; 5) the stomach and intestines, which digest food; 6) the heart, which circulates the blood. (Only five are needed.)

6. List the ten systems that make up the human body. What is the function of each system?

   Ten systems making up the human body are: 1) the integumentary system, which functions as a protective covering and contains sensory receptors; 2) the skeletal system, which serves as a means of support, movement, and protection; 3) the muscular system, which produces all movement of the body; 4) the nervous system, which controls and coordinates the functions of all other body systems; 5) the circulatory system, which supplies blood throughout the body; 6) the endocrine system, which secretes hormones into the bloodstream; 7) the excretory system, which eliminates waste from the body; 8) the respiratory system, which supplies oxygen to the body; 9) the digestive system, which changes food into substances that can be used by the body cells; 10) the reproductive system, which allows humans to reproduce.

7. What are four ways in which muscles are stimulated?

   Muscles are stimulated by: 1) massage; 2) electric current; 3) light rays; 4) heat rays; 5) moist heat; 6) nerve impulses; 7) chemicals. (Only 4 are needed.)

8. What are four areas of muscles that are affected by the nail technician during the massage?

   Four types of muscles that are affected by massage are: 1) shoulder and upper arm; 2) forearm; 3) hand; 4) lower leg and foot.

9. Name the three divisions of the nervous system and the function of each division.

   Three divisions of the nervous system and their functions are: 1) the central nervous system, which controls the voluntary actions of the five senses; 2) the peripheral nervous system, which carries messages to and from the central nervous system; 3) the autonomic nervous system, which regulates the activities of smooth muscles, glands, blood vessels, and the heart.

10. What are the chief functions of the blood?

    The chief functions of the blood are: to carry water, oxygen, food, and secretions to cells; to carry away carbon dioxide and waste products; to help equalize body temperature; to aid in protecting the body from harmful bacteria and infection; and to clot, preventing the loss of blood.

CHAPTER 7

1. What are the six basic parts that make up the nail unit?

   The nail unit is made of: 1) matrix bed; 2) nail plate; 3) cuticular system; 4) nail bed; 5) specialized ligaments; and 6) nail folds.

2. What is the only part of the nail unit that produces the nail plate?

   The matrix bed.

3. Define nail disorder.

   A nail disorder is a condition caused by injury to the nail, disease, or an imbalance in the body.

4. What is the golden rule for dealing with nail disorders?

   The golden rule states that if the nail or skin to be worked on is infected, inflamed, broken, or swollen, a nail technician should refer the client to a doctor.

5. What does the term "pterygium" mean as it relates to a nail disorder?

   The term "pterygium" relates to a nail disorder when there is an abnormal scarring of the proximal nail fold (eponychium) or the distal nail fold (hyponychium) to the nail plate.

6. Are the terms "cuticle" and "pterygium" interchangeable?

   No, the words "cuticle" and "pterygium" are not interchangeable. Pterygium as it relates to the nail is an abnormal disorder, while cuticle formation is a normal process.

7. Why should a nail technician not aggressively push back or cut cuticles during a nail service?

   Any small injuries to the eponychium or hyponychium that breaks the seal between these structures and the nail plate creates openings for a fungus or bacteria to enter the nail unit and cause an infection.

8. List five nail disorders that can be serviced by a nail technician.

   Five nail disorders that can be serviced by a nail technician are: 1) hangnails; 2) discolored nails; 3) eggshell nails; 4) furrows; 5) leukonychia; 6) onychatrophia or atrophy; 7) onychauxis; 8) onychophagy; 9) onychorrhexis; 10) pterygium (Only five are needed.)

9. List five nail disorders that cannot be serviced by a nail technician.

   Five nail disorders that cannot be serviced by a nail technician are: 1) onychia; 2) onychogryposis; 3) onycholysis; 4) onychoptosis; 5) paronychia; 6) pyrogenic granuloma. (Only five are needed.)

CHAPTER 8

1. What are the characteristics of healthy skin?

   Healthy skin is characterized by being slightly moist and acidic, soft, and flexible. Healthy skin also has elasticity, a smooth, fine-grained texture, and is free of blemishes and diseases.

2. What are five functions of the skin?

   Five functions of the skin are: 1) protection; 2) prevention of fluid loss; 3) response to external stimulus; 4) heat regulation; 5) secretion; 6) excretion; 7) absorption; 8) respiration. (Only five are needed.)

3. Describe the epidermis and dermis.

   The epidermis is the outermost protective covering of the skin. It contains no blood vessels, but does contain many small nerve layers. The dermis is the deep layer of the skin. It contains blood vessels, lymph vessels, nerves, sweat glands, and oil glands in an elastic network made up of collagen.

4. How is the skin nourished?

   The skin is nourished by blood and lymph.

5. What are the functions of sweat glands?

   The functions of sweat glands are to regulate body temperature and eliminate waste products through perspiration.

6. Name five type of lesions.

   Five types of lesions are: 1) bulla; 2) crust; 3) cyst; 4) excoriation; 5) fissure; 6) macule; 7) papule; 8) pustule; 9) scales; 10) scars; 11) stain; 12) tubercule; 13) tumor; 14) nodules; 15) ulcers; 16) vesicles; 17) wheals. (Only five are needed.)

7. What are the characteristics of eczema and psoriasis?

   Eczema is characterized by itching, burning, and the formation of scales and oozing blisters. Psoriasis is characterized by a chronic inflammation with round, dry patches covered with coarse silvery scales.

CHAPTER 9

1. What is the purpose of a client consultation?

   The purpose of a client consultation is to discuss the client's general health, the health of his or her nails and skin, and the client's lifestyle in order to select the most appropriate nail service.

2. What are the parts of the consultation?

   There are two parts of the consultation: 1) the analysis—the information gathering portion; 2) the recommendations—the service to be performed that will aid the client in achieving her goals.

3. What are the characteristics of healthy nails?

   Healthy nails are not inflamed, infected, swollen, or broken. They are slightly pink in tone and flexible.

4. How would your services differ for a runner and a guitar player?

   A guitar player may need short nails on the left hand and longer nails on the right. He or she will also need calluses on the fingertips of the left hand. A runner may have calluses on the feet that protect feet while running.

5. Under what circumstances would you refer a client to a physician?

   If an infection, swelling, broken skin, or an inflammation is evident, one should refer a client to a physician.

6. What are the three types of information on the client health/record form?

   The general information asks for the client's name, address, telephone number, and best appointment hours. The client profile asks for information regarding the type of work and leisure activities the client participates in. The medical record asks for information about the client's general health. This information will help you determine whether it is safe to perform hand and foot massage on the client.

7. Why do you maintain a client health/record form and the client service and product records?

   It shows your client you are a professional and that you care about their health and safety, as well as the quality of the service they receive. Knowing if your client has any health or safety concerns, what products were used during a service, and what services were performed, illustrates your interest and concern.

CHAPTER 10

1. Identify the four types of nail technology tools used in manicuring.

   Four types of nail technology tools used in manicuring are: 1) equipment; 2) implements; 3) materials; 4) nail cosmetics.

2. Describe procedures for sanitizing nail implements.

   Wash all implements thoroughly with warm soapy water. Rinse completely with warm water to remove any traces of soap or debris. Dry thoroughly with a clean, laundered towel. Metal implements must be completely immersed in a disinfectant container filled with an approved disinfectant. Follow the directions for the required sanitation time. Remove the implements from the container (using tongs or tweezers to avoid contaminating the disinfectant by allowing your fingers to come in contact with the solution). Rinse the implements with water and dry them thoroughly with a clean, laundered towel. Store the dry, sanitized implements in a sealed container, a sealed plastic bag, or a cabinet sanitizer until ready for use.

3. Briefly describe the procedures for handling blood in a salon.

   Immediately put on gloves. Blot the cut with cotton and sanitarily apply an antiseptic. Apply powered alum or styptic powder using the end of a cotton-wrapped orangewood stick. Complete the manicuring service if applicable. Properly dispose of the blood-contaminated material, implements, and gloves.

4. List two types of nail polish remover and suggested use for each.

   Two types of nail polish remover are: 1) acetone—used to dissolve and remove nail polish from natural nails; 2) non-acetone—used to remove polish from sculptured nails, or nails having wraps, tips or other artificial applications.

5. Why is having a material safety data sheet for all products used in a salon important?

   MSDSs provide access to the required and necessary information about the products you use.

6. List the five basic nail shapes.

   The five basic nail shapes are: 1) square; 2) squoval; 3) round; 4) oval; 5) pointed.

7. What should be considered when selecting the nail shape?

   Areas to consider include: 1) the shape of your client's hands; 2) the length of your client's fingers; 3) the shape of your client's cuticles; 4) your client's occupation and hobbies.

8. List and discuss the three-part procedure sequence required in manicuring.

   The three-part procedure sequence is: 1) *Pre-service:* sanitize your hands, greet your client, perform your client consultation, have your client remove jewelry and place it in a safe, secure place; 2) *Perform actual procedure;* 3) *Post service:* schedule client's next appointment, sell retail products to your clients, clean up and sanitize your work area, implements, equipment, supplies, and materials.

9. Describe the correct procedure for nail polish application.

   Start in the center of the nail and brush toward the free edge. Using the same technique, cover the left side of the nail, then the right side. The polish should be applied to the nail in three strokes.

10. What is the purpose of a reconditioning hot oil manicure?

    It is beneficial for clients who have ridged and brittle nails or dry cuticles.

11. Discuss the basic difference between a female manicure and a male manicure.

    The basic difference is the deletion of the colored polish application on the male manicure.

12. List three safety precautions that should be taken when using an electric file.

    Safety precautions include: 1) do not hold any attachments in one place on the nail for extended periods; 2) do not apply too much pressure at the base of the nail; 3) make sure all attachments are properly sanitized; 4) replace any worn attachments when needed; 5) properly dispose of any disposable attachment. (Only three are needed.)

13. What are the benefits of a paraffin wax treatment?

    Paraffin will: 1) soften the cuticles allowing less time for treating the cuticle areas; 2) aid in making the skin appear smoother and softer; 3) benefit clients with arthritis.

14. List the suggested procedures for performing a paraffin wax treatment.

    Suggested procedures for performing a paraffin wax treatment are: 1) have client remove his or her jewelry; 2) have client wash his or her hands; 3) perform a client consultation; 4) check skin for opened wounds or skin disorders; 5) spray your client's hands with antiseptic spray; 6) apply moisturizing lotion to your client's hands and massage into your client's skin; 7) test the temperature of the paraffin wax; 8) position your client's hand for the procedure; 9) assist client in dipping hands into the paraffin wax; 10) repeat process on other hand; 11) wrap hands in plastic wrap and cover with a cloth mitt; 12) allow paraffin to remain on hands for approximately 10–15 minutes; 13) remove paraffin; 14) proceed with manicure if applicable.

15. Name five hand and arm massage techniques.

    Five hand and arm massage techniques are: 1) relaxer movement; 2) circular movement; 3) effleurage; 4) friction; 5) petrissage.

CHAPTER 11

1. Name five pedicure supplies.

   Five pedicure supplies are: 1) pedicure station; 2) pedicure stool and footrest; 3) client's chair; 4) rinse and soap baths; 5) toe separators; 6) foot file; 7) toenail clippers; 8) antiseptic fungal foot spray; 9) antibacterial soap; 10) foot lotion; 11) foot powder; 12) pedicure slippers; 13) toe nail nippers; 14) nail rasp; 15) curette. (Only five are needed.)

2. List the seven steps in the pedicure pre-service.

   The steps in the pedicure pre-service include: 1) pre-service sanitation procedure; 2) setting up the pedicure station; 3) spread one terry cloth towel on the floor in front of the client's chair, spread another over the stool to dry feet; 4) set up standard manicuring table in pedicure station; 5) both basins should be filled with warm water and antibacterial soap in one and antiseptic in the other; 6) greet client; 7) complete client consultation.

3. Briefly describe the pedicure procedure.

The pedicure procedure includes: 1) removing shoes and socks; 2) spraying feet; 3) soaking feet; 4) rinsing feet; 5) drying feet; 6) removing polish; 7) clipping nails; 8) inserting toe separators; 9) filing nails; 10) using foot file to remove dry skin and callus growths; 11) rinsing the foot; 12) repeating steps 7-11 on other foot; 13) brushing nails; 14) applying cuticle solvent; 15) pushing back the cuticle; 16) brushing the foot; 17) applying lotion; 18) massaging foot; 19) proceed with steps 13-19 on other foot; 20) remove traces of lotion; 21) apply polish; 22) powder feet.

4. Describe the proper technique to use in filing toenails.

Toenails are filed straight across, rounded slightly at the corners to conform to the shape of the toes. Do not file into the corners of nails. Rough edges are to be smoothed with the fine side of the emery board.

5. Describe the proper technique for trimming toenails.

Use the toenail nippers like a pair of scissors, trimming the nail in a number of cuts to avoid flattening out the nail plate and injuring the hyponychium. The corners of the toenail may be trimmed at a 45-degree angle to prevent them from penetrating the soft tissues.

6. List the six steps in the pedicure post-service.

Post service pedicure steps include: scheduling another appointment; advising client about foot care; selling retail products; cleaning pedicure area; discarding used materials; sanitizing table and implements.

7. Name six foot massage techniques.

Six foot massage techniques include: 1) relaxer movement to the joints of the foot; 2) effleurage on the top of the foot; 3) effleurage on heel; 4) effleurage movement on toes; 5) joint movement for toes; 6) thumb impression-friction movement; 7) metatarsal scissors; 8) fist twist compression; 9) effleurage on instep; 10) percussion or tapotement movement. (Only six are needed.)

8. What is a safety caution for pedicuring?

A safety caution for a pedicure is to ask clients if they are being treated for high blood pressure, heart condition, or diabetes.

CHAPTER 12

1. Are electric files safe?

Yes, when used correctly.

2. What type of electric file has grown in popularity?

Micromotor

3. What is torque?

Resistance

4. What are RPMs

Revolutions per minute

5. What is a diamond bit?

Diamond particles are glued on a shank.

6. What grits does a carbide bit come in?

Fine, medium, and coarse

7. What application techniques ensure safety?

Proper control, balance, and pressure

8. How do you disinfect bits?

Clean out the dust, wash in warm water and soap, then soak in a disinfection solution for the recommended amount of time, remove, and store properly.

CHAPTER 13

1. What is aromatherapy?

The literal translation of aromatherapy is "therapy through aromas."

2. How are essential oils used?

The use of essential oils is limitless. You can use them in manicures, pedicures, massage, reflexology, and facials. They can be used to soften cuticles or in hand creams as a hand conditioner. Use them in light rings or diffusers to help clear the mind, for a quick lift, or to change the mood of a room. Essential oils can be used anywhere your nose goes.

3. List five basic essential oils and give their uses.

Essential oils include: 1) lavender—overall first-aid, antiviral and antibacterial, boosts immunity, antidepressant, anti-inflammatory, relaxant, balance and antispasmodic; 2) chamomile—anti-inflammatory, digestive, relaxant, PMS, soothes frayed nerves, migraine, stamina, and antidepressant; 3) marjoram—antispasmodic, anti-inflammatory, headaches, comfort, menstrual cramps, and antiseptic; 4) rosemary—stimulating to circulation, relieves pain, perception, and decongestant; 5) tea tree—antifungal and antibacterial; 6) cypress—astringent, stimulating to circulation, antiseptic; 7) peppermint—digestive, clears sinuses, antiseptic, energy, decongestant, and stimulant; 8) eucalyptus—decongestant, antiviral, antibacterial, and stimulant; 9) bergamot—antidepressant, antiviral, antibacterial, water retention, and anti-inflammatory; 10) geranium—balancing to mind and body, tranquility, antifungal, and anti-inflammatory. (Only five are needed.)

4. Why is a carrier oil sometimes necessary?

It lessens the concentration of the essential oil and adds slippage for the massage, making it easier to perform.

5. Why is aromatherapy a helpful tool in our industry?

By using aromatherapy and essential oils, you give clarity to the mind, healing and care to the hands and feet, and relaxation to the body.

CHAPTER 14

1. List the four supplies, in addition to your basic manicuring table, that you need for nail tip application.

Four supplies needed for nail tip application, in addition to the basic manicuring table, are: 1) abrasive; 2) a buffer block; 3) nail adhesive; 4) nail tips.

2. Name the two types of nail tips.

Two types of nail tips are plastic, nylon, and acetate. (Only two are needed.)

3. What portion of the natural nail plate should be covered by a nail tip?

Nail tips should cover no more than one-half the natural nail plate.

4. What type of tip application is considered a temporary service? Why?

Applying a tip without an overlay, such as a fabric wrap or acrylic nail, is considered a temporary service because a tip without such a service is very weak.

5. Briefly describe the procedure for a nail tip application.

The procedure for nail tip application is as follows: 1) remove all polish; 2) push back cuticle; 3) buff nail to remove shine; 4) clean nails; 5) size tips; 6) apply nail antiseptic; 7) apply adhesive; 8) slide on tips; 9) apply adhesive bead to seam; 10) trim nail tip; 11) blend tip into natural nail; 12) buff tip for perfect blend; 13) shape nail; 14) proceed with desired service.

6. Describe the proper maintenance of nail tips.

The proper maintenance for nail tips is to follow with weekly or biweekly manicures for regluing and rebuffing. Non-acetone polish remover should be used because acetone dissolves the tips.

7. Describe the procedure for the removal of tips.

The procedure for removing tips is as follows: 1) complete nail tip application pre-service procedure; 2) soak nails; 3) slide off tip; 4) buff nail; 5) condition cuticle and surrounding skin; 6) proceed with desired service; 7) complete nail tip application post-service if no further service is performed.

CHAPTER 15

1. List four kinds of nail wraps.

Four kinds of nail wraps are 1) silk; 2) linen; 3) fiberglass; 4) paper wraps.

2. Explain the benefits of using silk, linen, fiberglass, and paper wraps.

The benefits for silk, linen, fiberglass, and paper wraps are as follows: 1) silk wraps are strong, lightweight, and smooth when applied to nails; 2) linen is thicker than silk or fiberglass; linen is strong and lasts a long time; 3) fiberglass has a loose weave, which makes for easy penetration of the adhesive; it's especially strong and durable; 4) paper wraps are temporary.

3. Describe the procedure for fabric wrap application.

The procedure for fabric wrap application is as follows: 1) remove old polish; 2) clean nails; 3) push cuticle back; 4) buff nail to remove shine; 5) apply nail antiseptic; 6) apply glue; 7) cut fabric; 8) apply fabric adhesives; 9) apply fabric; 10) trim fabric; 11) apply fabric adhesive; 12) apply fabric adhesive dryer; 13) apply second coat of adhesive; 14) apply second coat of adhesive dryer; 15) shape and refine nails; 16) buff nails; 17) apply hand lotion; 18) remove traces of oil; 19) apply polish.

4. Explain how a fabric wrap is used as a crack repair.

A fabric wrap is used as a crack repair by cutting a repair patch to completely cover the crack or break.

5. Describe how to remove fabric wraps and what to avoid.

The fabric wrap removal procedure is as follows: 1) complete nail wrap pre-service; 2) soak nails; 3) slide off softened wraps; 4) buff nails; 5) condition cuticles. Avoid damaging the nail plate when removing fabric wraps.

6. Describe the purpose of paper wraps and explain why they are not recommended for very long nails.

The purpose of paper wraps is to provide a temporary method of strengthening the nail. Paper wraps are not recommended for very long nails because they do not provide the strength that long nails require.

7. List the materials used for paper wraps.

The materials used in paper wraps are mending tissues, mending liquid, and ridge fillers.

8. Define liquid nail wrap and describe its purpose.

Liquid nail wrap is a polish made of tiny fibers designed to strengthen and preserve the natural nail as it grows. After it has been brushed on the nail in several directions and allowed to harden, it creates a network that protects the nail.

CHAPTER 16

1. Describe the origin of acrylic nail chemistry and what makes it work.

   Ethyl methacrylate monomer and special additives are put through a chemical reactive process that transforms the liquid into a powder. When reunited with monomer, the pliable combination hardens.

2. List the supplies needed for acrylic nail application.

   Supplies include: 1) basic manicuring set up; 2) acrylic monomer; 3) dappen dish: 4) acrylic polymer; 5) antiseptic nail prep; 6) primer; 7) abrasives; 8) nail tips; 9) adhesive; 10) forms; 11) brush; 12) safety glasses; 13) safety mask; 14) plastic gloves.

3. Describe the procedures for application of acrylic nails over forms, over tips, on natural nails, and on bitten nails.

   Whether using tips to create an extension or placing forms properly at the fingers edge (at the hyponychium), always: 1) perform the acrylic pre-service; 2) remove polish; 3) clean nails; 4) push back cuticles; 5) buff nail to remove shine; 6) apply nail antiseptic; 7) position nail form or apply tip; 8) apply primer; 9) prepare liquid and powder; 10) dip brush into liquid; 11) form acrylic ball; 12) place ball of acrylic on free edge of the natural nail, the extension of the tip, or on the nail form; 13) shape free edge; 14) place second ball of acrylic; 15) shape second ball of acrylic; 16) apply acrylic beads; 17) apply acrylic to remaining nails; 18) remove forms if used; 19) shape nails; 20) buff nails; 21) apply cuticle oil; 22) apply hand cream and massage hand and arm; 23) clean nails; 24) apply polish; 25) perform acrylic post-service.

4. Describe the safety precautions for applying primer.

   The safety precautions for applying primer are: 1) never use primer without plastic gloves and safety glasses; 2) offer a pair of safety glasses to the client; 3) check primer on a regular basis to make sure it is not contaminated with bacteria; 4) to avoid over priming, always release the excess liquid in the primer brush back into the bottle before dotting the natural nail surface; 5) avoid touching the skin area.

5. Describe the proper procedure for maintaining healthy acrylic nails.

   The proper procedure for maintaining healthy acrylic nails is: 1) create a routine appointment for each customer that suits her nail growth pattern; 2) encourage speedy repairs and good hygiene practice at home; 3) always sanitize both your hands and your client's; 4) keep your work area neat and clean with disinfected instruments and new abrasives for each client.

6. How does the procedure for acrylic nail application over bitten nails differ from other acrylic nail procedures?

   The application of acrylics onto bitten fingernails requires more attention at the stress area and cuticle than on unbitten nails. Bitten nails have shorter nail beds that usually sit lower than the fingertip and heavier cuticle growth. Shorter nails are preferred in the first few services to ensure adhesion success.

7. Describe how to perform regular maintenance on acrylic nails.

   Regular maintenance for refilling acrylic nails requires: 1) complete acrylic application pre-service; 2) preparation and filling in at the new growth area by the cuticle; 3) shortening; 4) reshaping and rebalancing the stress area; 5) buff nails; 6) apply cuticle oil; 7) apply hand cream and massage hand and arm; 8) clean nails; 9) apply polish; 10) complete acrylic application post-service.

8. Describe the proper procedure for the removal of the acrylic product.

   To remove acrylic product, use a warm acetone soak. As the acrylic softens, gently scrape off the layers until completely removed. Wash and moisturize hands.

9. Explain how the application of odorless and light-cured acrylics differs from the application of traditional acrylics.

   Odorless and light-cured acrylics pick up three to five times more powder than traditional acrylics. These two systems require more of a patting method than a brush on method of application. Most odorless and light-cured products require the removal of a sticky residue prior to filing. Light-cured acrylics need exposure under a U.V. lamp to harden. Traditional acrylics pick up less powder and are used wetter. The surface is dry when hardened and can be immediately filed.

10. How does the dipping method of using acrylics differ from all other methods?

    With most acrylic applications, the liquid and powder are combined on the brush, then brought to the nail surface for application. The dipping method does not use a brush. Instead, adhesive is applied to the nail surface, then the entire nail is dipped into the powder to bring the two products together.

CHAPTER 17

1. Describe the chemistry difference between U.V. gel and a no-light gel.

   U.V. gels with photo initiators require a U.V. lamp to complete the hardening and bonding process. No-light gels are thickened adhesives that either air dry or use spray activators.

2. Identify the supplies needed for gel application.

   The supplies needed for gel application are light-cured gel, curing light, brush, nail forms, primer (if recommended by the manufacturer), block buffer, nail tips, and adhesive.

3. Demonstrate the proper procedure for applying light-cured gels using forms, over tips, and natural nails.

   The proper procedure follows: 1) perform gel application pre-service; 2) remove polish; 3) clean nails; 4) push back cuticles; 5) buff nails to remove shine; 6) apply nail antiseptic; 7) apply forms or tips if desired; 8) apply primer if recommended; 9) apply gel; 10) cure gel; 11) repeat steps 9 and 10 on the other hand; 12) apply second coat of gel to the first hand; 13) cure gel; 14) repeat steps 12 and 13 on the other hand; 15) apply third coat of gel on both hands, one then the other; 16) cure respectively; 17) apply cuticle oil; 18) apply hand cream and massage hand and arm; 19) clean nails; 20) apply polish or gel coat; 21) perform gel application post-service.

4. Demonstrate the proper procedures for applying no-light gel over tips and natural nails.

   The proper procedure follows: 1) perform gel application pre-service; 2) remove polish; 3) clean nails; 4) push back cuticles; 5) buff nails to remove shine; 6) apply nail antiseptic; 7) apply tips, if desired; 8) apply gel; 9) cure gel with activator of choice; 10) repeat steps 8 and 9 on the other hand; 11) apply second coat of gel and cure with activator; 12) shape and refine nails; 13) buff nails to remove shine; 14) apply cuticle oil; 15) apply hand cream and massage hand and arm; 16) clean nails; 17) apply polish; 18) perform gel application post-service.

5. Explain how both kinds of gels are removed.

   U.V. gels cannot be removed with chemicals. To remove, allow application to grow off or gently file each layer until all layers are removed. To remove no-light gels, use a warm acetone soak. As the layers soften, gently scrape off until completely removed. Wash and moisturize hands.

CHAPTER 18

1. Why should you develop nail art skills?

   You should develop nail art skills because nail art is a creative part of a nail technician's job. It turns nails into small canvasses on which you can paint pictures, designs, and collages with tiny gems, foils, or tapes.

2. List the three basics of nail art.

   The three basics of nail art include: 1) schedule ample time to perform the chosen art; 2) display your art; 3) be competitively priced; 4) invest in quality tools; 5) dedicate a small pair of scissors solely for nail art; 6) let the polish dry before applying most types of nail art. (Only three are needed.)

3. What is the technique called for airbrushing two or more colors on the nail at the same time?

   This technique is called a color fade or color blend.

4. List four nail art services.

   Four nail art services include: 1) gem application; 2) foiling; 3) striping tape application; 4) gold leafing; 5) gold bullion application; 6) flat nail art; 7) airbrushing. (Only four are needed.)

5. List four of the classifications of color on the color wheel.

   The four of the classifications of color on the color wheel are: 1) primary colors; 2) secondary colors; 3) tertiary colors; 4) complimentary colors.

6. How does the finished airbrushed French manicure differ from the traditional application?

   The airbrushed French manicure has no bumps or unevenness at the white tip. The application is very smooth and the white tip has a perfect shape every time.

7. Describe the parts of the airbrush and how they work together to release the paint.

   Each airbrush has a small cone shaped fluid nozzle, also called a tip, that a tapered needle fits into. When the needle fits snugly in the fluid nozzle, no paint is released when the trigger is depressed. When the needle is drawn back, the airbrush begins to release paint. The further the needle is drawn back, the more paint is released.

8. Describe the best airbrush to use for nails.

   An airbrush that is designed for small quantities of paint, is gravity-fed (gravity pulls the paint into the airbrush) and mixes the paint with the air inside the airbrush (internal mix). This type of airbrush usually has a well or small color cup for the paint to be placed in the airbrush.

9. What is the most common choice for an air source for airbrushing nails?

   The most common choice for airbrushing nails is a small compressor.

10. What is the most common air pressure used by nail technicians when airbrushing?

    Most nail technicians work at a pressure between 25 to 35 pounds per square inch.

11. Describe the procedure for an airbrushed version of a French manicure.

    The procedure for an airbrushed French manicure is as follows: 1) apply a clear base coat to the nails; 2) choose your French manicure airbrush paint and mist the French manicure color over the nail lightly; 3) optional: add a shimmer to your French manicure paint by misting a gold highlight or shimmer evenly over the French beige; 4) French tip application with a stencil; 5) using the stencil, roll the finger sideways and carefully line up the stencil with the white tip already sprayed; 6) optional: mist the lunula slightly lighter than nail tip color; 7) apply your nail paint bonder and let it dry for three minutes, then apply the airbrush paint protective glaze for durability.

CHAPTER 19

1. What are the advantages and disadvantages of working in the four types of salons?

   Full service salon: *Advantage*: You automatically get all the nail care business in the salon and it is convenient for clients to have their nails done when they are there for hair care or other services. *Disadvantage*: There are no other nail technicians to share information, ideas, and experience. Also, no one will be able to fill in for you if you become ill or go on vacation.

   Nails-only salon: *Advantage*: You have other technicians to share ideas and experiences. You could increase your business by serving their clients when they are sick, on vacation, or they retire. The client is coming to this salon specifically for a nail service, no prompting is necessary for your particular expertise. Clients who patronage this type of salon may take nail care more seriously, have special nail problems or want more creative artificial nail services. If this is the case, you will gain valuable experience. A nails-only salon is a good place for a nail technician to establish a serious clientele. *Disadvantage*: There could be more competition for clients.

   Tanning salon: *Advantage*: This type of salon has tanning clients coming in every fifteen to thirty minutes, giving you the opportunity to present your services to many people during the day. *Disadvantage*: You could be the only nail technician in the salon so you might have little opportunity to share new ideas. Continuing education is critical in this type of environment.

   Salon spa/day spa: *Advantage*: This salon offers varied services to attract clients. It may have whirlpool pedicure thrones enabling you to give a pampered pedicure. Natural nail care is usually a priority. *Disadvantage*: The range of nail enhancements and coverings might be limited.

2. What are ten questions that will help you determine if a salon is right for you?

   Ten questions that will help you determine if the salon is right for you are: 1) Will the salon provide additional training? 2) Will the salon help you build clientele? 3) Will you be considered an employee or an independent contractor who rents a booth? 4) If you are an employee, how will the salon pay you? 5) Will the salon provide nail care products or will you have to bring your own? 6) Does the salon offer benefits? 7) Are there fixed or flexible working hours? 8) What is the dress code? 9) Does the salon close for regular vacation periods or does each employee take a separate vacation? 10) What is the salon's reputation? 11) Does the salon have safe working conditions? (Only ten are needed.)

3. What are eight questions that will help you determine if a salon has safe working conditions?

   Eight questions that will help you determine if a salon has safe working conditions are: 1) Does it have proper ventilation? 2) Does it provide separate refrigerators for food and nail product storage? 3) Are MSDSs on display or within easy access to employees? 4) Are work stations well-equipped and clean? 5) Are nail technicians required to wear dust masks? 6) Are nail technicians required to wear safety glasses? 7) Are aerosol cans used or are safer application methods used? 8) Are salon workers ready for emergencies?

4. Explain the difference between income and expenses and give two examples of each.

   Income is the money you make. It includes salary, commission from services, commission from retail product sales, and tips.

   (Only two are needed.) Expenses are what you spend. They include equipment, supplies, books explaining techniques, comfortable shoes, uniforms, and tuition for courses on nail techniques. (Only two are needed.)

5. List four types of salon compensation.

   Four types of salon compensation are: 1) hourly wage; 2) salary; 3) commission; 4) salary/hourly plus commission.

6. List four practical uses for business records that are required by local, state, and federal laws.

   Four practical uses for business records required by local, state, and federal laws are: 1) determining income, profits, losses, or expenses; 2) providing the value of your clientele, or the salon's worth to prospective buyers; 3) getting a bank loan; 4) computing income tax, social security, unemployment, and disability insurance.

7. Explain the difference between an employee and a booth renter.

   An employee of a salon has appropriate taxes withheld from their paycheck. Most salons furnish the

ANSWERS

employee with supplies. A booth renter pays the salon owner rent for space in the salon. They also pay their own taxes and purchase their own supplies.

8. List seven questions a successful interviewer might ask.

   Seven questions that might be asked by a successful interviewer include: 1) Why did you choose this career? 2) Why should I hire you? 3) What interests you about our salon? 4) Describe your problem solving skills. 5) What motivates you? 6) What are your short-term and long-term goals? 7) What are your strengths and weaknesses?

9. List five types of information that a salon can gather by keeping accurate business records.

   Five types of information that can be gathered by keeping accurate records are: 1) profit and loss comparisons with other weeks, months, or years; 2) changes in demands for services; 3) inventory; 4) net income; 5) material and supply levels.

10. Discuss the advantages of keeping proper service, inventory, and personal appointment records.

    The advantages of keeping proper service, inventory, and personal appointment records are that service records can help another nail technician fill in for a client's usual technician; service records can record client's personal information; inventory records should be kept for use and retail value; personal records will help you arrange your work time for the client's convenience.

11. List nine guidelines that should be followed in booking appointments.

    Nine guidelines that should be followed in booking appointments are: 1) keep a supply of appointment books, pencils, erasers, pens, a calendar, and message pad within reach; 2) be prompt; 3) identify yourself and the salon when answering the phone; 4) be pleasant; 5) take the client's home phone number, type of service to be performed, and date and time of appointment when scheduling appointments; 6) speak clearly; 7) be tactful and courteous when speaking; 8) if you have appointments made in advance, call the night before to remind clients; 9) at the end of the appointment, ask clients if they wish to reschedule.

12. List six sources of support for nail technicians.

    Six sources for nail support are: 1) trade magazines; 2) professional organizations; 3) product distributors and their sales consultants; 4) manufactures; 5) world wide web; 6) mentors.

CHAPTER 20

1. What are the five principles of selling products and services?

   Five basic principles of selling are: 1) knowing your products and services; 2) knowing the needs and wants of your clients; 3) presenting your products and services; 4) answering your client's questions and objections properly; 5) close the sale.

2. What is the difference between a product or service feature and a benefit? List examples of each.

   A product's or a service feature is a specific fact about it that describes the product. The benefits of a product (or service) are what it will do for you client or how it will fulfill your clients wants and needs. For example: Hand cream comes in a 6 oz. size and contains lanolin-feature. It softens hands, conditions cuticles, and makes hands look younger.

3. What are three methods of marketing in the salon. Give examples of each.

   Marketing methods include: 1) salon literature: a tri-fold pamphlet listing services and descriptions; 2) outside advertising: hours and services in newspapers, church bulletins, etc.; 3) on-going promotions: have six pedicures in six months get the seventh free; 4) salon newsletter: direct mail to clients updating them on specials, new products, and salon business; 5) birthday cards with a special "Thank you" inside: sending a client a birthday card with an add-on service or offering them two products for the price of one as a gift on their next visit. (Only three are needed.)

4. Discuss how to set prices for products and services.

   The general rule for pricing the professional products is to double the salon cost of those products. Base your service prices on both your market and the cost of doing that service.

5. What is the least expensive, most effective form of advertising?

   It is word of mouth. Do great work and people will tell other people.

6. List several monthly events and give examples of promotions for each.

January	New Year's – A book of coupons to use throughout the new year.
February	Valentines Day – Two-for-one sweetheart deals.
March	First Day of Spring – Pedicure specials.
April	Prom Season – Nail art and polish to match your dress.

ANSWERS

May	Mother's Day – Gift Certificates for any service plus complimentary paraffin.
June	Weddings – Bridesmaid party discounts and added value, the groom is complimentary.
July	Independence Day – Beat-the-heat service specials like a pedicure with a cool mint masque.
August/ September	Back to School – Promote larger sizes of maintenance products for the college bound.
October	Breast Cancer Awareness Month – Organize a fundraiser among your clients.
November/ December	Holidays – Promote gift certificates, baskets, and stocking stuffers.

7. What are three ways to fill open time slots in your daily schedule?

Three ways to fill you daily schedule are: 1) do add-on services on the client already at your table; 2) pre-book your client's maintenance appointments; 3) use the time to do things that will get clients in the door and into your chair—call to confirm appointments for the next day or send out appointment reminders.

8. Calculate the client retention rate of a nail technician that has 23 regular clients out of 35 total clients of the week.

Divide the amount of regular clients you had by the amount of clients you saw.

23 divided by 35 = 66% retention rate for the week.

INDEX

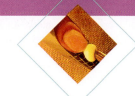